Fitness & Health

SEVENTH EDITION

Brian J. Sharkey, PhD

Steven E. Gaskill, PhD

University of Montana

Human Kinetics

Library of Congress Cataloging-in-Publication Data

Sharkey, Brian J.
  Fitness and health. -- Seventh edition / Brian J. Sharkey, Steven E. Gaskill.
    pages cm
  Includes bibliographical references and index.
  1. Physical fitness. 2. Health. I. Gaskill, Steven E., 1952- II. Title.
  RA781.S527 2013
  613.7--dc23

                              2012030825

ISBN-13: 978-0-7360-9937-0

The web addresses cited in this text were current as of September 14, 2012, unless otherwise noted.

Acquisitions Editor: Amy N. Tocco; **Developmental Editor:** Judy Park; **Assistant Editors:** Brendan Shea, PhD, and Casey A. Gentis; **Copyeditor:** Joy Wotherspoon; **Indexer:** Susan Danzi Hernandez; **Permissions Manager:** Dalene Reader; **Graphic Designer:** Fred Starbird; **Graphic Artist:** Dawn Sills; **Cover Designer:** Keith Blomberg; **Photograph (cover):** Dennis Welsh/UpperCut Images RF/age fotostock; **Photographs (interior):** © Human Kinetics, unless otherwise noted; **Photo Asset Manager:** Laura Fitch; **Photo Production Manager:** Jason Allen; **Art Manager:** Kelly Hendren; **Associate Art Manager:** Alan L. Wilborn; **Art Style Development:** Joanne Brummett; **Illustrations:** © Human Kinetics, unless otherwise noted; **Printer:** Walsworth

Printed in the United States of America   10 9 8 7 6 5 4

The paper in this book was manufactured using responsible forestry methods.

Human Kinetics
Website: www.HumanKinetics.com

United States: Human Kinetics
P.O. Box 5076
Champaign, IL 61825-5076
800-747-4457
e-mail: info@hkusa.com

Canada: Human Kinetics
475 Devonshire Road Unit 100
Windsor, ON N8Y 2L5
800-465-7301 (in Canada only)
e-mail: info@hkcanada.com

Europe: Human Kinetics
107 Bradford Road
Stanningley
Leeds LS28 6AT, United Kingdom
+44 (0) 113 255 5665
e-mail: hk@hkeurope.com

Australia: Human Kinetics
57A Price Avenue
Lower Mitcham, South Australia 5062
08 8372 0999
e-mail: info@hkaustralia.com

New Zealand: Human Kinetics
P.O. Box 80
Mitcham Shopping Centre, South Australia 5062
0800 222 062
e-mail: info@hknewzealand.com

E5250

To Ann and Kathy, perfect companions for the active life.

Contents

Preface

In 1974, Brian Sharkey published his first book, *Physiological Fitness and Weight Control*. According to the Centers for Disease Control and Prevention (CDC), if followed, this sound advice could save thousands of lives annually! That information has been around for decades, yet the population is far less active. We now face an epidemic of overweight and obesity. All this has occurred during a period in which we have learned a great deal more about physical activity, fitness, and health. These exciting research developments led to a new book, *Physiology of Fitness* (1979), and then second and third editions in 1984 and 1990. The editions of that book chronicled new developments and the author's journey from fitness enthusiast to performance advocate and, finally, to campaigner for the benefits of the active life.

In 1997, the fourth edition was retitled *Fitness and Health*. Epidemiological studies demonstrated that people can achieve many health benefits with regular, moderate physical activity and can earn even greater rewards by improving their level of fitness. But the greatest gains for personal and public health come when people move from sedentary living to an active lifestyle. The fifth edition of the book was published in 2002.

After 30 years of solitary effort, Brian decided to seek the assistance of a friend and colleague, Steve Gaskill, for the sixth edition. They met in 1980 when Steve was a coach and Brian was sport physiologist for the U.S. Nordic ski team. In the late 1980s, their lives took separate directions, but they remained friends and kept in touch. In 1998, after completing his doctorate in exercise physiology, Steve applied for a position at the University of Montana just as Brian was preparing to retire from there. Since then, they have renewed their professional and personal association, conducting research and development activities in the Human Performance Laboratory and in the field. Steve brought new ideas and energy to the book.

This totally revised seventh edition focuses on how you can bring about changes in important health behaviors and change your life. It also revives a chapter popular in earlier editions, titled Physiology of Fitness: Muscles, Oxygen, and Energy. It presents exciting new information on physical activity and brain health and about how the active life improves learning, high-order brain processes, and academic achievement. Finally, to help readers incorporate the active life, the authors have increased the information on behavior modification and purposeful exercise. This edition includes new information, charts, and graphs, as well as a clear focus on how you can achieve the many benefits of activity and fitness.

Written for adults of all ages, this book is especially intended for the person who wants to develop a deeper understanding of fitness and health, for the enthusiast who wants to know why and how the body responds, for the newcomer who needs motivation, and for the skeptic who needs proof. The authors have always sought to write a thinking person's fitness book, and they hope you'll find that this edition meets that description. Together, they plan to make this the best and most useful source available, one that will add purpose and meaning to involvement in regular, moderate physical activity.

HOW THIS BOOK IS ORGANIZED

Part I conveys the importance of regular, moderate physical activity. It describes how active habits contribute to health, vitality, and the quality of life. The added benefits associated with improved aerobic and muscular fitness are also discussed. Part II focuses on the psychology of behavior and how you can change behavior. Part III deals with aerobic and muscular fitness and the underlying physiology. Part IV presents proven ways to achieve aerobic and muscular fitness. Part V presents new information in the areas of nutrition and weight control, information that could reverse the current epidemic of obesity. Part VI shows you how to improve your performance in sport and work and how to cope with the environment.

Each chapter includes useful information in tables and figures, and some contain testing procedures and proven fitness programs. The special inserts (shaded boxes) provide additional background and details concerning fitness and health.

INSTRUCTOR RESOURCES

Developed for instructors of *Fitness and Health, Seventh Edition*, the instructor guide, test package, and presentation package plus image bank will assist you in developing courses that inspire students. All ancillary materials are free to course adopters and can be accessed at www.HumanKinetics.com/FitnessAndHealth.

- The **instructor guide** includes sample lecture outlines, key points, and student assignments for every chapter in the text, along with sample laboratory exercises and direct links to a range of detailed sources on the Internet.

- The **test package** features a bank of questions, including true-or-false, fill-in-the-blank, essay and short-answer, and multiple-choice. The test package is available for use through multiple formats, including a learning management system, Respondus, and rich text.

- The **presentation package plus image bank** includes PowerPoint slides of text, photos, and artwork from the book that instructors can use for a class discussion and illustration. The slides in the presentation package can be used directly within PowerPoint or printed to make transparencies or handouts for distribution to students. Instructors can easily add, modify, and rearrange the order of the slides as well as search for slides based on key words.

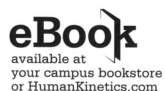

eBook
available at
your campus bookstore
or HumanKinetics.com

Join us as we enter a new era of physical activity and fitness, an era in which benefits are great compared to effort expended. Enjoyment and satisfaction will replace guilt and failure. Soon, activity and fitness will be recognized and practiced as vital contributors to health and the quality of life.

Brian and Steve

Introduction to the Active Life

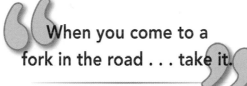

> ❝ When you come to a
> fork in the road . . . take it. ❞
>
> *Yogi Berra*

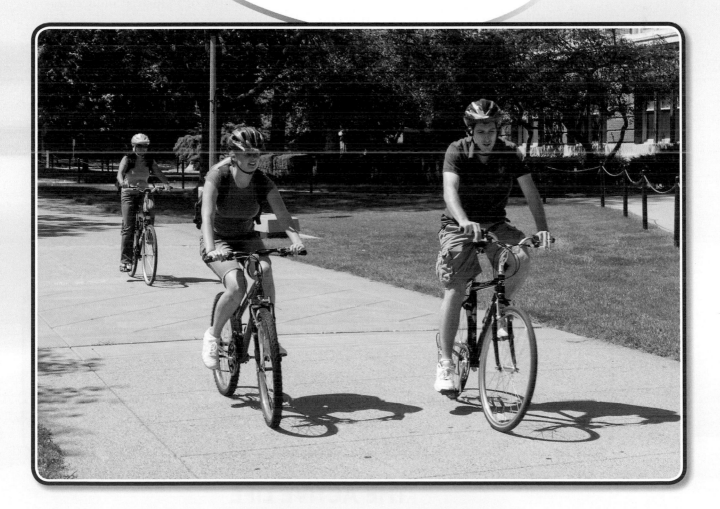

You've come to a fork in the road. One path shows evidence of heavy traffic, whereas the other, the one less traveled, is faintly etched into the land. One travels downhill, the route of least resistance, while the other rises slowly to distant heights. Will you be seduced by the easy route or motivated by the high road and the view from above? Sadly, many choose the easy route. Consequently, Americans have lost their identity as a vigorous, vital people. Along the way, they have become the fattest nation in the world, beset with chronic **fatigue**, **depression**, degenerative diseases of the heart, cancer, and **diabetes**. Our goal is to convince you to take the road less traveled, the active life, knowing that it will make all the difference in your **health** and vitality.

What is the road less traveled? Simply stated, it is the active life, a way of living based on regular physical activity and a cluster of related behaviors, including healthy food choices, weight control, stress management, abstinence from tobacco and drugs, moderate use of alcohol, attention to safety (wearing seat belts and helmets), and disease prevention. It is the path of individual responsibility that leads not only to health, vigor, and vitality, but also to self-respect and control of your destiny. This family of health-related behaviors has proved to be a profound paradox for our society, simple to comprehend but difficult to adopt.

People led active lives before society achieved the benefits of industrial modernization—technological developments, the automobile, labor-saving devices, television, and computers. These marvels of ingenuity now make it possible to minimize daily **energy expenditure** by using buttons, keystrokes, and voice commands to meet survival, work, and entertainment needs. Parallel to the decline in the need for human energy expenditure has been an increase in the consumption of highly processed, calorie-rich products, such as convenience and fast foods. Calorie-rich refined sugar has replaced complex **carbohydrate**, such as corn, rice, beans, and whole-grain breads and pasta. Food chemists added hydrogen to vegetable oils (hydrogenated fat, also known as trans-fatty acids) to prolong shelf life, but the final product does not prolong human life. Low-cost palm and coconut oils have replaced other ingredients to cater to our demand for tasty food in a hurry. Restaurant and fast-food servings grew larger while physical activity declined. Individually, the decline in activity or the rise in food consumption may not have been such a problem. Coming together as they have in recent years, the potential exists for alarming growth in the epidemic of diseases caused by the way we live. Fortunately, we can change these behaviors.

This introduction will help you do the following:

- Understand the dimensions of the active life
- Determine the benefits of active living and **fitness**
- Define the amount of activity needed for health
- Compare your current level of activity with recommended values

---

THE ACTIVE LIFE

Our species, *Homo sapiens*, emerged in central Africa more than 50,000 years ago. Genetic information indicates that our ancestors spread across the face of the earth as hunter–gatherers. Agriculture emerged some 10,000 years ago. Throughout this migration and until recently, by necessity, we humans have lived an active life. But that has changed, slowly at first, until the last few decades when we accelerated our transformation to sedentary ways. In 2001, less than 30 percent of the U.S. population was getting the minimum amount of exercise associated with health (150 minutes of moderate activity, such as brisk walking, per week) (Booth and Chakravarthy 2002). Only 10 years later, the U.S. Centers for Disease Control and Prevention (CDC 2011) report that barely 20 percent achieve the physical activity health guidelines and that 30 percent of American adults do no moderate physical activity at all. Very few people (about 10%) engage in sufficient activity for improving fitness and achieving additional health benefits. Few of us understand and appreciate the pleasures and benefits of the active life. The sedentary lifestyle has spread across the United States with the greatest level of inactivity in the southeast, as shown in figure I.1.

Sedentary behavior is bad for your health, leading to overweight and **obesity** for two-thirds of the adult population of the United States. The excess weight is associated with diabetes, heart disease, and some cancers, all of which are non-communicable diseases partially attributed to lifestyle. When people, even active ones, do too much sitting (in front of the TV, at the desk or computer, or driving in a car), the risk for premature mortality rises. We need to be more active and to break up sedentary time with periods of activity (Owen et al. 2010).

Sport psychologist William Morgan (2001) suggests that part of the reason people don't start or drop out of exercise programs is that the physical activity presented to the population lacks purpose and the exercise prescription focuses on measuring **heart rates** and **duration** instead of enjoyment or accomplishment.

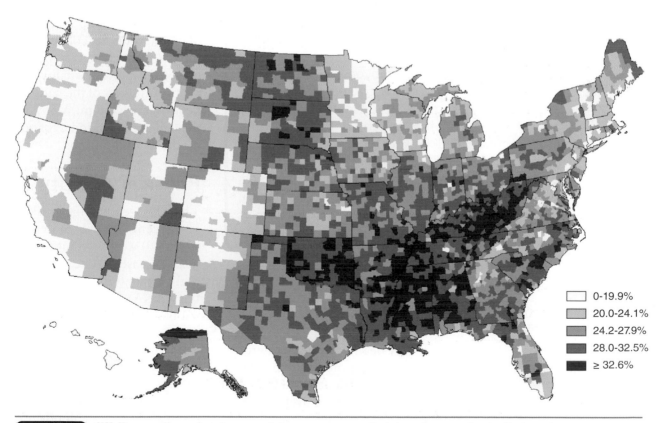

0-19.9%
20.0-24.1%
24.2-27.9%
28.0-32.5%
≥ 32.6%

FIGURE I.1 CDC age-adjusted estimates of the percentage of adults who are physically inactive.

Reprinted from http://apps.nccd.cdc.gov/DDT_STRS2/NationalDiabetesPrevalenceEstimates.aspx?mode=PHY

> **W**hy do strong arms fatigue themselves with frivolous dumbbells? To dig a vineyard is worthier exercise for men.
>
> **Marcus Valerius Martialis (38–103 AD)**

Morgan presents evidence of lifelong exercisers who engage in meaningful activity almost every day of their lives (as do your authors). Stone and Klein (2004) have found that long-term exercisers did so for fitness and health, but more importantly, for the powerful feelings generated by their regular participation (e.g., energy, enjoyment). Their activity had purpose, and yours should, too. Keep that in mind as we explore the active life.

The Cost of Physical Activity to Your Business or Community

The CDC, working with East Carolina University, provides a free, scientifically based web calculator to estimate the cost of physical activity in your community or business (www.ecu.edu/picostcalc). We (the authors of this book) decided to check on our local community of Missoula, Montana. We were staggered to learn that sedentary behavior is probably costing Missoula about $19 million in health care, $230,000 in workers' compensation, and $87 million in lost productivity. Furthermore, the calculator suggested that if we can get 5% of the inactive community members to become active, it would help the economy by about $5 million every year!

Of course, being scientists, we did a minicheck with a local business that has promoted physical activity for their employees. We used their numbers from 4 years earlier when they started their physical activity program. Of 26 employees, 19 (73%) were initially inactive. Eight of those (42% of inactive employees) participated fully in the activity program. The average salary was $29,000. The calculator suggests that sedentary lifestyles were costing the company around $50,000. After four years of the activity program, annual medical costs have dropped by $2,100 per person, per year. The business, with only 24 current employees (60% now meet physical activity health guidelines), has grown profits by $34,000 per year, well exceeding the predicted calculations. Not bad.

HEALTHY BEHAVIORS

The active life is at the core of a cluster of behaviors or habits that, viewed one at a time, seem too simplistic to be of much value. Yet collectively, they are our greatest hope for personal health and vitality and for the integrity of the nation's health care system. Many of the behaviors remind us of our mothers' admonitions.

Physical Activity

The CDC reports that in 2009, 37 percent of all U.S. deaths (897,000) were attributable to heart disease, stroke, and diabetes, all of which can be reduced with physical activity (CDC 2009). The National Alliance for Nutrition and Activity (NANA) further suggested that nearly 400,000 deaths were directly attributable to diet and physical inactivity (Wootan and Hailpern 2005). Stated another way, 18.1 percent of total U.S. deaths can be attributed to physical inactivity and poor diet. Compare those numbers to the lives lost annually in the United States in automobile accidents (~40,000), from unprotected sexual intercourse (~30,000), or from drug overdoses (~20,000). Lack of physical activity is now considered as much a contributor to heart disease as high blood cho-

As many as 300,000 lives are lost annually because of lack of regular, moderate physical activity.

lesterol, high blood pressure, and cigarette smoking, not because inactivity is more potent, but because so many of us are inactive or sedentary. Activity can reduce heart disease and control heart disease risk factors—elevated cholesterol, high blood pressure, diabetes, and obesity. Inactivity contributes to a substantial number of deaths annually. While physical activity is nearly free, the medical costs of chronic disease as a result of physical inactivity is estimated at $147 billion a year for obesity and $116 billion a year for treating diabetes in the United States (Finkelstein et al. 2008, Chenoweth 2005). Even more alarming is a report (Fincham 2011) noting that the cost of physically unfit and overweight people to American productivity and earning cost the United States more than $998 billion in 2010.

Healthy Food Choices

Poor food choices contribute directly to overweight, obesity, heart disease, diabetes, and cancer, and they contribute indirectly to other problems such as depression. After years of health education, average Americans still get 30 to 40 percent of their daily calories from **fat**. A substantial portion of their carbohydrate calories comes from highly processed **simple sugar** instead of from fruits, vegetables, and grains.

Understanding the importance of **nutrition** and food choices becomes even more important as greater numbers of Americans enter the workforce, work longer hours, and rely more on convenience foods, take-home meals, and eating out. Along with healthy food choices, the modern urban warrior needs to develop eating survival techniques. Poor diet, coupled with lack of exercise, causes at least 400,000 deaths a year, mostly from heart disease, and contributes to an increased risk of diabetes, cancer, and other ills. We'll say much more about food and nutrition in part V.

The World Is Fatter, Not Better Fed

Just because people are gaining weight does not mean the world is better fed or healthier, says the environmental group Worldwatch Institute. The institute reports that the share of adults worldwide who are overweight jumped from 1.5 billion in 2002 to nearly 2 billion in 2010, an increase of 25 percent, at the same time that the number of chronically hungry increased to well over 1 billion people. Being obese or underweight often results from the same problem—malnutrition. In the United States and other wealthy countries, the richer and the better educated people tend to eat well, whereas the poor often balloon from a diet of cheap and fatty fast foods. "Often, nations simply have traded hunger for obesity, and diseases of poverty for diseases of excess," said Worldwatch researchers. In the United States, well over 60 percent of the population is overweight; one in three adults is considered obese (Centers for Disease Control 2011c).

Weight Control

Dieting for weight loss is the most unsuccessful health intervention in all of medicine. More than 90 percent of people who have lost 25 pounds (11 kg) or more will return to their previous weight within the year. Worse yet, many weight-loss programs (diets) contribute to obesity. The truth that has emerged from the last decade of research is that diet alone won't help people achieve permanent weight loss. What will? The active life, combined with healthy food choices, and **behavior therapy** if necessary, is the answer to lifelong weight control. Activity maintains or builds the lean tissue (muscle) that has the capability to burn calories. Diet, by itself,

> **D**ieting for weight loss is the most unsuccessful health intervention in all of medicine.

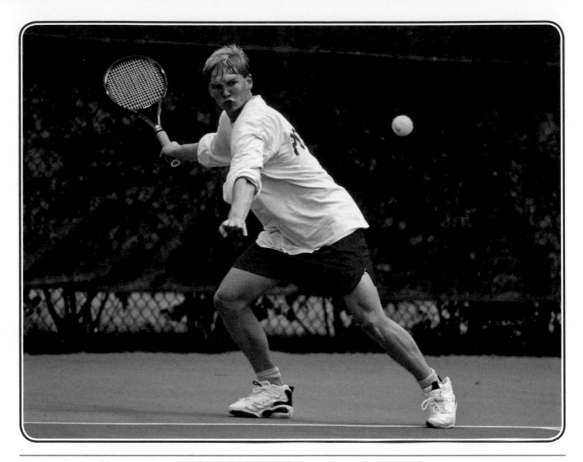

■ Activity builds lean tissue and is a lifelong solution to weight control.

leads to loss of muscle and a reduction in daily caloric expenditure, resulting in increased storage of fat.

Stress Management

Stress is our emotional response to events in life. What one person perceives as stress may be stimulating to another. Stress management implies the learning of effective coping strategies, or ways to deal with the many sources of stress in modern life. Stress has been linked to heart disease, cancer, ulcers, immunosuppression, and other ills. The link is uncertain, however, because of the difficulty in measuring stress and because some ills have been found to have other causes (e.g., ulcers are caused by bacteria). What is certain is that people can learn to cope with minor irritations and most major threats. The best results come when a person combines learned **behavior changes** with an arsenal of coping skills. Regular, moderate activity is the ideal way to cope with stress because it is effective, long lasting, much less expensive than drugs, and

Moderation Is Fun!

One of the enjoyable little moments that Brian has daily is sitting down to watch the evening news with a light beer and some low-fat pretzels. The beer provides a tasty way to relax, reduce stress, and lower the risk of heart disease. Likewise, Steve joins his wife for what she terms "booze and news" when they enjoy the evening news on TV and a small glass of red wine.

provides other health benefits. As you'll see in chapter 2, activity can be psychologically therapeutic as well as preventive.

Other Healthy Behaviors

Another important aspect of the active life includes eliminating negative behaviors, such as addiction to tobacco and other drugs, and moderating the use of alcohol. According to the Public Health Service's Office for Disease Prevention and Health Promotion, tobacco causes more than 400,000 deaths annually, including 30 percent of cancer deaths, 85 percent of all lung cancer deaths, and 21 percent of **cardiovascular** deaths. Illegal drug deaths total 20,000 per year, including overdose, suicide, homicide, AIDS (HIV infection), and more. Alcohol misuse causes 100,000 deaths a year, including almost half of all deaths from motor vehicle accidents (USDHHS and Public Health Service 1991). Yet one or two drinks of alcohol each day, whether wine, beer, or the hard stuff, are associated with reduced risk of heart disease. Who says disease prevention and health promotion have to be boring?

Safety habits such as the use of seat belts and child restraints in automobiles contribute to health and longevity. Bicycle, motorcycle, and skiing helmets reduce the severity and cost of accidents. Those who refuse to use safety devices should consider the effect on family, friends, and themselves.

The final category of health behaviors that we want to mention is the habitual practice of preventive measures appropriate to your age, sex, medical condition, and family history. These measures include vaccinations and other preventive measures such as **blood pressure** and **cholesterol** checks and tests for glaucoma and prostate, breast, and skin cancer (see chapter 3). The fact is that you, not your doctor, are responsible for your health. By combining personal responsibility with prevention and early detection tests, you have a cost-effective strategy for survival. The strategy is cost effective because prevention is always cheaper than treatment, because you use lower-cost health providers, and because you need to see physicians less frequently. If your employer has a comprehensive employee health or **wellness** program, use it. If not, create your own as you assume personal responsibility for your health.

> **B**y combining personal responsibility with prevention and early detection tests, you have a cost-effective strategy for survival.

Integration

By now, you've noticed how many facets of the active life interact in a reciprocal manner. Activity maintains muscle, which burns **calories**, helps maintain a healthy weight, and reduces the risk of heart disease, diabetes, and cancer, while also serving as the centerpiece of the stress management program. Of course, activity helps you look better, improves vitality, and reduces fatigue. Healthy food choices help you maintain or lose weight, lower cholesterol, make physical activity more enjoyable, and reduce the risk of heart disease, cancer, and other ills. The active life is not a hodgepodge of unrelated habits; it is a highly integrated family of behaviors that become more potent in combination than each is individually.

THE ROAD LESS TRAVELED

Some 30 percent of the U.S. population is completely sedentary (getting no physical activity), and another 78 percent does less than the minimum recommended activity (30 min of moderate activity most days of the week). Therefore, only 22 percent get the minimum recommended activity (CDC 2011b), and probably less than 10 percent achieve the

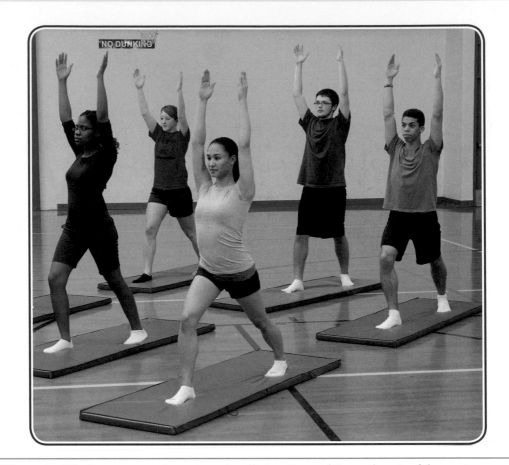

■ The active life does not require pain and suffering. Instead, it can be a joyful experience.

Institute of Medicine recommendation (1 hr moderate activity, most days) and are active enough to ensure the physical and mental benefits of regular physical activity. Most people deprive themselves of the joys and benefits of the active life and are likely to burden their families and the health care system. According to the CDC, sedentary habits vary by state and county, ranging from a low of 10.1 percent (Boulder County, Colorado) to a high of 43 percent (Carter County, Kentucky). Activity differs by age, education, sex, and race (Macera et al. 2003). Related data show that adult overweight and obesity increased in the United States from 55.9 to 64.5 percent between 1992 and 2002 (Flegal et al. 2002). It continued to increase to 72 percent in 2011, including 35 percent who are obese (CDC 2011a). Indeed, the active life is the road less traveled. Isn't it time that you joined the ranks of the few informed, resolute people who have the good sense and conviction needed to take the fork in the road, take personal responsibility, and embark on the active life?

Some view the active life and its associated behaviors as a medieval torture or religious rite, replete with fasting, denial, and mortification of the flesh. These folks are unwilling to give up the pleasures of rich (fatty) foods and unable to break addictions to tobacco, drugs, or alcohol. Because behaviors are often interrelated in a pattern of self-indulgence, these same people are likely to disdain the pleasures and rewards of the active life. Sadly, they do so at considerable cost to themselves and to society. Although few admit sorrow or repent their indulgences, they are destined to suffer a penance of fatigue, the purgatory of depression, and in time, frailty, disease, and early death. And the rest of us are expected to pay their bills and pick up the pieces of their lives.

Zealous fitness instructors have been heard to say, "No pain, no gain," "Go for the burn," or "It has to hurt to be good." Of course, none of these statements is true for health and fitness. Any pain, burn, or hurt should be seen as an identifiable end point during exercise. The active life is not one of denial and deprivation, nor is it one of pain and suffering. It is a joyful experience, an affirmation of what we can be—physically, mentally, socially, and spiritually. The active life provides the energy to begin, the vigor to pursue, and the vitality to persist, to go the distance. It replaces overindulgence with moderation, substitutes **positive addictions** for negative ones, and yields health, energy, and the capacity to live.

BENEFITS OF PHYSICAL ACTIVITY AND FITNESS

If you were regularly active, you would face each day with the energy to carry out daily tasks without undue fatigue. You would have vigor and alertness, ample energy and the **muscular fitness** to carry out work and leisure pursuits, a reserve to meet unforeseen emergencies, and the **flexibility** and **balance** to perform well and avoid injury. If you are like many active people, your first thoughts focus on the physical activity you will do, including when and where you will do it. When you become addicted to exercise, regular physical activity becomes an indispensable part of life. Physical activity and fitness do more than improve performance; they elicit other benefits that improve your physical and psychological health, benefits that enhance vigor and extend the prime of life.

Activity and fitness accomplish the following:
- Reduce the risk of heart disease, hypertension, stroke, and other vascular problems
- Burn calories and lower risk of overweight, obesity, diabetes, metabolic syndrome, and some cancers
- Reduce the likelihood of **osteoporosis**, osteoarthritis, and lower back pain
- Improve the function of the immune system
- Add years to your life, reduce frailty and infirmity, and extend the prime of life

These impressive benefits are achieved at little or no cost while you engage in enjoyable pursuits. And the benefits dramatically reduce reliance on medicine and the costs associated with the health care system. Additional psychological benefits even exist!

Psychological benefits of activity and fitness include the following:
- Diminished **anxiety** and depression
- Controlled stress and minimized adverse effects on the body
- Improved self-esteem, **self-concept**, and body image
- Increased life and vigor
- Enhanced interest in intimate behavior

In recent years, studies have identified cognitive improvements as another important contribution of physical activity, one with benefits for both kids and elders.

Cognitive benefits across your lifespan include the following:
- Improved cognition and problem solving
- Improved memory
- Improved attention span and reduced attention-deficit/hyperactivity disorder (ADHD)
- Reduced risk of dementia and Alzheimer's disease

It is true that activity and fitness are important aids to learning and cognition. Students learn better when active, and activity lowers the risk of dementia for senior citizens.

Our bodies were designed to move, not to sit in front of a desk, computer, video game, or television set. Physical activity and fitness focus the movement and ensure that you are likely to receive this impressive list of benefits. Other benefits include improvements in posture, **muscle tone**, and appearance. Some people even report a spiritual dimension associated with fitness.

PHYSICAL ACTIVITY RECOMMENDATIONS

The public and some fitness instructors are confused. For years, they thought that exercise had to be intense if it was to yield desired benefits. For competitive performance and to achieve high levels of fitness, that recommendation still holds true. But what if your interest is in improving or maintaining health? In the summer of 1993, a group of world-renowned experts came together with the American College of Sports Medicine (ACSM) and the CDC to develop recommendations for physical activity and health. They reviewed the latest scientific evidence and reached consensus that every American should accumulate 30 to 60 minutes of moderate to intense physical activity on most days of the week in at least 10-minute segments.

In 2008, the U.S. Department of Health and Human Services published revised physical activity guidelines for Americans. The new guidelines note that the substantial health benefits gained by doing physical activity can be achieved by following these recommendations.

- Adults should do 2 hours and 30 minutes a week of moderate intensity, or 1 hour and 15 minutes (75 min) a week of vigorous-intensity **aerobic** physical activity, or an equivalent combination of moderate- and vigorous-intensity aerobic physical activity. Aerobic activity should be performed in episodes of at least 10 minutes, preferably spread throughout the week.

- Additional health benefits are provided by increasing exercise to 5 hours (300 min) a week of moderate-intensity aerobic physical activity, or 2 hours and 30 minutes a week of vigorous-intensity physical activity, or an equivalent combination of both.

Adults should also do muscle-strengthening activities that involve all major muscle groups, performed on 2 or more days per week (USDHHS 2008).

Note that the recommendation of 150 minutes per week is the minimum. More health benefits are possible if you do more and add resistance training and flexibility exercises (Blair, LaMonte, and Nichaman 2004). From a public health perspective, we gain more if millions become active than we do if a few become superbly fit.

Subsequent chapters document the benefits of exercise and provide evidence to support the latest physical activity guidelines.

ACTIVITY INDEX

Before we move on, you may want to gauge your current level of activity using the following simple assessment tool (Activity Index). Developed in the 1970s, the index proved to be related to a laboratory test of aerobic fitness (maximal oxygen intake). As you increase **exercise frequency**, intensity, and duration, your index score and fitness both go up. How much activity do you need? You'll make that decision as you become better acquainted with the pleasures and benefits of activity. A score of 40 or more on the activity index is an indication that you are active enough to earn some of the health benefits associated with

Using your regular daily activity, circle the corresponding score. Then, calculate your activity index by multiplying your score for each category (score = intensity × duration × frequency).

	Score	Daily activity
Intensity	5	Sustained heavy breathing and perspiration
	4	Intermittent heavy breathing and perspiration—as in tennis, racquetball
	3	Moderately heavy—as in recreational sports and cycling
	2	Moderate—as in volleyball, softball
	1	Light—as in fishing, walking
Duration	4	More than 60 min
	3	30–60 min
	2	20–30 min
	1	Less than 20 min
Frequency	5	Daily or almost daily
	4	3–5 times a week
	3	1–2 times a week
	2	Few times a month
	1	Less than once a month

Evaluation and Fitness Category

Intensity_____ × duration _____ × frequency_____ = _____

Score	Evaluation	Fitness category*
100	Very active lifestyle	High
80–100	Active and healthy	Very good
60–80	Active	Good
40–60	Acceptable (could be better)	Fair
20–40	Not good enough	Poor
Under 20	Sedentary	Very poor

*Index score is associated with aerobic fitness.

From B.J. Sharkey and S.E. Gaskill, 2013, *Fitness and health, seventh edition* (Champaign, IL: Human Kinetics). Adapted from Kasari 1976.

regular activity. By increasing the amount or intensity of exercise, you will earn additional health benefits as you raise your aerobic fitness.

If your index score is below 40, you should begin today to increase your daily activity. Then, when we get into a discussion of the extra benefits associated with improved fitness (chapter 13), you will be ready to make a reasoned response to the question "Am I satisfied with my current level of activity and fitness, or do I feel the need to undertake a training program?"

SUMMARY

This introduction began with a description of the active life as the road less traveled, described how the health behaviors of the active life interact, and finished with a simple assessment of your level of activity. Along the way, it documented the fact that less than 15 percent of the U.S. population is active enough to get the physical and mental benefits of regular activity, and defined the amount of activity needed to achieve health benefits. This question remains: How did Americans reach such a dramatic level of inactivity?

The United States began as a vigorous nation of farmers, miners, loggers, laborers, and merchants. Americans survived a revolution, a civil war, and the industrial revolution. They migrated across the continent and continued to thrive in spite of two world wars, a depression, and current world conflicts. Yet today, they are gaining the reputation of being an overweight, lazy, complacent people, content to waste away the hours with fast food, television, video games, and computer chat rooms. The United States has become the fattest nation in the world, with one-third of their adult citizens classified as obese. It is the only developed country that has ignored the need for universal health care. Many Americans have lost a sense of responsibility for their acts, expecting others to bear the cost of their personal habits and mistakes.

Will the active life change all that? Probably not, but it is a positive way to begin exercising individual responsibility, to lighten our burden on society, and to lead family and friends along the road less traveled. With the active life, you'll feel better, look better, and improve your physical and psychological health. Your energy level will increase, along with your productivity. You'll be more attractive, even sexier. And if you stick with the active life, you'll delay chronic illness and prolong the period of adult vigor. You'll be able to romp with your grandchildren and, years later, have the vitality to enjoy your great-grandchildren. You might as well make plans to live for 85 years, give or take a few. If you adopt the active life, you could live with vigor and vitality until the end of your years.

There is no path. You make the path when you walk.

Antonio Machado

Physical Activity, Fitness, and Health

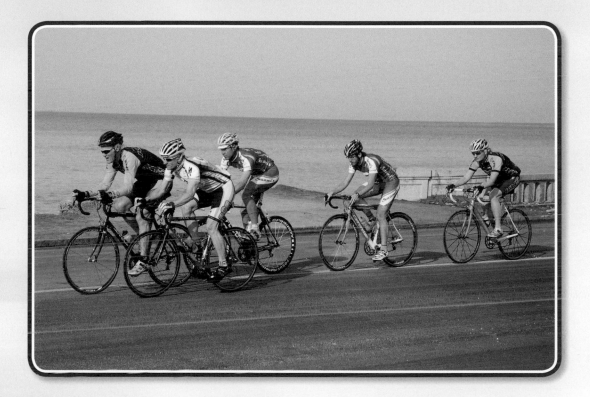

Would you be upset to learn that according to the U.S. Department of Health and Human Services, unhealthy eating and physical inactivity causes 310,000 to 580,000 deaths every year in the United States? That these lives are lost by simply failing to apply a medically proven therapy? It's true. Our high-cost health care system has ignored a simple, low-cost health treatment with the capacity to save hundreds of thousands of lives and billions of dollars. This miracle treatment goes unused in favor of expensive drugs, costly operations, and even organ transplants. How could this happen? One contributing factor is that physicians are compensated for performing procedures rather than providing the counseling that leads to improved health habits. Additionally, with the development of penicillin and other wonder drugs, we patients have sought a quick fix for problems and have relinquished personal responsibility for our health. Hospitals, drug and insurance companies, and yes, even lawyers, have reaped enormous profits in this so-called health care system while simple, inexpensive health habits have gone unused.

Fortunately, the times are changing. As we work to rebuild our ailing health care system, we are searching for ways to reduce costs and the reliance on drugs and medical procedures. At the same time, researchers are questioning the value of certain operations and drugs, and confirming the contributions of physical activity and related habits to health, longevity, and the quality of life. Finally, local, state, and federal organizations are moving to increase physical activity and curb the rise in sickness and death associated with inactivity. This section reviews studies that provide the modern foundation for the relationship of physical activity and fitness to physical and psychological health. It discusses the benefits and risks of activity, catalogs the extra benefits of fitness, and provides advice to help you begin your transformation to health, vitality, and the active life.

1

Activity and Fitness
Health Benefits

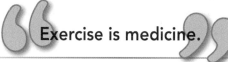

"Exercise is medicine."

*American College of Sports
Medicine (ACSM) and the American
Medical Association (AMA)*

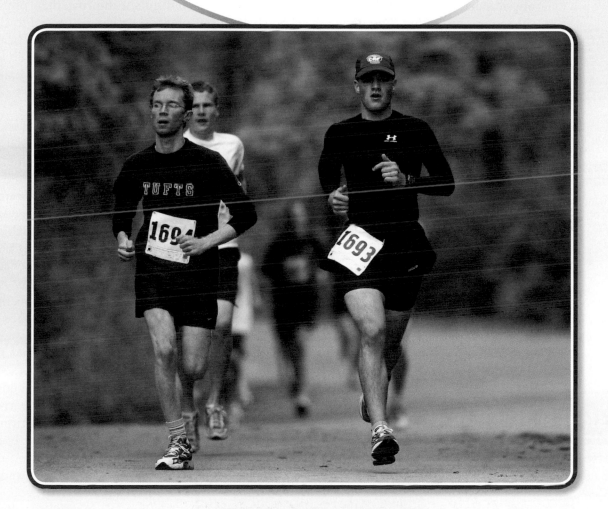

The idea that physical activity is associated with good health is not new. The Chinese have long practiced tai chi and other forms of activity to prevent diseases associated with sedentary living. In Rome more than 1,500 years ago, the physician Galen prescribed exercise for health maintenance. References to the health values of exercise appear throughout recorded history, usually with little measurable effect on the populace. Why, then, do we invest time and energy to provide the latest evidence on the relationships among physical activity, physical fitness, and health? One reason is that we are devout optimists, the product of many years of professional experience and numerous success stories. Another reason is that never before have so many studies demonstrated so much about the health benefits of activity and fitness.

The Exercise is Medicine initiative was launched by the American College of Sports Medicine (ACSM) and the American Medical Association (AMA) in 2007. It calls for physical activity to become a standard component of disease prevention and medical treatment. The initiative urges health care providers to assess and review patient's physical activity programs, and include exercise clearance, exercise prescription, and referrals to qualified health and fitness professionals in standard office visits. Patients are encouraged to discuss physical activity with their doctors and to learn how to continue or improve their physical activity programs. The initiative acknowledges that physical activity is crucial to the prevention, management, and treatment of numerous chronic conditions, including heart disease, type 2 diabetes, obesity, high blood pressure, and some cancers. While exercise clearly benefits the function and appearance of the body, the **Exercise is Medicine campaign** focuses on the internal benefits and how these benefits contribute to longevity and the quality of life (for more information, consult www.exerciseismedicine.org).

We concur that exercise is powerful medicine, but you don't need to visit your doctor in order to get started on a program of regular, moderate physical activity. The goal of this book is to encourage a lifetime commitment to activity, fitness, and the active life.

Epidemiology, the study of epidemics, is a fitting way to study the modern epidemic—diseases of lifestyle—that is responsible for more than half of all deaths in the United States. The epidemiologist studies populations to determine relationships between behaviors, such as physical activity, and the incidence of certain diseases. Researchers look at **morbidity** (sickness) and **mortality** (death). Studies can be **retrospective**, looking back at past behaviors, or **prospective**, following a group into the future. **Cross-sectional research** looks at chronological slices of the population. Lack of solid information on activity, fitness, and other health habits often confound retrospective studies, whereas prospective studies face problems such as changing habits and dropout among participants. Issues of access to medical records (confidentiality) plague many studies, but the major problem is that of self-selection. Critics argue that subjects are physically active because they are well, not necessarily well because they are active.

Risk Ratio

In a study of Harvard alumni, those with the least activity had 78.8 cardiovascular deaths per year per 10,000 study participants versus 43.0 for the most active, yielding a **risk ratio** of 54 percent (43.0 ÷ 78.8 = .54). Stated another way, the risk was 46 percent lower (100 − 54 = 46%) for the active alumni (Paffenbarger, Hyde, and Wing 1986).

Because self-selection confounds the results of retrospective and cross-sectional studies, only carefully controlled prospective studies, involving random assignment of participants to levels of activity (or inactivity), allow cause-and-effect conclusions. Because these studies are difficult to conduct and are most likely unethical because inactivity is dangerous to health, we may never have absolute proof of the value of activity and fitness. But when the preponderance of studies confirm the health benefits of activity and when the risks and costs of being active are minimal, recommending a prudent, if not totally proven, course of action seems reasonable.

Space does not permit a comprehensive review of the role of activity and fitness in health and disease, so this chapter reviews several classic studies and provides a summary of epidemiological research. To avoid endless details, it summarizes the effects of activity and fitness with reference to the risk ratio (RR), the ratio of morbidity or mortality for the active members of the population to that for the inactive members. Then, it discusses plausible mechanisms or reasons that activity may have beneficial effects and provides guidelines for recommended activity.

This chapter will help you do the following:

- Determine the health benefits of physical activity and fitness
- Understand the relationships among physical activity, fitness, and health
- Appreciate how activity reduces the risk and severity of chronic diseases such as heart disease, diabetes, and some cancers
- Assess the role of activity in arthritis, osteoporosis, and lower back problems
- Compare your current level of activity with recommended values
- Define the amount of activity needed for health

ACTIVITY REDUCES THE RISK OF CORONARY ARTERY DISEASE

In spite of tremendous progress in the past 30 years, heart disease (more specifically, **coronary artery disease**, or **CAD**), remains the nation's number-one killer for men and women. Diseases of the heart and blood vessels and strokes kill almost one million people in 1 year in the United States, far more than all the American lives lost in the four major wars of the last century (636,282). CAD is responsible for over half of those deaths, often in a sudden dramatic event called a **heart attack**. But this seemingly sudden event is actually the product of **atherosclerosis**, a process that narrows the arteries and restricts the blood flow to the heart.

Atherosclerosis begins to develop during childhood. The process is accelerated by a number of primary risk factors. In 1993, in recognition of the important role of activity, the American Heart Association (AHA) raised lack of physical activity to the level of a primary risk factor, along with cigarette smoking, elevated cholesterol, and high blood pressure (hypertension). Figure 1.1 presents CAD risk factors and the possible influence of physical activity.

Positively influenced by physical activity	May be influenced by physical activity	Not influenced by physical activity
Overweight and obesity High blood glucose Elevated blood lipids High blood pressure Physical inactivity	Electrocardiographic abnormalities Elevated uric acid and C-reactive protein Abnormalities in pulmonary (lung) function Some cancers Personality or behavior patterns (being hard driving, time conscious, aggressive, competitive, hostile) Psychic reactivity (reaction to stress)	Family history of heart disease Sex (men at greater risk until age 55) Cigarette smoking Poor food choices

FIGURE 1.1 CAD risk factors.

Adapted from B.J. Sharkey, 1974, *Physiological fitness and weight control* (Missoula, MT: Mountain Press), 11. By permission of B.J. Sharkey.

Atherosclerosis may be initiated by inflammation of the lining of the coronary artery, a protective response to injury, or even an infection. Thereafter, high levels of circulating fats in the blood infiltrate the lining of the artery, aided perhaps by high blood pressure and chemicals, such as those in cigarette smoke. Cholesterol (**low-density lipoprotein cholesterol, or LDL**) becomes oxidized, leading to further damage to the artery. A scablike **plaque** forms and grows until it blocks the flow of blood or until it ruptures and clogs the artery (see figure 1.2). C-reactive protein, a marker of inflammation, is correlated to CAD risk. Some medical experts think that viruses may accelerate atherosclerosis or stimulate immune system responses that contribute to plaque formation and clotting. Gradual narrowing reduces blood flow (**ischemia**) and often leads to exertional pain (**angina**) experienced in the chest, left arm, or left shoulder.

Some plaque is hard and some is soft. The soft plaque has the potential to burst and cause a clot that can immediately interrupt blood flow and cause a heart attack (**myocardial infarction**). Lack of blood and oxygen can damage heart muscle if it isn't treated quickly. This soft, or vulnerable (unstable), plaque may be the major cause of lethal heart attacks. The size, composition, and local inflammation processes may predispose a plaque to rupture. Biomechanical or thermodynamic forces, including increased blood pressure and heart rate, adrenalin, and even physical exertion, sometimes trigger rupture and an acute heart attack. Ten percent of heart attacks are associated with physical activity; 90 percent are not. Inactive people are 50 times more likely to have a heart attack during exertion. In contrast, the risk for those who engage in habitual vigorous activity increases only 5 times during exercise. The overall risk for the active people was only 40 percent that of sedentary people (Siscovick et al. 1984). To lower the risk of a heart attack during exercise for inactive people, it is important to start a program slowly. For more details, see chapter 10.

Autopsy studies show that atherosclerosis is under way in some young adults, and surveys have confirmed the presence of CAD risk factors in children of all ages, especially when they are overweight. When doctors examined teenage hearts donated after accidental deaths, they found that 1 in 6 already showed the blockage and plaque deposits characteristic of coronary artery disease (Tuzac 1999). Studies link atherosclerosis in youth to sedentary living, excess caloric consumption, and obesity. Thus, a program of risk-factor identification and early intervention seems prudent, especially for those with a strong family history or multiple risk factors for heart disease. The active life can slow, stop, or reverse

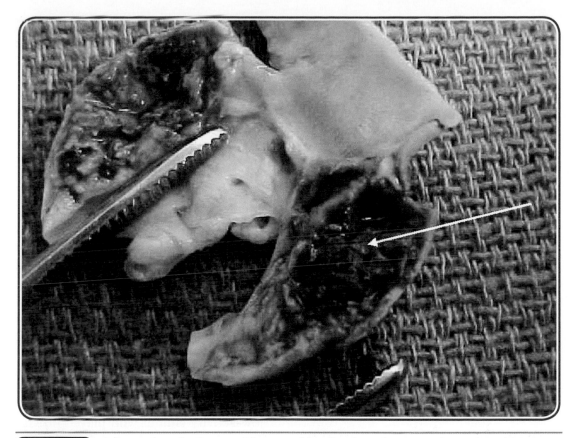

FIGURE 1.2 Atherosclerosis plaque with recent bleeding into the center (arrow), making it more unstable and likely to cause a clot.

Courtesy of Vascular Disease Foundation – www.vdf.org.

atherosclerosis. Indeed, a demanding intervention program consisting of activity, a low-fat diet, and medication, if needed, may halt and even reverse the process (Ornish 1993).

Inactivity and CAD

The landmark London bus driver study published in 1954 (Morris and Raffle) focused world attention on inactivity as a factor in heart disease. The study compared the incidence of CAD between bus drivers and conductors who went up and down the stairs of the double-deck bus. The more active conductors were found to have a rate 30 percent below that of the drivers. The disease appeared earlier in drivers, and their mortality rate was more than twice as high following the first heart attack. In spite of confounding factors (e.g., the stress of driving, drivers being more likely to be overweight), the study sparked interest in the role of activity.

In a classic epidemiological study, Paffenbarger and associates (1986) studied thousands of Harvard alumni to determine the influence of activity, vigorous activity, and sports on cardiovascular illness and death. In comparison with less active subjects (those who engaged in less than 1,000 cal of activity per week, the equivalent of walking 30 min/day), those who participated in moderate and high levels of activity had mortality risk ratios (RR) of .71 and .54, respectively. Risk ratios are a method to compare the risk of different people to some standard. In this case, the standard was the mortality rate in less active people across a period of time. The relative risk of .54 for the high activity group means that they had only 54 percent of the mortality rate as the less active.

Less active	<1,000 calories per week	RR = 1.0
Moderate	1,000–2,500 calories per week	RR = .71
High activity	>2,500 calories per week	RR = .54

Moderate activity yielded a 29 percent reduction, and high levels of activity (2,500 cal/week is equivalent to 25 mi, or 40 km, of jogging per week) yielded a 46 percent reduction in risk.

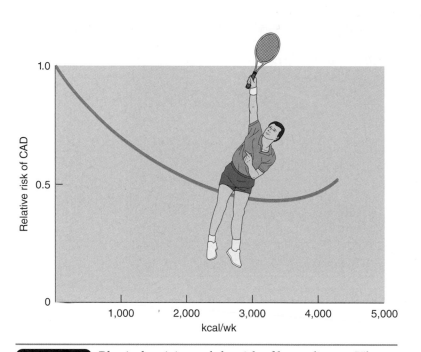

FIGURE 1.3 Physical activity and the risk of heart disease. The risk declines up to 3,500 calories per week and then begins to rise. This unexplained tendency for the risk to go back up may be the result of the small number of cases that report more than 3,500 calories (or the equivalent of walking about 35 mi, or 56 km) per week.

Those who played light or moderately vigorous sports had mortality ratios of .79 and .63 when compared with those who played no sports. Risk ratios for mortality as well as first attacks of coronary artery disease were inversely related to physical activity, as indicated by calories of weekly exercise. The mortality ratio approached .5 when activity exceeded 2,500 calories per week, but when activity exceeded 3,500 calories per week, the contribution of activity seemed to diminish (see figure 1.3). The data of Paffenbarger and associates indicates that moderately vigorous activity and sport were more effective in reducing the risk of CAD. The risk for low-activity alumni who played no vigorous sports was 2.4 times that of active alumni who engaged in vigorous sports.

Most other studies have shown similar results—that heart disease risk is inversely related to the amount of regular physical activity, be it occupational, leisure time, or vigorous sports. They show that the activity must be current or contemporaneous to be beneficial, and that participation in high school or college sport did not confer protection later in life. In fact, regularly active adults maintain a lower risk of CAD whether or not they had been physically active during their youth. One study concludes that favorable long-term stabilization of most coronary risk factors is achievable with energy expenditure due to physical activity above 1,000 calories per week. Burning 2,000 calories per week is associated with additional benefits, especially with favor-

Women's Risk

A study of 84,129 women participants in the Nurses' Health Study found that adherence to lifestyle guidelines involving diet, exercise, and abstinence from smoking is associated with a very low risk of CAD. Women in the low-risk category were those who engaged in moderate to vigorous exercise for at least 30 minutes a day, did not currently smoke, had a favorable **body mass index (BMI)**, consumed half a drink of alcohol daily, and scored in the top 40 percent on a diet high in fiber and low in saturated fats and trans-fatty acids and low on the **glycemic index**. They had a relative risk for CAD 17.8 percent below the population average (Stampfer et al. 2000).

able modification of HDL cholesterol and maintenance of weight (Drygas et al. 2000).

Autopsy studies conducted on American soldiers killed in the Korean conflict showed an alarming number (77%) with evidence of CAD, indicating that the pathology of atherosclerosis is developing by the age of 22 years (Enos, Beyer, and Holmes 1955). As previously mentioned, the Tuzac analysis of deceased teenage hearts concluded that heart disease, and therefore prevention, must begin much earlier than first believed (1999). Autopsies of older men (45 to 70 years) found that the incidence of scars, infarcts, and occlusions in the arteries were

Calories per Week

Throughout this book, the term *calorie* refers to the kilocalorie, defined as the amount of heat required to raise 1 kilogram of water (1 L) 1 degree centigrade. We use *calorie* because it is the common usage, the one that you see when you read food labels or diet books. By familiarizing yourself with the caloric cost of activities as well as the calories consumed in food, you will become an informed consumer of food and activity and will see how excess caloric intake requires an increase in caloric expenditure.

In general, you burn about 100 calories when you jog 1 mile (or about 62.5 cal when you jog 1 km). To burn 2,500 calories per week, you would need to jog 25 miles (40 km). Alternatively, you could play singles tennis 3 hours each week (8 cal\min × 50 min = 400 cal [with a 10 min rest per hr]; 400 × 3 hr = 1,200 cal), walk briskly for 60 minutes (6 cal\min × 60 min = 360 cal), and jog 3 miles (4.8 km) three times (9 mi × 100 cal\mi, or 14.5 km × 62.5 cal\km, = 900 cal), for a total of about 2,500 calories of vigorous activity per week.

30 percent less for those who had been moderately active and even lower for those who were heavily active (Morris and Crawford 1958).

Animal studies agree that moderate activity is beneficial, but suggest that exhaustive or stressful effort may somehow accelerate the development of CAD. Exhaustion may be stressful for an animal, and stress provokes a hormonal response that suppresses the immune system and may accelerate the atherosclerotic process in both animals and humans. No evidence exists that enormous amounts of activity, such as that performed by ultra-endurance athletes, is detrimental to those athletes' health.

Physical Activity Versus Fitness

If activity and sport can lower the risk of CAD, what about the contribution of improved fitness? Do people earn extra benefits by raising their level of fitness? Physical fitness, specifically aerobic fitness, has long been associated with better health. The issue was raised in 1988 at the annual meeting of the ACSM. Doctors Steven Blair and Harold Kohl reported on their study of more than 10,000 men. They analyzed all-cause death rates for sedentary and active men whose fitness had been assessed in a treadmill test. The surprising results have influenced the way we view activity, fitness, and the amount of exercise required to achieve public health benefits.

The all-cause death rate was almost three times higher for the sedentary men. And within the sedentary classification, aerobic fitness level made a difference only at the lowest level, where the least fit had twice the risk of other sedentary subjects (five times the risk for active men) (Blair and Kohl 1988). Among the active subjects, the death rates were not significantly different, regardless of the level of aerobic fitness! These findings suggested that, for the male subjects in this study, becoming physically active conferred most of the health benefits, and that higher levels of aerobic fitness didn't provide greater protection from all-cause mortality (heart disease contributes more than one-half of all-cause mortality) (see table 1.1).

Table 1.1   Physical Activity Versus Fitness: Age-Adjusted Death Rates per 10,000 Men

Fitness group	Lowest	2	3	4	Highest
Sedentary (inactive) men	74	31	35	28	33
Active men*	13	8	14	16	13

*While the death rates for the active men vary slightly between fitness levels, there is no significant difference. Within the sedentary men, the lowest fitness group had twice the death rate compared to the other sedentary men. Remaining active reduces your overall mortality risk to one-third that of inactive people (Blair and Kohl 1988).

Does this mean that physical fitness is not associated with better health? No, it does not. In fact, when the sedentary and active subjects were analyzed together, a trend toward a reduced death rate with increasing fitness is present (Blair et al. 1989).

Fitness level	Death rate*	Relative risk
1 Lowest	64.0	1.0
2	25.5	.40
3 Medium	27.1	.42
4	21.7	.34
5 Highest	18.6	.29

*All-cause deaths per 10,000.

Although higher levels of fitness are associated with only minor reductions in all-cause death rate, they are correlated with fewer risk factors and they probably do provide added protection, especially for those with elevated risk (family history, elevated cholesterol, triglycerides, hypertension, diabetes, obesity).

Are you wondering why some sedentary subjects are more fit than others? Physical fitness is a product of heredity and training. With good heredity, a sedentary person could have a higher level of fitness than an active friend. The good news is that moving from sedentary to active living imparts a sizable drop in health risk and all-cause mortality. When already active people improve their fitness, the decrease in risk is more subtle but is still important, especially for someone with inherited risks.

A study of fitness and CAD risk factors in 4,631 healthy Norwegian men and women confirmed that low levels of aerobic fitness were associated with a much higher prevalence of cardiovascular risk factors, including obesity, hypertension, and unfavorable levels of blood **lipids**, when compared with median or higher levels of fitness (Aspenes et al. 2011). The authors conclude, "Together with the evidence from clinical experimental studies, these cross-sectional data suggest that, by increasing peak oxygen uptake ($\dot{V}O_2$peak), the risk of cardiovascular disease may be reduced."

A study conducted in Finland offers further proof of the extra benefits of fitness. The authors concluded that higher levels of both leisure-time physical activity and fitness had a strong inverse relationship with the risk of heart attack. The study supports the conclusion that lower levels of physical activity and of fitness are independent risk factors for coronary artery disease in men (Lakka et al. 1994).

Cardioprotective Mechanisms

Numerous studies have shown that physical activity and fitness are associated with a lower risk of CAD. Yet because of self-selection, most of the studies do not allow cause-and-

Public Health and Exercise: In Review

Let us emphasize one of the most important public health messages of our time: Regular, moderate physical activity conveys many, if not most, of the important health benefits associated with exercise. From a public health standpoint, an increase in physical activity will provide millions of Americans with some level of protection from heart disease, hypertension, adult-onset diabetes, certain cancers, osteoporosis, depression, premature aging, and more. Improved aerobic fitness provides added benefits (see figure 1.4). The studies showed that moderate physical activity is necessary to achieve most of the gains and that a large segment of the population can attain protection from many chronic diseases. Indeed, epidemiologist Dr. Steven Blair (2009) has concluded that "physical inactivity is one of the most important public health problems of the 21st century, and may even be the most important."

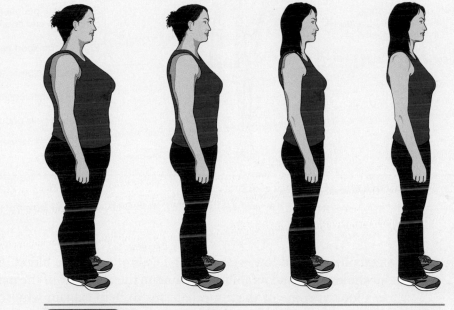

FIGURE 1.4 Exercise is medicine. Physical activity conveys health benefits, as well as the key to weight control. At what level of fitness, from sedentary to fit, would you place yourself?

effect statements and the level of assurance desired in scientific and medical research. To conduct further investigations about the influence of activity on cardiovascular health, researchers have explored a number of hypotheses concerning cardioprotective mechanisms (see figure 1.5).

Among the many possible ways in which activity may prevent or minimize the process of atherosclerosis, the major benefits are not directly related to the heart itself. But physical activity does improve the function of the heart through reduced workload, improved **cardiac contractility**, increased blood volume, lower resting and exercise heart rates, and higher stroke volume. Other benefits of physical activity include slight increases in the concentration of **aerobic enzymes**, an increase in arterial diameters, an increase in the number of arterioles and **capillaries**, and a decrease in plaque formation. In our opinion, two of the major benefits of activity in reducing atherosclerosis are its ability to

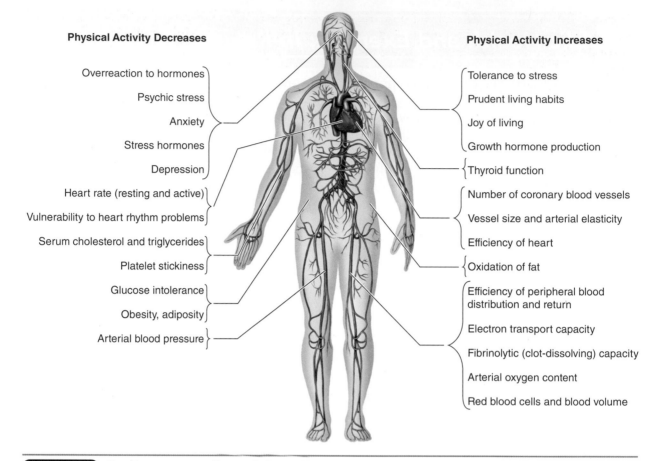

Physical Activity Decreases

Overreaction to hormones
Psychic stress
Anxiety
Stress hormones
Depression
Heart rate (resting and active)
Vulnerability to heart rhythm problems
Serum cholesterol and triglycerides
Platelet stickiness
Glucose intolerance
Obesity, adiposity
Arterial blood pressure

Physical Activity Increases

Tolerance to stress
Prudent living habits
Joy of living
Growth hormone production
Thyroid function
Number of coronary blood vessels
Vessel size and arterial elasticity
Efficiency of heart
Oxidation of fat
Efficiency of peripheral blood distribution and return
Electron transport capacity
Fibrinolytic (clot-dissolving) capacity
Arterial oxygen content
Red blood cells and blood volume

FIGURE 1.5 Cardioprotective effects of physical activity.

Adapted from B.J. Sharkey, 1974, *Physiological fitness and weight control* (Missoula, MT: Mountain Press), 15. By permission of B.J. Sharkey.

> *The major benefits of activity are its ability to metabolize fat and lower circulating levels of fat in the blood and its ability to maintain the elasticity of the major arteries.*

metabolize fat and lower circulating levels of fat in the blood (triglycerides and cholesterol) and its ability to maintain the elasticity of the major arteries. Let's look at some of these mechanisms to help explain why something as simple as regular, moderate activity is good for your health.

Vascular Changes

Your vascular system, which delivers blood carrying oxygen, food, and hormones to the cells of your body, is the first line of defense against disease. It also removes waste products and heat. Physical activity provides beneficial changes in blood clotting, blood pressure, and blood distribution, along with the specific benefits previously noted for your heart.

• *Blood clotting.* Blood is designed to form a clot and stem the flow of blood when we are injured. But a clot (called a **thrombus**) that forms within an uninjured vessel is dangerous, and a clot in a narrowed coronary artery could be disastrous. Clots form when the soluble protein fibrinogen is converted to insoluble threads of **fibrin**. Normally, we are able to dissolve an unwanted thrombus by dissolving the fibrin (fibrinolysis). Exercise enhances this process, but the effect lasts only a day or two. The stress of exhaustive or highly competitive exercise seems to inhibit this system, allowing more rapid clotting time. Regular, moderate, or even vigorous activity is the way to enhance the ability of the body to dissolve unwanted clots (Molz et al. 1993). Chronic aerobic exercise training may cause favorable adaptations that contribute to decreased risk for ischemic events (inadequate oxygen delivery to heart or skeletal muscle), both at rest and during exertion (Womack, Nagelkirk, and Coughlin 2003). In fact, a review of the literature concludes that regular exercise is the most practicable approach known to decrease plasma fibrinogen levels (Ernst 1993).

• *Large-artery elasticity.* Aging and sedentary living contribute to a loss of large-artery compliance (elasticity). This loss of compliance increases **systolic blood pressure** and increases the risk of plaque rupture and heart attack. Research (Seals 2003) has shown that regular aerobic exercise favorably attenuates age-associated decreases in arterial compliance. People who begin and maintain a moderate exercise program can improve arterial compliance and reduce their risk of myocardial infarction (heart attack). Regular exercisers, even those who show no improvement in fitness, have greater arterial elasticity than sedentary people do (Ferreira et al. 2002).

• *Blood pressure.* High blood pressure, or **hypertension**, increases the workload of the heart by forcing it to contract against a greater resistance. Anything that lowers blood pressure also reduces the workload of the heart. Regular, moderate physical activity has been shown to reduce blood pressure in middle-aged or older people, especially those with elevated levels. Walking, but not weightlifting, has been shown to reduce **systolic** blood pressure in elderly people (Rejeski et al. 1995). Of course, changes in blood pressure could also be the consequence of weight loss or reduced stress, both known outcomes of regular activity.

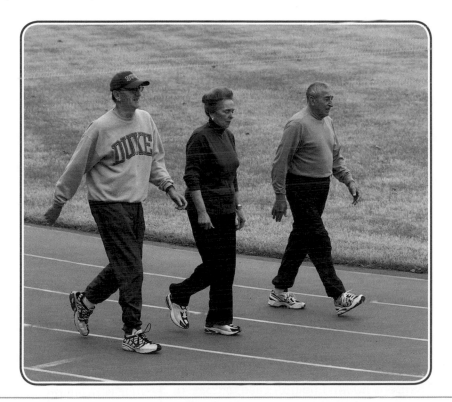

■ Regular, moderate exercise, such as walking, provides many benefits for the vascular system, including reduced blood pressure.

• *Blood distribution.* Regular physical activity improves the body's ability to distribute blood to muscles during exercise, further reducing the workload of the heart. Vessels leading to digestive and other organs are constricted, and vessels that serve working muscles open (dilate) to allow blood to flow where it is needed during exercise.

• *Blood volume.* The 10 to 15 percent increase in blood volume that comes with **endurance** training enhances the performance of both the heart and skeletal muscles. These changes serve to lower the heart rate and blood pressure during physical activity. Because the oxygen needs of heart muscle are directly related to the product of heart rate and blood pressure, these improvements serve to reduce the likelihood that you'll exceed the ability to supply oxygen to **cardiac** muscle. As with most other effects of activity and training, the benefits depend on regular, not occasional, activity.

Metabolic Changes

The metabolic changes that result from activity may be the most important in the fight against CAD as well as several other disorders. The changes include increased fat mobilization and **metabolism**, reduced blood lipids and body fat, and changes in **insulin** sensitivity. The metabolic changes associated with physical activity contribute significantly to reductions in heart disease risk.

• *Fat metabolism.* If you eat too much, you will gain weight in the form of stored fat. Excess fat is a health risk for heart disease, hypertension, diabetes, and some forms of cancer. You can diet (starve) to get rid of fat, but there is a hitch: The starving breaks down muscle tissue for energy, so you lose the only tissue that is capable of burning large amounts of fat. Muscular activity is the proven way to mobilize fat from **adipose tissue** and then to burn it for energy in skeletal muscles. Exercise burns fat and avoids loss of muscle **protein**. Regular activity can build additional muscle, thereby enhancing your ability to burn fat.

The body of a physically fit person is an efficient fat-burning furnace.

Regular activity burns calories, helping you maintain a desirable body weight and percent body fat and resulting in a leaner, healthier figure. **Aerobic fitness** training enhances the ability to mobilize and metabolize fat. Training increases the proportion of energy derived from fat (versus carbohydrate) at rest and during moderate activity. Physically fit people also burn more calories during and after vigorous exercise (Knab et al. 2011), making their bodies efficient fat-burning furnaces. This enhanced ability to use fat as an energy source leads to even greater benefits that are closely tied to reduced risk of

Aspirin

Studies have shown that one small aspirin (81 mg) a day reduces the risk of unwanted clots associated with heart disease and stroke. The aspirin reduces the stickiness of platelets, small particles in the blood that are caught in the fibrin threads of a developing clot. Most people tolerate one small aspirin a day, taken with a meal. This practice is an inexpensive way to reduce the risk of CAD and stroke, and it may help reduce the risk of colon cancer. The small tablet reduces the risk of gastrointestinal problems. Some people, however, may require a higher dose (Kong 2004). Concurrent use of ibuprofen may decrease the heart benefit of aspirin (Gaziano and Gibson 2006), but a study of 3,859 patients found no increase in heart attacks among those who took aspirin and ibuprofen compared with those who took aspirin alone (Patel and Goldberg 2004). In either case, a coated aspirin may be a wise choice for long-term therapy.

atherosclerosis and CAD (see following section on blood lipids). Physical activity has even been found to decrease the risk of developing gallstones, independent of other risk factors such as obesity and recent rapid dietary weight loss (Leitzmann et al. 1999).

• *Blood lipids. Lipid* is another word for fat. The **blood lipids** include cholesterol and triglycerides, and each is related to the risk of heart disease. The level of cholesterol in the blood is an important predictor of the risk of heart disease. Total cholesterol includes low-density **lipoprotein** (LDL) cholesterol and **high-density lipoprotein (HDL) cholesterol**. Regular activity can lead to a modest decline in total cholesterol, but that is only part of the story. LDL is the dangerous subfraction of cholesterol found in the plaques that clog coronary arteries. Activity, diet, and weight loss all contribute to a drop in LDL. Regular activity, particularly prolonged or vigorous activity, and weight loss both contribute to a rise in HDL cholesterol, the beneficial subfraction that collects cholesterol from the arteries and transports it to the liver for removal from the body. So, exercise reduces total cholesterol (especially the LDL portion), raises HDL, and greatly improves your total cholesterol-to-HDL ratio, one of the best predictors of heart disease risk.

Triglycerides, consisting of three fatty acids and a molecule of glycerol, constitute a transport and storage form of fat. High blood levels are associated with heart disease, obesity, and hypertension. Regular activity is a proven way to lower circulating levels of triglycerides. Levels decline after exercise, and the effect persists for 1 or 2 days. Several days of exercise lead to progressive reduction of triglyceride levels. The final plateau depends on diet, body weight, intensity and duration of exercise, and genetic tendencies. Clearly, regular, moderate activity leads to a significant reduction in triglycerides.

• *Other metabolic mechanisms.* A number of additional metabolic mechanisms support the value of activity as a cardioprotective therapy. Regular activity and training have been shown to increase insulin sensitivity and **glucose** tolerance. This effect of exercise is particularly important for people who are obese and those with adult-onset diabetes (also called **type 2 diabetes** or non-insulin-dependent diabetes mellitus—NIDDM). High levels of circulating fat inhibit the ability of insulin to transport glucose into muscles. Exercise enhances the transport of glucose into muscles, even in the absence of insulin. Thus, regular activity helps by reducing body weight and fat levels and by increasing insulin sensitivity and glucose transport. All these improvements reduce the risk of heart disease and NIDDM.

Electrolytes, including potassium, sodium, and calcium, are essential to the function of muscles, including the heart. During exertion, the untrained heart may experience diminished oxygen supply, which can trigger an imbalance of electrolytes, electrical instability, and disturbances in heart rhythms. Death can result from lethal rhythm disorders, such as tachycardia (rapid beating) or fibrillation (irregular, uncontrolled, unsynchronized beating). Fitness training minimizes this likelihood by reducing the workload of the heart, improving oxygen supply and efficiency, and correcting electrolyte imbalances.

Cholesterol-to-HDL Ratio

Before training and weight loss, Bill had an elevated risk of CAD and a cholesterol level of 240 and an HDL of 40, for a ratio of 6 (240/40). Training and weight loss reduced the cholesterol to 200 and raised the HDL to 50, yielding a much improved ratio of 4. He could further improve his lipid profile and reduce his risk of CAD by continuing training, maintaining or lowering his body weight, and reducing his consumption of total and saturated fat. Lowering cholesterol to 180 and raising HDL to 60 produces a favorable risk profile. Subsequent chapters say more about cholesterol.

ACTIVITY REDUCES
THE RISK OF CHRONIC DISEASES

We have taken much time and space to establish the role of activity and fitness in reducing the risks of heart disease. Now we will briefly sketch how activity can protect you from a growing list of chronic diseases and disorders.

Hypertension and Stroke

People with very high blood pressure (greater than 160/95) are three times more likely to experience CAD and four times more likely to experience congestive heart failure than others. Resting blood pressure values above 130/85 are associated with an increased risk of CAD in middle-aged and older people, and the risk increases with age (Vasan et al. 2001). Hypertension also increases the risk of stroke and kidney failure. The causes of hypertension are still under investigation. But we do know that inactivity increases the risk of developing hypertension by 35 percent, and that unfit subjects have 52 percent greater risk than the fit. Regular endurance exercise lowers resting systolic and diastolic pressures by about 10 millimeters of mercury, with even greater benefits during activity. Active hypertensive patients have half the risk of death from all causes than inactive hypertensive patients do (Paffenbarger 1994).

A **stroke**, which is a clot or hemorrhage (bleeding) of a blood vessel in the brain, can result in loss of speech or muscle control, or even death. The risk factors are similar to those for CAD. In most studies, the risk of stroke decreases as activity increases. But with activity that is more vigorous and, possibly, with heavy lifting, the trend may reverse, especially in unfit people. Transient ischemic attacks (TIAs) are sudden, brief periods of weakness, vertigo, loss of vision, slurred speech, headache, or other symptoms that sometimes precede a stroke. Similar symptoms have been associated with heavy weightlifting exercises, especially in those with elevated blood pressure. Repeatedly, we find compelling arguments for moderation.

Cancer and Immunity

In recent years, evidence has been accumulating that an active lifestyle is associated with lower risk of certain types of cancers. Most often studied is the link between activity and lower risk of colon cancer. Some researchers hypothesize that regular activity shortens intestinal transit time for potential carcinogens in fecal material. If that is the mechanism, it is hard to understand why the incidence of rectal cancer isn't lower as well. But lack of physical activity is causally related to colon cancer: 12 to 14 percent of colon cancer can be attributed to lack of frequent involvement in vigorous physical activity (Slattery 2004). Some studies suggest that activity may help reduce the risk of prostate cancer. When activity was examined by intensity of effort, vigorous activity decreased prostate cancer risk by 30 percent (Friedenreich et al. 2004).

Women who were active in their youth have fewer cancers of the breast and the reproductive system (Frisch et al. 1985). These authors noted that body fat was lower in the previously active women. In fact, a study of more than 25,000 women found that the risk was lowest (RR was .28) in lean women who exercised at least 4 hours per week (Thune et al. 1997). One study found that sustained activity throughout life, and particularly activity done later in life, may provide the greatest benefit in reducing the risk of breast cancer (Friedenreich, Courneya, and Bryant 2001). The role of dietary fat and obesity in

Metabolic Syndrome

Defined as a clustering of metabolic abnormalities related to insulin, metabolic syndrome includes the following:

- Blood pressure greater than 130/85 millimeters of mercury
- Serum triglycerides greater than 150 milligrams per deciliter
- HDL cholesterol less than 40 milligrams per deciliter
- Fasting blood glucose greater than 110 milligrams per deciliter
- Central adiposity (waist circumference greater than 35 in., or 89 cm, for females or 40 in., or 102 cm, for males)

The presence of three of these metabolic markers is associated with obesity, diabetes, and heart disease (see figure 1.6). Low levels of aerobic fitness are associated with increased clustering of the metabolic abnormalities of the syndrome in men and women (Whaley et al. 1999). A sedentary lifestyle and especially poor fitness are not only associated with metabolic syndrome, but could be considered features of the syndrome. A low level of fitness may provide a means of identifying those who would benefit from interventions to prevent the syndrome and its dire consequences (Lakka et al. 2003). Excess central or abdominal fat, as indicated by waist circumference, is a predictor of the metabolic syndrome. High levels of visceral abdominal fat are also associated with measures of inflammation, which predict several chronic diseases, including heart disease (Despres 2004).

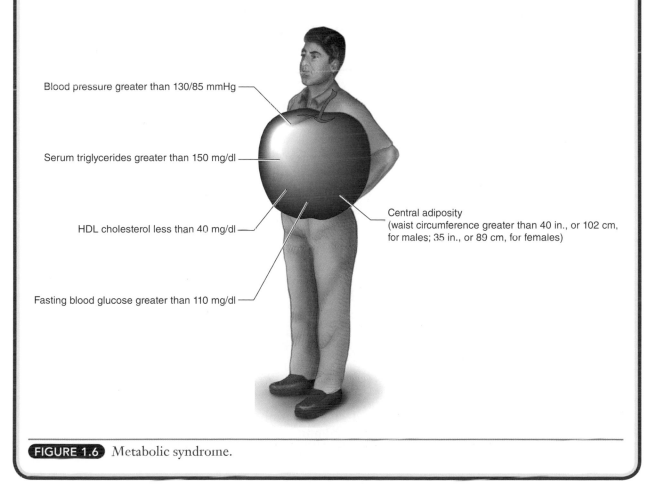

Blood pressure greater than 130/85 mmHg

Serum triglycerides greater than 150 mg/dl

HDL cholesterol less than 40 mg/dl

Fasting blood glucose greater than 110 mg/dl

Central adiposity
(waist circumference greater than 40 in., or 102 cm, for males; 35 in., or 89 cm, for females)

FIGURE 1.6 Metabolic syndrome.

the development of cancer continues to interest researchers. Increased body weight was associated with increased death rates for all cancers combined and for cancers with multiple specific sites (Calle et al. 2003).

A substance that causes genetic damage (e.g., carcinogens in meat or cigarette smoke) may initiate cancers. Promoters (such as estrogen in the case of breast cancer) then stimulate cell proliferation. A healthy immune system may play a role in the control of initiators or the suppression of transformed cells or their by-products. On the other hand, a compromised immune system may allow initiation and promotion to go unchecked. You will be glad to know that regular, moderate physical activity enhances the function of the immune system, whereas high levels of stress or exhaustive exercise seem to suppress the system (Nieman 2003).

Diabetes and Obesity

There is a recognized link among NIDDM, CAD, and hypertension, specifically that all three share **insulin resistance** and that obesity and lack of activity are part of the problem (Alberti et al. 2009). Insulin-resistant cells can't take in glucose, so glucose levels rise and the body secretes more insulin, which tends to increase blood pressure (through increased blood volume and **vasoconstriction**). Obesity and high levels of blood lipids seem to foster a resistance to insulin, whereas exercise increases insulin sensitivity and the movement of glucose into working muscles. Regular activity has returned to a place of prominence in the treatment of NIDDM. For some, it removes the need for diabetes medication. In general, regularly active adults have a 42 percent lower risk of NIDDM (RR equals .58).

Arthritis, Osteoporosis, and Back Problems

This group of musculoskeletal problems accounts for significant pain and suffering, as well as massive sums of money for often unnecessary treatments. Activity can treat or prevent all these problems. Osteoarthritis (painful joint degeneration, as in the knees), doesn't seem to be caused by exercise unless a previous injury has occurred. In addition, regular, moderate activity is an essential part of treatment for most forms of arthritis.

Osteoporosis is the progressive loss of bone mineral that occurs faster in women, especially after menopause. Cigarette smoking, low body weight—especially from dieting—and lack of activity accelerate the decline in bone density. With age, the condition can lead to brittle bones, hip fractures, and the characteristic dowager's hump caused by the collapse of vertebrae in the neck. Adequate calcium intake can slow the loss of bone mineral. Weight-bearing exercise helps maximize bone mass during youth, maintain bone mass in middle age, and slow age-related loss in later years. Regular exercise also helps older people avoid crippling falls (Beck and Snow 2003). Two years of intense exercise helped retain bone density in postmenopausal women (Kemmler et al. 2004). Weight-bearing exercises must serve upper and lower body sites. Running and calcium intake stimulated lower body bone mass of women runners at the expense of bone mass from upper body sites (Nevill et al. 2003). Continued participation in impact activities is also beneficial for the skeletal health of males, especially after the age of 40 years (VanLangendonck et al. 2003).

Back problems result from the acute or chronic assault to underused and undertrained bodies. Regular attention to abdominal and back exercises and flexibility of the back and hamstring muscles can minimize the risk of back problems or can rehabilitate the back. Among the many therapies used on back problems, including surgery, manipulation, injections, and drugs, none has proved more effective than rapid return to physical activity and early ambulation. Chapter 11 provides specific suggestions for **core training** and back health.

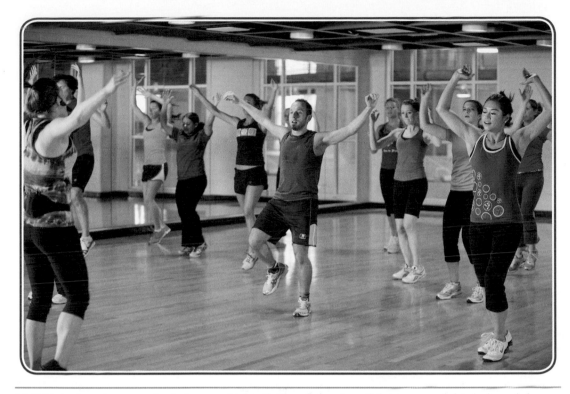

■ Weight-bearing exercise helps maximize the bone density of the young, and it helps adults maintain their bone density.

ACTIVITY INCREASES LONGEVITY

By decreasing the risk of CAD, cancer, and other diseases of lifestyle, regular activity extends the period of adult vigor and compresses the period of sickness that precedes death. In a real sense, activity adds life to your years and years to your life. When Paffenbarger (1994) analyzed the effects of changing to more favorable health habits, moderate activity (1,500 cal/week) conferred an average of 1.57 years above less active living, and vigorous sports provided 1.54 years over no sports participation. Data on Harvard alumni indicated that vigorous activity (defined as more than 6.5–7.5 cal/min, the equivalent of a brisk walk) was associated with reduced mortality. Mortality declined with increasing levels of vigorous activity up to about 3,500 calories per week, but not for nonvigorous activity (Lee, Hsieh, and Paffenbarger 1995).

A report from the Institute for Aerobics Research (Blair et al. 1995) confirmed that fit folks live longer. Data on 9,777 men aged 20 to 82 showed that those who were unfit when they entered the study were 44 percent less likely to die over the 18-year period of the study if they improved their fitness. Those who were fit at the start of the study and remained fit were 67 percent less likely to die than were those who remained unfit. The benefits were found across all age groups, and the most fit people had the lowest risk of premature death. Chapter 6 says more about aging and how to live better and longer.

SUMMARY

For more than 60 years, epidemiologists have studied the relationships of occupational and leisure-time activity with health, and an impressive list of benefits has emerged. The studies clearly show how activity enhances health while it reduces the risk of CAD, hypertension, and stroke, as well as some cancers, diabetes, osteoporosis, obesity, and other chronic disorders. We have presented evidence of additional health benefits associated with vigorous activity and fitness and have shown how regular, moderate physical activity extends the length and quality of life. Now we will turn our attention to the topic of mental or psychological health to see how the active life contributes to mental health, cognitive abilities, and the joy of living.

Mental and Cognitive Health

A Sound Mind in a Sound Body

> "A sound mind in a sound body
> is a short but full description
> of a happy state in this world."
>
> *John Locke*

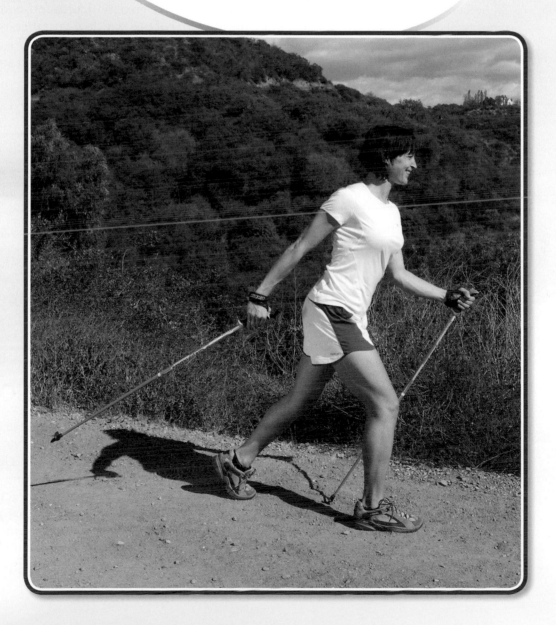

Y ou have heard of **psychosomatic illness**, a physical ailment caused or exacerbated by the state of mind. But few have heard the term *somatopsychic*, which suggests the effect of the body (*soma*) on the mind. This chapter describes how use of the body, specifically with regular, moderate physical activity, has a beneficial effect on the mind and mental health. Although the research in this area is still in its infancy and many questions remain, reviewing the case for what may be the most significant role for activity and fitness is important. As with activity and physical health, we must wonder about self-selection: Does activity promote mental health, or does mental health promote activity? Do happy, less anxious, or less depressed people have the interest, vigor, and energy to be active?

Evidence from epidemiological studies indicates that the level of physical activity is positively associated with good mental health, when mental health is defined as positive mood, general well-being, and relatively infrequent symptoms of anxiety and depression (Stephens 1988). As you will see, in intervention studies, activity has reduced levels of anxiety and depression. If it is true, as some have estimated, that at any given time as many as 25 percent of the population suffer from mild to moderate anxiety, depression, and other emotional disorders, we should not ignore the potential of this safe, low-cost therapy. The second part of this chapter focuses on how activity is associated with improved learning and cognition throughout the life span. One study showed that participants who are both active and maintain high lifelong levels of cognitive activity achieve the maximal protection against dementia (Cracchiolo et al. 2007).

This chapter will help you do the following:

- Understand how activity reduces anxiety and depression
- Appreciate how activity helps us deal with stress
- Recognize positive aspects of an addiction to activity
- Determine the influence of activity on learning
- Assess the effect of regular, moderate physical activity on the risk of dementia and Alzheimer's disease

ACTIVITY REDUCES ANXIETY AND DEPRESSION

If activity were a drug and it could be proved effective in the prevention and treatment of anxiety and depression, it would be hailed as a modern miracle, worth billions to the company with legal rights to the formula. Well, activity isn't a drug, but is rather a learned behavior that requires **motivation** to begin a program and **persistence** to adhere to it.

Anxiety has been defined as a diffuse apprehension of some vague threat, characterized by feelings of uncertainty and helplessness. It is more than ordinary worry in that people can perceive it as a threat to their self-esteem. **State anxiety** is a transitory emotional response to a specific situation, characterized by feelings of **tension**, apprehension, and nervousness. **Trait anxiety** is a relatively stable level of anxiety proneness, a predisposition to respond to threats with elevated anxiety. Studies have investigated the effects of acute and chronic physical activity on state and trait anxiety.

Activity such as walking has been shown to reduce state anxiety, as have meditation, biofeedback, and some other forms of mental diversion (see list that follows). So, if you are tense and apprehensive about an upcoming responsibility, meeting, or presentation, go for a walk. Doing so certainly can't hurt, and it probably will help. A study showed that resistance training or aerobic exercise significantly reduces state anxiety. The effect was similar in both forms of effort, and the benefit remained throughout 8 weeks of training (Hale and Raglin 2002). If you become anxious about physical threats such as a steep ski slope or white-water rapids, instruction, practice, and improved skill will help diminish future anxiety. Of greater importance is the question about whether regular activity or training reduces trait anxiety.

Anxiety exercise prescription

Mode	Aerobic activities, such as walking or resistance training
Frequency	Regular (almost daily), especially when needed
Intensity	Moderate, such as a brisk walk
Time	Not established, but 30-60 min should work

Studies of police, firefighters, athletes, and even patients indicate that physical training and improved fitness are associated with reductions in trait anxiety. A comprehensive review of the research found that activity was statistically related to a reduction in state and trait anxiety as well as psychophysiological measures of anxiety. The effects ranged from small to moderate (Landers and Petruzzello 1994). Studies show that moderate exercise is more effective than high-intensity exercise, that activity-induced reductions seem to persist for many weeks, and that reductions occur independently of age and health status (Weinberg and Gould 2003).

Depression is characterized by sadness, low self-esteem, pessimism, hopelessness, and despair. Symptoms range from fatigue, irritability, lack of direction, and withdrawal, to thoughts of suicide (see form 2.1). Whereas mild depression may resolve without treatment and moderate depression may go away in 6 months, severe cases, in which suicide is a real risk, are usually treated with drugs. Most activity studies have been conducted on mild to moderate nonclinical subjects.

A comprehensive statistical review of studies related to activity and depression concluded that activity significantly decreased depression for all age groups and fitness levels, and that larger decreases were associated with more sessions and longer exercise programs (North, McCullagh, and Tran 1990). A study evaluated the effects of treadmill exercise and found substantial rapid improvement in mood in patients with major depression (Bauer et al. 2001). Physical activity seems to work across all ages; more active children (Crews, Lochbaum, and Landers 2004) and teens are less depressed (Motl et al. 2004), and activity reduces the risk of depression in older adults (Strawbridge et al. 2002).

Although some researchers have hypothesized that exercise must lead to improvements in aerobic fitness in order to decrease depression, results have not supported that theory. A study of women found that even low levels of activity (one or two times per week) have a positive effect on mental health (depressed feelings and psychological disorders) (Kull 2003). We may safely say that those with mild to moderate depression may experience at least as much relief from activity and training as they do from conventional forms of therapy (see following list). Let's consider some reasons why this may be so.

Depression exercise prescription

Mode	Aerobic exercise or light resistance exercise with multiple repetitions
Frequency	Almost daily, with acute and long-term benefits
Intensity	Light to moderate, with improved benefits associated with increased intensity, duration, and frequency
Time	30 min or longer

A number of hypotheses have been advanced to explain the effect of activity and training on mental health. They range from simple behavioral strategies to complex biochemical theories.

Form 2.1   Self-Evaluation for Depression

The following statements, suggested by the National Institute of Mental Health, can help you determine whether you may be suffering from depression. Indicate whether you agree or disagree with the following:

_____I feel downhearted, blue, and sad.

_____I don't enjoy the things that I used to.

_____I feel that others would be better off without me.

_____I feel that I am not useful or needed.

_____I notice that I am losing weight.

_____I have trouble sleeping at night.

_____I am restless and can't keep still.

_____My mind isn't as clear as it used to be.

_____I get tired for no reason.

_____I feel hopeless about the future.

Total the number of statements with which you agreed. If you agreed with at least five, including one of the first two, and if you have had the symptoms for at least 2 weeks, you may need professional help. If you agreed with the third statement, seek help immediately.

From B.J. Sharkey and S.E. Gaskill, 2013, *Fitness and health, seventh edition* (Champaign, IL: Human Kinetics).

Coping Strategies

Regular activity serves as a positive coping strategy, a diversion, distraction, or time-out from the problems and stressors of everyday life. Activity occupies the mind, allowing the passage of time during difficult periods. It allows the substitution of good habits for bad ones, positive addictions for negative ones. Activity is a form of meditation, providing the benefits of other approaches along with improvement in health and fitness. It provides a sense of control over one's life and environment. People can be separated into two groups—internals, who believe that they can control outcomes in their lives, and externals, who believe that chance or other people control their lives. Internal controllers are more likely to adhere to healthy behaviors. Can a person change this locus of control? Can one become an internal and improve adherence to healthy behavior?

The perception of acquiring mastery in a particular area influences coping behavior. Perception of mastery also influences performance, and it is theorized that experience alters perception. Thus, successful experience may reinforce a coping behavior, thereby ensuring continuation of the behavior. Some have even suggested that this enhanced **self-efficacy** (defined as a sense of one's ability to organize and execute actions required to achieve designated outcomes) may generalize to other areas of performance. We have much to learn

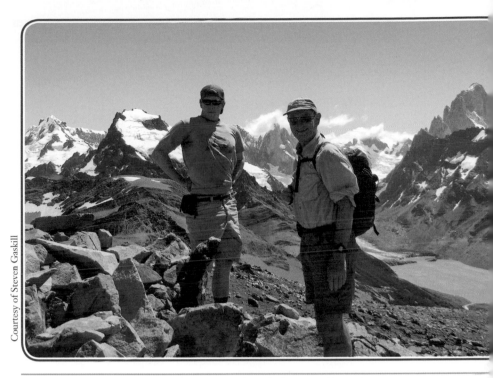

Courtesy of Steven Gaskill

■ The authors both enjoy getting out for a hike or walk in the mountains as part of their coping strategy: Steve (right) on a hike in Patagonia.

concerning these theories. We can say that regular activity provides a sense of control and mastery over one dimension of life, and it may improve control and mastery over others.

Does activity measure up to other therapies? One study found that fitness training, embedded in a cognitive-behavioral program, was associated with positive changes in other relevant aspects of patient function, including coping strategies, sustained efforts to continue activities, and improved physical well-being. Other therapeutic efforts and drug therapy were associated with ambivalent patterns of positive as well as negative emotional and behavioral characteristics (VanderVliet et al. 2004).

Self-Esteem, Self-Concept, and Body Image

Can regular activity or improved fitness have a beneficial effect on self-esteem (self-approval) and self-concept, and could that reduce or prevent anxiety or depression? Self-concept is our knowledge, assumptions, and feelings about ourselves. A widely used test of self-concept employs 100 statements and a 5-point answering scale to determine five components of self-concept: personal self, social self, family self, moral and ethical self, and physical self (body image). You might not expect activity and fitness to alter all the scales, but changes in physical and personal self seem possible.

An extensive review of research on children indicated that activity was associated with a positive self-concept, participation in activity programs contributed to self-esteem, and fitness activities were more effective than other components of the physical education program in developing self-concept (Gruber 1986). Research on adults agrees that activity and fitness improve self-concept (see form 2.2). When you take control of your life, lose weight, improve **strength** and endurance, and enhance your appearance, you feel better about yourself and your body. This new confidence may alter your outlook on life, even

Form 2.2   Self-Concept

Are you generally

__ relaxed or __ anxious?

__ in good shape or __ poor shape?

__ adventurous or __ conservative?

__ trim or __ overweight?

__ hardworking or __ lazy?

__ ambitious or __ aimless?

__ strong or __ weak?

__ physically attractive or __ unattractive?

__ persistent or __ not persistent?

__ extroverted or __ introverted?

__ self-confident or __ insecure?

__ a leader or __ a follower?

Do you want to improve some aspect of your self-concept? Select one or two attributes and find ways to make improvements.

From B.J. Sharkey and S.E. Gaskill, 2013, *Fitness and health, seventh edition* (Champaign, IL: Human Kinetics).

your personality. As activity and fitness alter the self-image, this renewed confidence in the body can be an important step toward improved personal—even intimate—relations.

Self-esteem can be enhanced through participation in physical activity, perhaps by enhancing physical ability and self-estimation. Runners and other athletes identify with other participants. We define ourselves as runners, cyclists, swimmers, and so on, and we derive social acceptance from the group. One fear associated with injury is the loss of identity and social acceptance.

Biochemical Mechanisms

Activity and training can influence metabolism and a number of hormones. Regular participation provides biofeedback that leads to changes in heart rate, blood pressure, and other measures. Activity temporarily raises body temperature and induces relaxation and mild fatigue, factors related to the tranquilizing effect of exercise. A study by deVries and Adams (1972) showed that a single bout of exercise (walking) was as effective in reducing tension as a tranquilizer, and that the effect of the exercise lasted longer. Fitness training

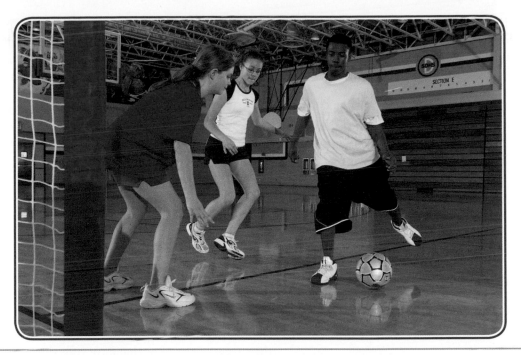

■ Activity has been shown to improve self-concept in children and adults.

leads to profound metabolic effects that include increased efficiency and responsiveness to hormones, such as insulin. Training has a favorable influence on hormones and neurotransmitters associated with depression. Of course, activity also enhances blood circulation, improving cognitive and even intimate performance. Studies show that activity and fitness increase interest, involvement, and satisfaction in sexual activity (Bortz, Wallace, and Wiley 1999, Bortz 2010).

Exercise also seems to enhance and protect brain function. Animals engaged in voluntary wheel running showed evidence of gene-expression changes in the brain. Animals that exercised showed an increase in a molecule (neurotrophic factor) that increases neuronal survival, enhances learning, and protects against cognitive decline (Cotman and Engesser-Cesar 2002). Researchers have also measured improved learning and delayed cognitive decline in active older adults. New research indicates that older people who exercise three or more times per week are less likely to develop Alzheimer's and other types of dementia. People who exercised regularly had a 30 to 40 percent lower risk of dementia. Even light activity such as walking helps to delay the onset of symptoms (Larson et al. 2006).

Some researchers also believe that activity increases levels of mood-altering substances called endorphins. Studies show that endorphins, morphine-like compounds produced in the brain, can reduce pain and induce a sense of euphoria. Runners whose levels of beta-endorphins in the blood increased after a marathon were quick to speculate that these opiates were responsible for the sensation known as the runner's high. Although blood-endorphin levels increase during and after an endurance effort, studies have shown that the levels do not correspond with mood states (Markoff, Ryan, and Young 1982). But a lack of correlation between blood levels and moods should not be surprising because a barrier between the blood and the brain prevents easy transport between the systemic circulation and the brain. Hence, blood levels of endorphins do not necessarily tell us what is happening to endorphin levels in the brain, where moods are formed. When rats exercised daily for 1 hour on a treadmill, beta-endorphin levels in their brains (**hypothalamus**) were much higher than they were in control animals (Asahina et al. 2003). Increased levels in the blood are probably a reflection of the role of endorphins as a narcotic. Running feels easier after about 20 minutes, which is when researchers have detected increased levels of beta-endorphin. So if you have tried running and found it uncomfortable, try to continue beyond 20 minutes. You may find that it becomes easier with the help of your natural painkillers.

Clearly, activity and fitness have the potential to improve mild to moderate cases of anxiety and depression, and improve self-concept and body image. But why wait until you are anxious or depressed to begin? Start now and you may be able to prevent or minimize assaults to your mental health.

ACTIVITY MINIMIZES STRESS

Many believe that stress has become one of the major health problems of the modern age. Physiological responses necessary for the survival of primitive peoples may be unhealthy in highly complex societies. Stress, tension, and reactive behavior patterns have been associated with heart disease, hypertension, suppression of the immune system, and a variety of other ills. Structures in the brain, including the hypothalamus, mediate the emotional response to life events. When something excites or threatens us, the hypothalamus tells the anterior pituitary gland to secrete adrenocorticotropic hormone (ACTH), a chemical messenger that travels to the adrenal cortex and orders the release of hormones such as cortisol (see figure 2.1). These hormones are necessary for the body to respond to stressful situations. Stress has been defined as anything that increases the release of ACTH or cortisol.

Stressful situations also elicit a response in the sympathetic nervous system that leads to secretion of hormones from the adrenal medulla, including **epinephrine** (adrenaline) and **norepinephrine**. These hormones mobilize energy and support the cardiovascular response to the stressor. This aspect of the stress response is called the fight-or-flight mechanism. The hormones prepare the body to fight or run, but they have other effects that can be harmful to health. Epinephrine makes the blood clot faster and increases blood pressure, an advantage in a fight but a disadvantage in the workplace, where it can increase the risk of a heart attack or a stroke.

The stress response is necessary to prepare an athlete for maximal effort in a physical challenge, but it can be unhealthy if it occurs too often in the wrong setting. If you become stressed on the job, when a natural physical catharsis is impossible or improper, circulating hormones can be a problem. Research has sug-

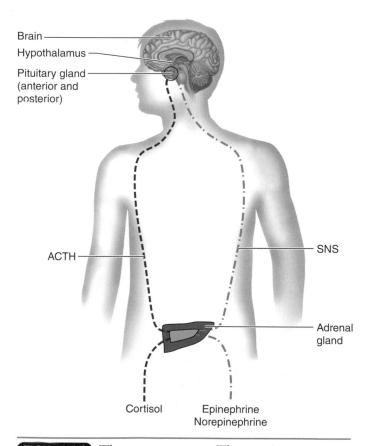

FIGURE 2.1 The stress response. The reaction starts in the hypothalamus, which then communicates with the anterior pituitary gland, triggering a release of ACTH. Likewise, the sympathetic nervous system signals the adrenal glands, where hormones for the 'flight or fight' response are secreted.

gested that some of us are hot reactors, exhibiting exaggerated blood pressure responses to everyday stressors. Hostile hot reactors become enraged when a driver cuts them off in traffic (road rage) or they experience other psychosocial stressors. This hostility elicits a flood of hormones designed for combat. Blood pressure and heart rate increase, arteries constrict, clotting time shortens, and blood flow to the heart drops off, contributing to increased risk of a heart attack. Hot reactors stew in their own juices, setting the stage for immediate or future health problems. Although occasional stress is not a threat, prolonged exposure to stress hormones eventually suppresses the immune system and reduces resistance to infection.

Some early animal studies suggested that exercise itself was a stressor (Selye 1956). Those results make sense when you realize that the researchers forced the animals to run on a treadmill and shocked them when they tried to rest, or forced them to swim to exhaustion in a deep tank with a weight tied around the tail. Electroshock and fear of drowning are stressful for most of us. For humans, exercise is stressful when it is highly competitive, exhausting, or threatening. Rock climbing, for example, is stressful for the neophyte but relaxing and exhilarating for the veteran. Stress is in the eye of the beholder.

Type A

The type A behavior pattern is characterized by extreme competitiveness, ambition, and a profound sense of time urgency. The type B personality, the opposite of type A, is relaxed, calm, and even phlegmatic. In studies by cardiologists Friedman and Rosenman (1973), type A subjects had higher cholesterol levels, faster blood-clotting times, higher adrenaline levels, more sudden deaths, and a sevenfold greater risk of heart disease. Subsequent studies, including the massive Framingham study, failed to find a link among the type A behavior pattern, stress, and heart disease. They did find a link between anger or repressed hostility and heart disease risk (Wilson, Castelli, and Kannel 1987).

Although most of us intuitively accept stress as a risk factor for heart disease, the type A personality, in the absence of anger and hostility, does not seem to be the problem. Studies of corporate structure suggest that employees, not hard-driving executives, face the most stress. Executives live fast-paced lives but retain a sense of control. Employees often feel that they have no control over their lives, a circumstance that is stressful. A high level of anger in young men (concealed anger, griping, and irritability) is associated with increased risk of CAD and heart attacks (Chang et al. 2002).

Ulcers?

Years ago, ulcers were thought to be a product of stress, which led to increases in stomach acid, which then eroded a hole in the stomach (gastric ulcer). Today we know that *Helicobacter pylori*, an acid-resistant organism that survives in the stomach, causes many ulcers. Eliminating the bacterium with antibiotics cures the ulcer (Sachs et al. 2003).

Regular, moderate activity minimizes the effects of stress. It is relaxing and tranquilizing, and it counters the tendency to form blood clots, lowers resting blood pressure, and reduces epinephrine and cortisol. Regular activity enhances the function of the immune system, whereas the exhaustion of running a marathon is immunosuppressive. Occasional exposure to stressful activity is fine if one has trained for the event. Regular, moderate activity and fitness contribute to health, in part by reducing the **diastolic blood pressure** response to stress (Hendrix and Hughes 1997). In one study, highly fit people experienced lower cardiovascular responses to stress than less-fit people did, even though the groups did not

Stress Test

Certain life events, both positive and negative, have been identified as stressful. A score of over 300 points gained in one year may indicate a serious illness will occur within 2 years. Here are some of the events and their relative stressfulness (Roth and Holmes 1985).

Death of spouse	100 points
Divorce	73
Separation	65
Jail term	63
Death of family member	63
Personal injury or illness	53
Marriage	50
Fired from job	47
Retirement	45
Marital reconciliation	45
Pregnancy	40
Death of friend	37
Mortgage	31
Personal achievement	28
Spouse starts or stops work	26
Trouble with boss	23
Change of residence	20
Vacation	13

differ in hostility (Alderman and Landers 2004). Another study correlated subclinical coronary artery disease, as measured by electron-beam computed tomography, to depression, anxiety, hostility, and stress. This study of 630 active-duty military personnel found no correlation between CAD and any of the psychological factors, including stress (O'Malley et al. 2000). Perhaps the soldiers used activity to minimize their stress.

We know that regular activity is a coping mechanism that serves to improve tolerance to psychological stress. Although meditation and other forms of stress management are useful, regular, moderate activity is the best form of stress management because it provides the benefits of meditation and relaxation while delivering added health benefits, including weight loss, control of anxiety and depression, improved appearance, vitality, and even longevity, as well as reduced risk of CAD, hypertension, cancer, diabetes, and other ills. Aerobic training is more effective than stress management in lowering heart rate and blood pressure during psychological stress (Spalding, Lyon, and Hatfield 2004).

Psychoneuroimmunology (PNI) studies the links among the brain, the nervous system, and the immune system. PNI focuses on how thoughts, emotions, and personality traits interact with the immune system and become manifest in sickness or health. Thoughts or emotions can enhance or suppress the immune system through neurotransmitters secreted by the sympathetic nervous system or through hormones released on command of the brain (e.g., ACTH). The immune system is immensely complicated, consisting of lymphocytes, T cells, natural killer cells, antibodies, immunoglobulins, and more. The immune system serves to protect the body from foreign assaults. When exposed to prolonged stress, however, the system tends to break down, allowing invading microorganisms to proliferate. PNI suggests that by altering your perception of the supposed threat and by reprogramming your thinking and your outlook on life, you can reduce exposure to stress and spare the immune system.

Another way to bolster the immune system is by participating in regular activity. Studies confirm the beneficial effect of activity and training on components of the immune system. The studies agree that regular, moderate activity and training contribute to a healthy immune system (Mackinnon 1992, Nieman and Pedersen 1999). Intensity, duration, or frequency of training greater than a person is accustomed to increases the risk of **overtraining**, a condition characterized by fatigue, poor performance, and suppression of the immune system. On the other hand, well-trained athletes and workers are able to complete full days of physically challenging work with no decline in immune function. Studies of wildland firefighters showed that the firefighters could sustain up to 14 hours of hard work without adverse effects on immune function (Ruby et al. 2002). Activity, relaxation, imagery, and other coping strategies help you deal in a rational way with difficult problems, freeing the immune system to function on your behalf.

> *I*f life is getting too stressful, slow the pace of change.

Physically active people tend to deal well with stress, contract fewer upper respiratory tract infections (colds and sore throats), and miss fewer work days because of illness. They can perform on the job or athletic field day after day. These health improvements appear related to improved immune function. In an ongoing study at the University of Montana, daily habitual activity levels appear to be inversely linked to levels of C-reactive protein, an inflammatory marker in the blood linked to increased risk for heart disease. In many ways, direct and indirect, the active life seems to reduce illness and increase vitality.

ACTIVITY IMPROVES COGNITIVE HEALTH

Is it possible that a somatopsychic effect exists in which the health of the body (*soma*) affects the health of our brain (*psychic*), thus influencing learning and cognitive function? In his book *Spark: The Revolutionary New Science of Exercise and the Brain*, John Ratey summarizes the positive affect that physical activity has on brain function (Ratey and Hagerman 2008). Current research has even demonstrated that physical activity can stimulate **neurogenesis** (the growth of new brain cells) while also increasing the number of neural connections (Bekinschtein et al. 2011). A growing body of knowledge shows that youth and adolescents who participate in regular moderate and vigorous physical activity do better at school in terms of academic achievement, attendance, attention, memorization, and integration. They also exhibit fewer disciplinary problems and incidences of attention-deficit/hyperactivity disorder (ADHD) (Gaskill, Miller, and Wambold 2012, Trudeau and Shephard 2008).

These studies make a strong case for increasing physical activity in schools rather than the current trend to reduce recess, cut physical education, and spend more time sitting in the classroom. The understanding that physical activity was related to brain health is not new. Ancient philosophers believed that bodily activity improved brain fitness. Plato, Hippocrates, and many others stressed the mind-body connection throughout their writings, yet it is only recently that both empirical evidence and mechanistic studies are beginning to document the basis for the body-mind connection. Let's take a look at some of the opinions and evidence.

In a study of 482 2nd- through 12th-grade students, we (Gaskill, Miller, and Wambold 2012) evaluated physical activity compared to both grade point average and standardized tests scores. The most active fourth of the students averaged nearly a full grade point higher and did significantly better on standardized tests than the quartile of least active students. The academic achievement gap increased with grade level. By high school, the GPA gap was nearly 1.5 grade points (3.52 for the most active versus 2.14 for the least active). Students in the Naperville, Illinois school district are all required to participate in nearly an hour of daily physical activity, which substantially raises their heart rates. They also placed 1st in the world in science testing and 6th in math. Additionally, their rates of overweight and obesity are less than 10 percent, nearly half of the rate of nearby communities and one-third of the national average (Ratey and Hagerman 2008).

During the last 5 years, more than 100 studies have documented the effect of physical activity or fitness on academic performance (Singh et al. 2012). In a number of studies, up to an hour of physical activity time replaced academic classroom time. In every study, academic performance measures either increased or at least did not decrease, even when time was taken from academic time for physical activity. In addition, attendance improved, and disciplinary referrals and attention deficit were reduced. What is generally not mentioned in these studies are all of the other benefits of physical activity: reduced obesity rates, decreased risk of chronic disease, improved self-efficacy, and all of the other benefits discussed in this book. In animal studies, and using new imaging techniques in humans, scientists have shown that increased physical activity helps our brains to grow new **neurons** and to increase the connections between neurons (Bekinschtein et al. 2011). This brain growth, termed *neurogenesis*, was previously believed not to occur in adults. Data suggest that coordinative and sustained aerobic exercise dramatically improve brain function. This is particularly true for youth, but adults and the elderly can also both improve cognition and slow the rates of decline.

The stimulus for neurogenesis and the associated improved memory, integration of information, and attention span that leads to higher cognitive function and academic achievement is the result of a number of hormones and brain chemicals that are increased or decreased by the exercise stimulus. Contracting muscles release growth factors such as *vascular endothelial growth factor* (VEGF) and fibroblast growth factor (FGF-2) and help stimulate blood vessel growth in both the body and the brain. Vascular diameter is enlarged by nitric oxide, increasing blood flow and decreasing hardening of the arteries, even in the brain. Exercise stimulates insulin-like growth factor, thus better regulating insulin while also improving synaptic plasticity in the brain. As blood glucose decreases

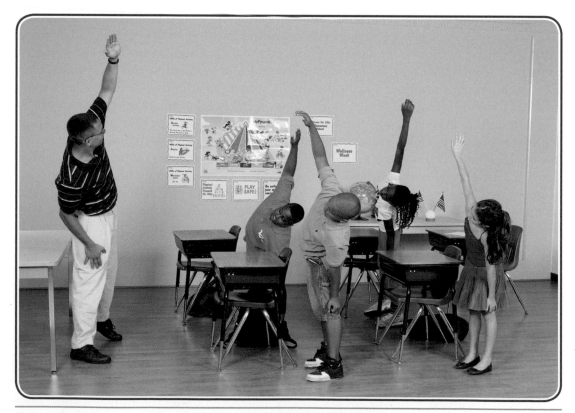

■ Regular 10-minute activity breaks during school improve academic success.

as a result of exercise, both exercise and lower blood glucose stimulate brain-derived neurotropic factor, which has been termed "Miracle Grow for the brain" by Dr. Ratey (Ratey and Hagerman 2008). Exercise also stimulates a number of neurotransmitters and neurotrophin to stimulate and encourage growth of the hippocampus area of the brain. These effects elevate our mood and reduce our chances for dementia. So, there really is a body–brain connection. Current research shows that an active lifestyle has many positive outcomes in our brains.

In the fall of 2011, the American College of Sports Medicine held the first conference dedicated to how physical activity affects cognition and learning. More than 400 scientists, teachers, administrators, doctors, and politicians attended. The exciting news is that many schools and communities are adapting new policies that encourage or require physical activity on a regular basis for school youth. Those schools are seeing improvements in learning, behavior, attendance, and graduation, as well as decreases in attention-deficit/hyperactivity disorder (ADHD). The following box lists best practices learned at this conference, along with some great resources that parents and school officials can use in order to change their schools.

Ideas for Initiating Physical Activity in Schools to Improve Learning

School districts are all struggling to meet the costs of providing an education. Luckily, schools that have added physical activity to their school day—before, after, and during (including added recesses, lunch-break activities, physical education classes, and in-class activities) the day—have seen improved education outcomes even when some time is taken away from classroom instruction. This has been accomplished with minimal costs that are less than adding more instructional time. Schools have done this by adapting these guidelines:

- No student should sit for more than 60 minutes at a time without at least 10 minutes of physical activity.
- Students achieve at least 50 minutes physical activity per day, and preferably more. The daily guideline for youth is a minimum of 60 minutes.
- Activities should engage both the brain and the body.
- Activities are low cost.
- The burden on teachers is low.
- Activities should be disconnected from motor skills (i.e., any activity the students like).
- Activities are appropriate for the age group.
- Students want to do the activities.
- Program is reproducible and transferable to other schools.
- Everyone participates at a comfortable intensity level.

Many web resources for parents and schools are available:

- www.take10.net
- www.letsmove.gov
- www.activelivingresearch.org
- www.catchinfo.org
- www.cdc.gov/healthyyouth/physicalactivity/facts.htm
- www.cdc.gov/obesity/downloads/CSPA_Synthesis_Brief.pdf

Form 2.3   Physical Activity and Brain Health

The most important thing is to get started, to do something. Start with a little more than you currently do and then work up to 30 minutes of brisk walking most days of the week. A simple method is to use a pedometer and gradually work up to 10,000 steps every day. Once you reach that goal, challenge yourself to become more physically fit. If your body and mind are worth caring for, isn't it worth spending less than 5 percent of your waking hours, about 6 hours a week, to gain all of the activity-related health benefits while also improving your brain and quality of life?

Here is a simple goal prescription for a week of exercise to help both your brain and body. When possible, this is best done earlier in the day. You choose the activities that you like:

Day 1: Moderate intensity*: 75 minutes in 10+ minutes at a time or 10,000 steps of walking.

Day 2: Higher intensity**: 30 minutes plus some resistance training (45 min total).

Day 3: Moderate intensity*: 75 minutes or 10,000 steps of walking.

Day 4: Moderate intensity*: 75 minutes or 10,000 steps of walking.

Day 5: Higher intensity**: 30 minutes plus some resistance training (45 min total).

Day 6: Moderate intensity*: 75 minutes or 10,000 steps of walking.

Day 7: Day off or moderate intensity*: 75 minutes or 10,000 steps of walking.

*For higher intensity (vigorous) activities, it is best to find activities that challenge you both physically and mentally, such as dancing, sports, or new skills. To estimate your heart-rate range, use the following formulas:

Heart rate at the bottom of vigorous = (220 – _____ [age] × .75) = _____

Heart rate at the top of vigorous = (220 – _____ [age] × .90) = _____

** For moderate intensity activities, you can walk briskly or wear a heart rate monitor. Keep your heart rate in the following range.

Heart rate at the bottom of moderate = (220 – _____ [age] × .60) = _____

Heart rate at the top of moderate = (220 – _____ [age] × .75) = _____

From B.J. Sharkey and S.E. Gaskill, 2013, *Fitness and health, seventh edition* (Champaign, IL: Human Kinetics).

You will hear us say, many times over, that 30 minutes of daily moderate physical activity is the **threshold** for adult health (60 minutes for youth up through age 18). This could also be said for brain health. There are some caveats. While much research has been completed, much remains to be done. A simple summary is to recommend that you become active and physically fit, stay active in physical activities, and engage in aerobic activities that are technically and physically challenging. While any physical activity, including walking, will help, the optimal exercise prescription for brain health is beyond the simple prescription for physical health. Rather, it is more related to improving fitness. Get your body in shape to improve your brain.

Our summary of recommendations to maintain brain health, to improve learning and academic achievement, and to reduce the likelihood of dementia are given in the box on page 45. Additionally, form 2.3 provides a simple exercise goal prescription for adults to help reduce dementia.

ACTIVITY AS A POSITIVE ADDICTION

Substance abuse with nicotine, alcohol, or prescription or recreational drugs presents a health and social dilemma that threatens to tear society apart. Each of these substances presents a staggering cost in health care, rehabilitation, and social services, not to mention loss of human potential. We don't pretend to have answers to this problem, but we do have some suggestions for prevention and individual responsibility.

In his book *Positive Addiction*, Dr. William Glasser contrasts positive and negative addictions (1976). Negative addictions such as drugs or alcohol relieve the pain of failure and provide temporary pleasure, but at a terrible cost in terms of family, social, and professional life. Positive addictions, such as physical activity, lead to psychological strength, imagination, and creativity. Dr. Glasser suggests that as people participate in meditation, yoga, or running, they eventually achieve a state of positive addiction. When they reach this state, their minds are free to become more imaginative or creative. The mind conceives more options in solving difficult or frustrating problems; it has more strength. Proof of addiction comes when guilt and anxiety accompany the early stages of withdrawal after a person is forced to abandon a habit.

Dr. Glasser suggested that positive addiction can be achieved from almost any activity you choose, as long as it meets the following criteria:

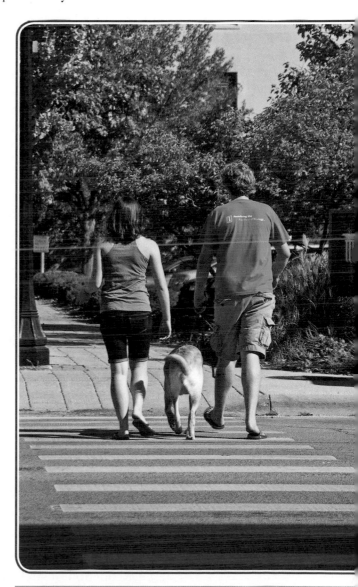

- The activity is not competitive.
- You do it for approximately 1 hour daily.
- The activity is easy to do and doesn't take much mental effort.
- You can do it alone or occasionally with others, but you don't rely on others to do it.
- You believe that it has some physical, mental, or spiritual value.
- You believe that if you persist, you will improve.
- You can do it without criticizing yourself.

In the chapter titled "Running—The Hardest but Surest Way," Glasser suggests that running, perhaps because it is our most basic solitary survival activity, produces the non-self-critical state more effectively than any other practice. He recommends running to everyone, from the weakest to the strongest. He feels that when people can run for an hour without fatigue, they will almost certainly achieve

■ A positive addiction to meditation or activity, such as an evening walk with your dog, can improve your creativity and help you deal with difficult problems.

positive addiction. If the runner avoids competition and runs alone in a pleasant setting, addiction should occur within the year.

We knew that we were addicted to running long before Dr. Glasser wrote his book. Over the years, the addiction to running has evolved to an addiction to activity; it works with hiking, cycling, cross-country skiing, swimming, and even **weight training**, as long as we keep it noncompetitive and uncritical. As interests change or injuries occur, we've been able to transfer the addiction to new activities. The addiction ensures that we will remain active for the rest of our lives.

Is it possible to be too dedicated to activity, fitness, or training—to be negatively addicted or dependent? Probably. An old friend, the eminent and venerable sport psychologist Dr. William Morgan, first called attention to the possibility, noting runners who were so addicted that they neglected family and work. Some continued to train in spite of an illness or injury (Morgan 1979). We, too, have seen runners with an obsessive compulsion for their sport. Closer inspection revealed that some lives seemed confounded with other problems and that these people had turned to running as therapy. Several studies have linked compulsive running with the eating disorder **anorexia nervosa**. Others, however, found that addicted runners fell within the normal range of behavior whereas those with anorexia nervosa did not.

For our part, we prefer a compulsion to running over a negative addiction to alcohol or drugs. The compulsive activity may alter family relationships and work performance, but it won't destroy the body and the mind. The obsession with running may serve as therapy, just as activity serves to reduce anxiety and depression. Dr. Glasser suggests that people can use positive addictions as replacements for negative ones. Imagine the health benefits of replacing smoking, alcohol, or drug use with daily activity! Although this replacement model clearly works for some people, the sizable dropout rates common in exercise programs and programs aimed at cessation of smoking, alcohol, or drug use seem to limit its application.

SUMMARY

Health has been called the first of all liberties. What some call optimal health or wellness implies a vitality and zest for living that is much more than the absence of disease. Our definition of health also embraces psychological, emotional, and mental health. Thus, healthy people are free from disease, anxiety, and depression. Their physical condition, nutritional state, and emotional outlook enable them to carry out daily tasks with vigor and alertness, without undue fatigue, and with ample energy to enjoy leisure-time pursuits and meet unforeseen emergencies.

The International Society of Sport Psychology (Tenenbaum and Singer 1992) believes that the benefits of regular vigorous activity include the following:

- Reduced state anxiety
- Decreased level of mild to moderate depression
- Reductions in neuroticism and anxiety
- Complement to professional treatment of severe depression
- Reduction of stress indices
- Beneficial emotional effects for all ages and both sexes
- Cognitive performance is enhanced and maintained throughout life

We have seen how regular, moderate activity serves to enhance physical, mental, and cognitive health. Now let's explore the role of health care in the active life.

Personal Health

It's Your Responsibility

> "A healthy state can exist only when the men and women who make it up lead clean, vigorous, healthy lives; when the children are so trained that they shall endeavor, not to seek ease, but to know how to wrest triumph from toil and risk."
>
> *Teddy Roosevelt*

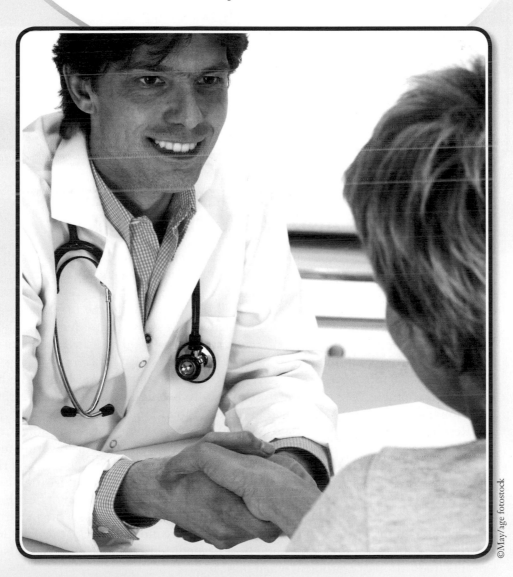

©May/age fotostock

The so-called American health care system is not about health, nor is it a system. It is a chaotic mixture of doctors, hospitals, drug and insurance companies, lawyers, and—oh, yes—patients, held together by market factors, mutual dependence, and self-interest. The arrangement does not focus on prevention or health, but on the treatment of illness, disease, and disabling injury. It isn't a system because it wasn't planned; it just grew. It defies economic theory. If demand goes down, prices go up, faster than wages or inflation. Worst of all, it has fostered an unhealthy attitude: Ignore commonsense health habits and become sick or injured, and the health care system will perform a miracle cure and insurance will pay much of the enormous cost.

Many Americans rely on their doctors to take care of their health. Of course, that approach doesn't work. Your doctor can't make you stop smoking, lose weight, eat less fat, fasten your seat belt, or get regular exercise. These simple habits have more to do with health and disease than all the influences of medicine. More than half of all diseases and deaths can be attributed to lifestyle. Granted, medical tests and treatments that prevent or minimize disease and disability are available, but not all the procedures require a physician.

This chapter will help you do the following:

- Recognize the values and limitations of both health screening and early detection
- Develop a schedule for periodic medical examinations
- Determine the need for a pre-exercise medical exam
- Understand the risks and benefits of regular, moderate physical activity

FUNCTIONS OF HEALTH SCREENING AND EARLY DETECTION

The senior author has had the pleasure of working in two bureaucracies—a university and a federal agency. Although they are different in many respects, both share an interest in the health of their employees and both offer employee health or wellness programs. Most wellness programs use a computerized health risk analysis as the first step in a comprehensive health-screening program. The analysis uses answers to questions about health habits and some basic information (age, sex, weight, blood pressure, and cholesterol) to calculate health risks and compute one's risk age. Overweight smokers with a family history of heart disease may have a risk age years above their chronological age. The health risk analysis is a simple, low-cost way to focus future health behaviors. A health risk analysis and longevity estimate are included in the form found in the appendix.

Results from a cholesterol test could lead to a class on healthy food choices, an activity program, or even a doctor's visit and a prescription for cholesterol-lowering medication. The principle is simple: Use low-cost approaches to identify health habits and risks, apply more expensive tests for those at risk, and reserve high-cost tests and treatments for those in real need. Years ago, testing advocates promoted broad application of health-screening tests. Now we realize that many tests should be reserved for those who, by virtue of age, risk factors, family history, symptoms, or exposure, are most in need of the test. Generalized testing is costly, wastes the time and effort of medical personnel, and risks **false positive** results (indication of a problem when none exists).

Age, sex, health risks, family history, and occupation determine the need for health screening. Young, apparently healthy people do well with infrequent tests, unless, of course, they have a family history, symptoms, or exposure, or they change habits. Regrettably, age alone increases the need for certain tests, such as mammography, colonoscopy (for colon cancer), and a digital prostate examination. A family history of glaucoma raises the need for a regular glaucoma test, and occupational exposure to noise or toxic chemicals calls for evaluation of hearing or lung function, respectively. A comprehensive worksite wellness program provides a wide range of health-screening procedures (see figure 3.1), along with appropriate immunizations (e.g., flu shots for retired employees) and booster shots.

Considerable interest exists in the development of tests to detect problems such as cancer. The idea is that early detection will improve the prognosis for recovery. Indeed, some studies

We're Number 2! (But Really Number 49 or 51.)

In 2009, the United States ranked number 2 in health care spending (behind Malta), as a percentage of GDP, but ranked 49th for infant mortality and 51st for life expectancy according to the CIA World Factbook (www.cia.gov). Why? One reason is that the United States had 44 million uninsured citizens amid a patchwork of private insurance and government programs. Americans spend billions on insurance, diagnostics, drugs, and procedures, but little on prevention. Japan, which spends less than $2,000 per person per year, beat the United States by 4.5 years in the category of how long people live in good health, not just how long they live (Doe 2009). If the effort to insure all uninsured Americans withstands political attacks, the ranking should improve somewhat.

showed that early detection was associated with extended survival. This notion is fine, so long as the extension of life exceeds the improvement in detection time. However, early detection is meaningless if no effective treatment for the disease is available. Of course, if the disease can be transmitted (e.g., AIDS) and its spread can be limited, early detection makes sense from a public health standpoint.

In recent years, medical opinion has changed concerning the course of treatment for several medical problems. For example, in older men, aggressive treatment of prostate cancer (surgery, radiation) is not always superior to watching and waiting. Survival time doesn't always improve with aggressive treatment, and quality of life is often impaired (incontinence, impotency). Back operations and heart surgery, even for patients with obvious symptoms, have been performed more often than necessary, leading one to question the accuracy of detection and diagnosis. But many tests are warranted, especially when they lead to changes in behavior. Low-cost blood pressure and cholesterol tests can identify problems while time is still available to slow, stop, or even reverse the disease process. So if your age, sex, race, family history, health habits, or exposure puts you at risk for a disease, use an early detection test, as long as the proposed test meets the following criteria:

- The disease has a significant effect on the quality of life.
- Acceptable methods of treatment are available.
- Treatment during the asymptomatic (no symptom) period significantly reduces disability or death.
- Early treatment yields a superior result.
- Detection tests are available at reasonable cost.
- The incidence of the disease in the population is sufficient to justify the cost of screening.

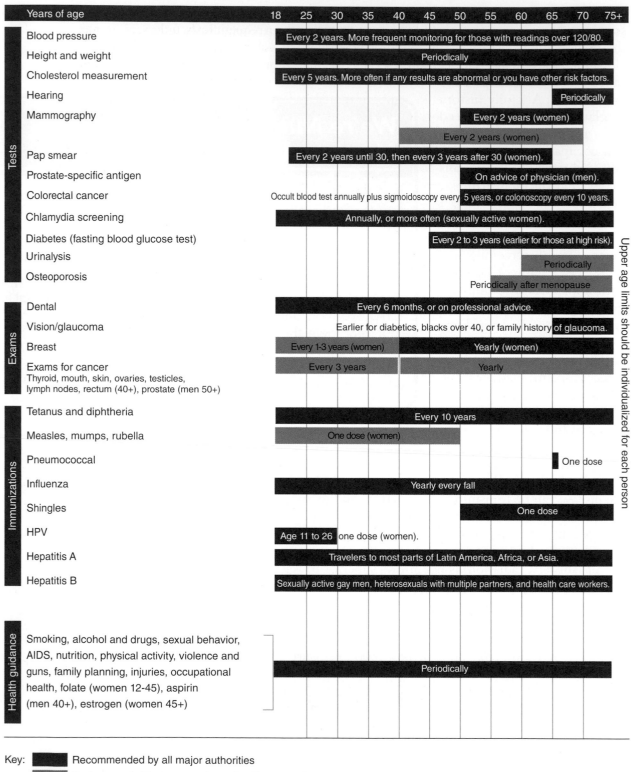

Years of age	18	25	30	35	40	45	50	55	60	65	70	75+

Tests

- **Blood pressure** — Every 2 years. More frequent monitoring for those with readings over 120/80.
- **Height and weight** — Periodically
- **Cholesterol measurement** — Every 5 years. More often if any results are abnormal or you have other risk factors.
- **Hearing** — Periodically
- **Mammography** — Every 2 years (women)
- **Pap smear** — Every 2 years until 30, then every 3 years after 30 (women).
- **Prostate-specific antigen** — On advice of physician (men).
- **Colorectal cancer** — Occult blood test annually plus sigmoidoscopy every 5 years, or colonoscopy every 10 years.
- **Chlamydia screening** — Annually, or more often (sexually active women).
- **Diabetes (fasting blood glucose test)** — Every 2 to 3 years (earlier for those at high risk).
- **Urinalysis** — Periodically
- **Osteoporosis** — Periodically after menopause

Exams

- **Dental** — Every 6 months, or on professional advice.
- **Vision/glaucoma** — Earlier for diabetics, blacks over 40, or family history of glaucoma.
- **Breast** — Every 1-3 years (women) / Yearly (women)
- **Exams for cancer** — Every 3 years / Yearly
  Thyroid, mouth, skin, ovaries, testicles, lymph nodes, rectum (40+), prostate (men 50+)

Immunizations

- **Tetanus and diphtheria** — Every 10 years
- **Measles, mumps, rubella** — One dose (women)
- **Pneumococcal** — One dose
- **Influenza** — Yearly every fall
- **Shingles** — One dose
- **HPV** — Age 11 to 26 one dose (women).
- **Hepatitis A** — Travelers to most parts of Latin America, Africa, or Asia.
- **Hepatitis B** — Sexually active gay men, heterosexuals with multiple partners, and health care workers.

Health guidance

- Smoking, alcohol and drugs, sexual behavior, AIDS, nutrition, physical activity, violence and guns, family planning, injuries, occupational health, folate (women 12-45), aspirin (men 40+), estrogen (women 45+) — Periodically

Upper age limits should be individualized for each person

Key:
■ Recommended by all major authorities
■ Recommended by some major authorities

FIGURE 3.1 Adult preventive care timeline: recommendations of major authorities.

Few tests meet these criteria; blood pressure tests, breast examinations, and Pap smears do, whereas **exercise stress tests**, diabetes screening, and X-rays for lung cancer do not. Surprisingly, the routine (annual) medical examination also fails to meet the criteria.

In the past, health was defined as the absence of disease, and that is how many people still think of the term. In the 1980s, the definition of health was expanded to include a state of complete physical, mental, and emotional well-being, not merely the absence of disease or infirmity. In that context, the relationship of activity to health becomes clearer.

Blood Pressure

High blood pressure, or hypertension, a silent killer with no obvious symptoms, is easy and inexpensive to test. Moreover, several acceptable methods of treatment are available, and successful control extends the quantity and quality of life. Systolic pressure is the pressure exerted against arterial walls when the heart contracts to send blood into the system. Diastolic pressure is the pressure against arterial walls between beats, when the heart is relaxed. Both measures contribute to the mean arterial pressure, and both have consequences for health. Use the information in table 3.1 to evaluate your blood pressure.

Borderline cases often respond to diet, weight loss, and exercise. Cases that remain elevated may require medication. Studies clearly show the value of controlling blood pressure. **Aerobic exercise** combined with weight loss is recommended for the management of elevated blood pressure in sedentary, overweight people (Blumenthal et al. 2000). High blood pressure can damage arterial walls and contribute to atherosclerosis, and excess pressure increases the risk of stroke. Although salt intake, excess weight, and stress may exacerbate the problem, the cause is poorly understood. More than 90 percent of all cases are idiopathic, arising spontaneously or from an obscure or unknown cause. Modern molecular biology will someday unlock the cause of these constricted arteries, but you can't wait for someday. Check your pressure regularly and never rely on a single measure. If the pressure is elevated in several checks, restrict salt and fat, lose weight, engage in regular, moderate activity, and learn how to manage stress. If all that isn't enough, or if the pressure is above 160, see your physician. New medications provide control of blood pressure with fewer side effects. But don't rely on medications for control; continue with diet, exercise, weight loss, and stress management.

Table 3.1　Blood Pressure (BP) Evaluation

Category	Systolic BP (mmHg)	Diastolic BP (mmHg)	Action
Normal BP	<120	<80	Retest annually.
Prehypertension	120–130	80–85	Retest in 6 mo.*
Hypertension	>130	>85	See physician.**

*Change diet (reduce salt intake), lose weight, reduce stress, increase physical activity.

**Possible medication.

Data from NHLBI 2012. Available: http://www.nhlbi.nih.gov/health/health-topics/topics/hbp/

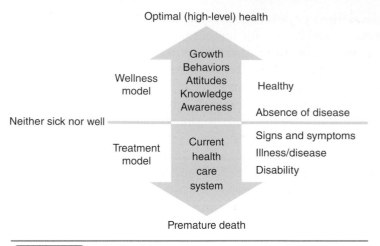

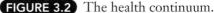

FIGURE 3.2 The health continuum.

The relationship of health and wellness is equally clear. Ardell (1984) defined wellness as "a conscious and deliberate approach to an advanced state of physical and psychological/spiritual health." So wellness defines movement toward an advanced state of optimal or high-level health (figure 3.2).

The old view of health placed illness on one side of a line and health on the other, with doctors and the treatment-oriented health care system defending the line. We now view wellness as a dynamic process in which you are personally responsible for your health. The health care system is treatment oriented. Workers in the system focus on correcting problems brought on by illness, disease, injury, or disability. Wellness involves disease prevention and promotion of behaviors that lower the risk of illness or injury. The treatment system employs an army of high-priced professionals and costs billions. Wellness relies on individual responsibility, low-cost helpers, and reduced reliance on costly specialists and procedures. The active life is the keystone of health and wellness.

ANNUAL MEDICAL EXAMINATION

The typical medical examination includes a history, physical examination, and tests dictated by the patient's age, sex, and the findings of the exam. In the past, we all assumed that the annual medical examination would help us stay healthy and reduce the likelihood of illness or premature death. But when researchers compared those who had annual exams with those who did not, they found an equal number of chronic diseases and deaths in the two groups. The study suggests that, for healthy adults, the benefits of an annual physical may not justify the financial cost (Mehrotra, Zaslavsky, and Ayanian 2007). A past president of the American Medical Association has said that he hasn't had a routine physical since he joined the army decades ago, and he asks patients who request a checkup, "What do you want one for?" The box 'A Clean Bill of Health?' discusses a typi-

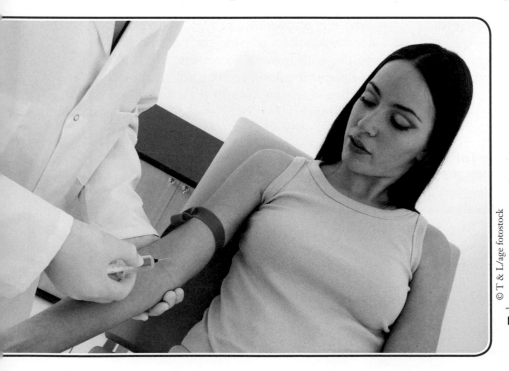

© T & L/age fotostock

- Use screening programs to monitor elevated cholesterol and blood sugar.

cal scenario that illustrates why the annual medical exam pays off for the doctor and the laboratory, but not for the patient.

If you have symptoms or are in doubt about the condition of your health, see your physician. If you or a member of your family has a history of hypertension, check your pressure regularly. Buy a home blood pressure device and check it at home, at the drugstore, or at your worksite wellness program. Check elevated cholesterol regularly at worksite screenings, health fairs, or walk-in clinics. Check your kids to see whether they need to use diet and exercise to minimize a family problem. Use screening programs to check blood sugar, and if problems arise, see your physician. Of course, women should have regular checkups throughout pregnancy. Studies fail to provide convincing evidence of the value of periodic medical examinations, let alone annual exams (Gordon, Senf, and Campos-Outcalt 1999). A reasonable frequency of medical examination includes the following:

- At around 18 and 25 years of age
- Every 5 years between ages 35 and 65
- Every 2 years after age 65 (Gordon, Senf, and Campos-Outcalt 1999)

> **I**f you have symptoms or are in doubt about the condition of your health, by all means, see your physician.

In our view, this schedule could be too intensive for apparently healthy adults who are willing to take charge of their health. We use the physician when necessary, but we employ other ways to get answers to medical issues, such as the *Merck Manual*, the book or website doctors use when they are stumped (www.merck-manuals.com). We have a wellness program blood panel every year to keep track of blood lipids (e.g., cholesterol), and we take advantage of other worksite wellness and community health-screening programs that fit our needs. We see the dentist often enough and have periodic eye exams to adjust prescriptions and test for glaucoma. Otherwise, our visits to the doctor's office are for specifics, to renew a prescription, to the dermatologist to check on a suspicious growth, or to the orthopedic surgeon for a major injury (we self-treat minor injuries or seek a friendly athletic trainer or physical therapist for advice). But, as we said, if you have symptoms or are in doubt about the condition of your health, see your physician.

CHOLESTEROL SCREENING

Cholesterol is a heart-disease risk factor. Although the risk rises with the level of cholesterol, some people with relatively low values experience problems with atherosclerosis (see table 3.2). Cholesterol is a fatlike substance found in all human and animal tissues, but not in plants. We ingest cholesterol in foods from animals (e.g., meat, eggs, fish, poultry, and dairy products), or we can synthesize it in the body. If you don't eat much cholesterol, the body will make all it needs from other fats. The blood transports cholesterol in low- or high-density lipoprotein packages.

The ideal total cholesterol level is below 150 milligrams. Values from 150 to 200 should respond to a moderate reduction of saturated and hydrogenated fats in the diet. Levels from 200 to 240 call for a concentrated effort to reduce the level of this **atherogenic** fat and take additional dietary measures, including increasing intake of bran and other natural foods to reduce cholesterol. Cholesterol levels that remain above 240 after dietary, exercise, and weight-loss interventions may require drug therapy, especially if other risk factors are present. Fortunately, cholesterol drugs have proved successful at lowering levels and the incidence of heart disease. Consult your physician for details.

A Clean Bill of Health?

Joe is a typical patient; he is 45, somewhat overweight and out of shape, smokes a pack a day, and indulges his love for meat and potatoes. His company pays for his annual medical exam, so the physician schedules a battery of tests, including a blood lipid panel, chest X-ray, resting **electrocardiogram (ECG)**, pulmonary function tests, and other procedures. Aside from somewhat elevated blood pressure and cholesterol and a low level of HDL cholesterol, Joe's ECG and other tests appear normal. So Joe goes out and celebrates his clean bill of health with a prime rib, a salad with lots of dressing, a baked potato with butter, sour cream, and bacon bits, and a slice of cheesecake. The next morning, he experiences a crushing pain in his chest and is rushed to the hospital with a heart attack.

This all-too-common scenario illustrates the fact that many tests lack the sensitivity to provide early detection. A resting ECG seldom predicts an impending myocardial infarction (heart attack). An exercise electrocardiogram (stress test) may have had a better chance of identifying Joe's problem, but the exercise test occasionally suggests heart disease when none is present. Pulmonary function tests and chest X-rays seldom detect lung cancer early enough to improve the prognosis (the X-ray actually increases the risk of cancer). And some tests increase the likelihood of surgery when it may not be needed. If Joe had complained of a back problem and the doctor had ordered an MRI (magnetic resonance imaging) that revealed a bulging disk, he might have been scheduled for an operation that could make things worse (Jensen et al. 1994). Does this mean that all tests and medical exams are a waste of time? Of course not; many valid reasons point to the need for a medical examination.

Why do we forget that we need to be responsible for our own health? If Joe had stayed within a normal weight and had met the physical activity guidelines for health, he would have been at a much lower risk of heart disease, diabetes, hypertension, and other chronic diseases. Tests help identify problems, but they are not infallible.

Low-density lipoprotein cholesterol (LDL) is the dangerous version that finds its way into the lining of the coronary arteries. It can combine with oxygen and enhance the development of plaques in arteries. High-density lipoprotein cholesterol (HDL) acts like a transport system that picks up excess cholesterol and delivers it to the liver for reprocessing or removal. Thus, higher HDL levels are protective, with a 1-milligram increase associated with a 2 to 3 percent reduction in CAD. Conversely, low values are an independent risk factor. So you can have a low total cholesterol level and still have some risk if your HDL is low. You should know all three numbers (total cholesterol, LDL, and HDL), as well as your cholesterol to HDL ratio. Table 3.2 shows the risk associated with blood lipids and displays how the risk declines as HDL levels rise.

Another way to assess your risk is to calculate your total cholesterol to HDL ratio. A ratio under 4 (e.g., 200 ÷ 50) is associated with a low risk of heart disease, whereas a ratio over 6 (e.g., 240 ÷ 40) is not. All adults should be tested every 5 years unless values are borderline or high, a circumstance that calls for annual testing and treatment.

Research has identified two additional tests to help determine one's risk of heart disease:

1. Homocysteine is often elevated in the blood of those at high risk for heart problems. A blood test will show if a problem exists. If it does, the solution is simple: an increase in

Table 3.2   CAD Risk Categories

Value	Risk category
TOTAL CHOLESTEROL (MG/DL)	
<200	Desirable
200–239	Borderline high risk
240 or over	High risk
LDL CHOLESTEROL (MG/DL)	
<100	Optimal
100–129	Near optimal
130–159	Borderline high
160–189	High
>190	Very high
HDL CHOLESTEROL (MG/DL)	
>60	Desirable
45 (men), 55 (women)	Average
<40	High risk
TOTAL CHOLESTEROL TO HDL RATIO (CHOLESTEROL/HDL)	
<3.5	Desirable
3.5–5	Average
>5	High risk
TRIGLYCERIDES (MG/DL)	
<150	Normal
150–199	Borderline high
200–499	High
>500	Very high

Source: American Heart Association. www.americanheart.org.

foods containing the B **vitamin** folate (or a folate supplement). Folate is also important for pregnant women or those planning to become pregnant.

2. **C reactive protein** (C-RP) is a sign of inflammatory activity that is associated with an increased risk of a heart attack (Ridker et al. 2000). C-RP may influence apoptosis or fragmentation of human coronary vascular smooth muscle cells, a key event in the development of atherosclerotic lesions, and the vulnerability of plaque to rupture (Blaschke et al. 2004). But because C-RP is also associated with chronic infections and arthritis, it is viewed as a relatively moderate predictor of CAD (Danesh et al. 2004). Studies indicate that cholesterol-lowering statin drugs may also lower C-RP, and that people with lower C-RP levels have a greater reduction in coronary risk (Nissen et al. 2005). A blood test can determine the level. Efforts to reduce the risk may include daily intake of an aspirin,

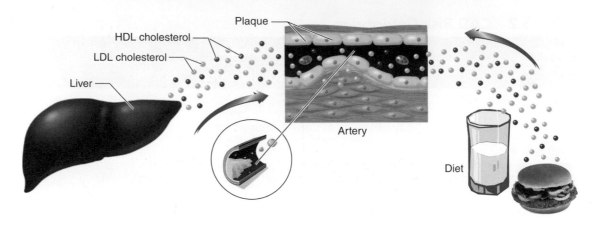

FIGURE 3.3 Your cholesterol levels are a reflection of both dietary cholesterol and cholesterol that your body makes. High LDL cholesterol results in the buildup of arterial plaque. We can reduce high LDL cholesterol by reducing dietary cholesterol, by increasing dietary fiber, and by exercising regularly.

vitamin E, or an alcoholic beverage, as well as weight loss, statin therapy, and, of course, physical activity (see the following list and figure 3.3).

Prescription for elevated cholesterol

Exercise	30 min of moderate daily aerobic activity lowers LDL a modest amount; higher intensity or duration exercise (e.g., jogging) further reduces LDL and improves HDL cholesterol.
Diet	Reduce animal and hydrogenated fat intake, increase fiber by eating bran and whole-grain products, increase vitamin C and E intake, and consume some alcohol (1 or 2 drinks a day).

In case you were wondering about triglyceride levels, some say that they do not provide clinically relevant information about CAD risk beyond that obtained with measures of cholesterol, LDL, and HDL (Avins and Neuhaus 2000). But elevated triglycerides may be a risk factor for CAD when cholesterol levels are low (see table 3.2). High triglycerides are often associated with low HDL and blood clotting, and they may lead to enlargement of the liver. Normal fasted levels should be below 150 milligrams per 100 milliliters. Later chapters explain more about the blood lipids, cholesterol, and triglycerides.

If your risk of heart disease is high, you can use new information to improve your health. The National Cholesterol Education Program has formulated new guidelines for LDL cholesterol. High-risk people (based on risk factors) should aim to get LDL cholesterol below 70, well below the previous goal of 100 milligrams per deciliter. Studies indicate that the lower the LDL cholesterol level, the better. Achieving this level probably requires use of prescription drugs (Grundy et al. 2004).

PRE-EXERCISE MEDICAL EXAMINATION

Should you see your doctor before you increase your physical activity? Here is the opinion of the eminent Swedish physician and exercise scientist, Dr. Per Olaf Åstrand (Åstrand and Rodahl 1970, 608):

As a general rule, moderate activity is less harmful to the health than inactivity. You could also put it this way: A medical examination is more urgent for those who plan to remain inactive than for those who intend to get into good physical shape!

Dr. Per Olaf Åstrand

The active life is certain to enhance—not threaten—your health if you are free of symptoms, if you make a gradual transition to a more active life, and if you follow a sensible program. On the other hand, you should consider a preparticipation medical examination if you have been sedentary, if you are concerned about your health, if you have one or several primary heart disease risk factors (hypertension, elevated cholesterol, cigarette smoking, or inactivity), or if you are over 45 years of age (55 for women) and plan to engage in a vigorous exercise program. The American Heart Association (AHA) and the American College of Sports Medicine (ACSM) recommend a preparticipation medical exam, including a progressive, ECG-monitored exercise test (stress test) for everyone with known cardiac, pulmonary, or metabolic disease, for patients with symptoms, and for those over 45 (55 for women) before participation in vigorous exercise (Balady et al. 1998).

A medical examination is more urgent for those who plan to remain inactive than for those who intend to get into good physical shape!

Health-Screening Questionnaire

For apparently healthy people under 45 years of age, the risk of participation in activity and fitness programs can be substantially reduced with inexpensive preparticipation health screening. Canadian researchers have developed the Physical Activity Readiness Questionnaire to identify the small number of adults for whom physical activity might be inappropriate or those who should seek medical advice before participating. We recommend a more comprehensive questionnaire (see form 3.1). The questionnaire was adapted from the AHA and the ACSM form that provides simple, self-administered preparticipation questions to identify heart-disease risk factors and some other health issues.

Exercise Stress Test

Severe chest pain (angina pectoris) or even a heart attack can sometimes be the first sign of coronary artery problems. A gradually increased exercise challenge, known as a stress test, can detect indications of previously undiagnosed heart disease. Narrowed coronary arteries may be able to supply the blood that you need for sedentary pursuits, but during exercise, the oxygen needs of heart muscle go up. Electrocardiographic abnormalities or physical symptoms may indicate a problem.

Maximal or near-maximal workloads may be needed to elicit the symptoms of previously undiagnosed heart disease. Many physicians choose to terminate the stress test when the heart rate reaches some percentage of the age-adjusted maximal heart rate, reasoning that it is unnecessary to risk a maximal test. Unfortunately, wide variability in maximal heart rates means that the test may be too strenuous for some and too easy for others (see table 3.3).

A physician uses a progressive ECG-monitored exercise test as a diagnostic tool to identify the presence of heart disease, as a pre-exercise test to reduce risks or set limits, as a postcoronary test to indicate the extent of damage and subsequent progress in therapeutic

History

Have you had any of the following?

- ☐ Heart attack
- ☐ Heart surgery
- ☐ Cardiac catheterization
- ☐ Coronary angioplasty (PTCA)
- ☐ Pacemaker or implantable cardiac defibrillator or rhythm disturbance
- ☐ Heart valve disease
- ☐ Heart failure
- ☐ Heart transplantation
- ☐ Congenital heart disease

If you marked any of the statements in this section, consult your health care provider before engaging in exercise. You may need to use a facility with a medically qualified staff.

Cardiovascular and other risk factors

- ☐ You are a man older than 45 years.
- ☐ You are a woman older than 55 years or you have had a hysterectomy or you are post-menopausal.
- ☐ You smoke.
- ☐ Your blood pressure is greater than 140/90.
- ☐ You don't know your blood pressure.
- ☐ You take blood pressure medication.
- ☐ Your blood cholesterol level is greater than 240 mg/dl.
- ☐ You don't know your cholesterol level.
- ☐ You have a close blood relative who had a heart attack before age 55 (father or brother) or age 65 (mother or sister).
- ☐ You have diabetes or take medicine to control your blood sugar.
- ☐ You are physically inactive (i.e., you get less than 30 minutes of physical activity on at least 3 days per week).
- ☐ You are more than 20 pounds (9 kg) overweight.
- ☐ You have chest pain brought on by physical activity.
- ☐ You developed chest pain in the past month.
- ☐ You take heart medications.
- ☐ You have musculoskeletal problems.
- ☐ You have concerns about the safety of exercise.
- ☐ You take prescription medications.
- ☐ You are pregnant.

If you marked two or more of the statements in this section, consult your health care provider before engaging in exercise. You might benefit by using a facility with a professionally qualified exercise staff to guide your exercise program.

If none of the above is true, you should be able to exercise safely without consulting your health care provider in almost any facility that meets your exercise program needs.

Note: If you have a temporary illness, such as a common cold, or are not feeling well at this time, postpone.

From B.J. Sharkey and S.E. Gaskill, 2013, *Fitness and health, seventh edition* (Champaign, IL: Human Kinetics). Adapted, by permission, from American Heart Association (www.heart.org).

programs, or after a coronary bypass or angioplasty procedure to establish extent of recovery, as well as work and activity limits. Although most stress tests are conducted on the treadmill, arm testing (cranking) may be required for people returning to jobs that require strenuous use of the upper body.

One reason for maximal testing is to evaluate functional capacity, or maximal attainable workload. The stress test can be used to clear patients for hard work and to establish their **work capacity**. When treadmill tests are used to predict aerobic fitness, subjects should not support their weight by holding the railing of the treadmill. This practice lowers the actual workload and invalidates the prediction of fitness and work capacity.

The stress test should end when the subject cannot continue or has symptoms of exertional intolerance (chest pain, intolerable fatigue) or distress (staggering, dizziness, confusion, pallor, labored breathing, or nausea), when significant electrocardiographic changes occur, or when blood pressure drops in spite of increasing workload. Termination of the test at some predetermined percentage of the assumed maximal heart rate, on the other hand, risks missing important signs or symptoms. As we have noted, maximal heart rate is highly variable. Using an age-related maximal heart rate (e.g., 220 beats per minute [bpm] – age = predicted maximal heart rate) can lead to substantial errors. For example, the maximal heart rate for 40-year-old patients may average 180 beats per minute (220 – 40 = 180), but the range goes from below 144 to above 216. So a test terminated at 85 percent of the predicted maximal heart rate (.85 × 180 = 153 bpm) may be too strenuous for a few and much too easy for others. For these reasons, we suggest

Table 3.3   Age and Maximal Heart Rates

Age	Average maximal heart rate
20	201
30	193
40	186
50	179
60	172
70	165

Maximal heart rate declines with age. The decline is slower among active and fit people (170 at 70 years). The decline is more rapid for those below average fitness (147 at 70 years). This measure has considerable variability.

Source: American Heart Association. www.americanheart.org.

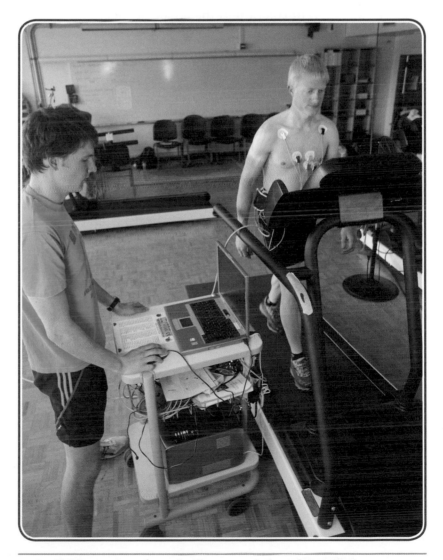

■ An ECG-monitored treadmill test can help reduce exercise risks.

Maximal Heart Rate

The variability in maximal heart rate, as defined by a statistic called the **standard deviation (SD)**, is plus or minus 12 beats per minute (bpm): 68 percent of all cases fall within plus or minus 1 SD, 95 percent within plus or minus 2 SD, and 99 percent within plus or minus 3 SD. So, for our example, it is likely that 1 in 100 40-year-olds will have a maximal heart rate below 144 or above 216. Incidentally, as chapter 10 shows, this variability in maximal heart rate complicates the use of the heart rate for the prescription of exercise. And to make matters more confusing, the standard deviation for maximal heart rate goes up to 15 bpm for older people.

continuing the stress test until the subject reaches fatigue or the termination criteria mentioned earlier.

Exercise Electrocardiogram

The electrocardiogram (ECG) is a strip of paper with a record of the heart's electrical activity. Each complete ECG cycle (see figure 3.4) represents one beat of the heart. The P wave shows the electrical activity that immediately precedes the **contraction** of the upper chambers, or atria. The QRS complex represents the electrical discharge of the lower chambers, or **ventricles**, and the T wave results when the depolarized ventricles are recharged. Because the ECG paper moves at a specified speed (usually 25 mm/sec), the timing and width of the waves can provide information about the rate of electrical conduction. For example, if conduction is slow or blocked, the base of the QRS will be broad. The physician, nurse, or exercise-test technologist administering a stress test pays careful attention to the ECG waveform and knows how to identify changes that suggest heart disease or other problems.

Conduction disturbances occasionally occur during stress tests, so emergency equipment and trained personnel should be available during evaluation of high-risk patients. Fortunately, most patients recover and are able to return to supervised activity after defibrillation. Tests conducted on apparently healthy people are not considered unsafe, but test administrators should know how to perform cardiopulmonary resuscitation (CPR) and other emergency techniques.

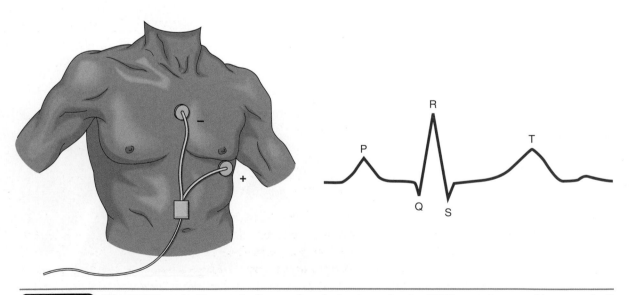

FIGURE 3.4 The ECG cycle. P wave indicates depolarization of atria. QRS wave is caused by spread of excitation through ventricles. T wave indicates repolarization of ventricles.

Test Results

When the exercise stress test results suggest heart problems (e.g., ECG abnormalities, chest pain, or abnormal blood pressure response), the test is called positive. Stress-test findings are verified when they are confirmed with **cardiac catheterization**, an invasive imaging technique. In this procedure, a catheter is inserted into a blood vessel in the leg and worked into position in the aorta. Injection of an opaque dye into each coronary artery allows X-ray detection of narrowing because of atherosclerosis. When narrowed arteries are found after a normal (negative) stress test, the test is called a **false negative**. Results of a positive stress test are considered false when the catheter test reveals normal coronary arteries (i.e., a false-positive stress test).

When cardiologists identify a positive test showing narrowed coronary arteries, the medical intervention is often a coronary bypass or angioplasty operation to repair one or more of the narrowed coronary arteries. In a **bypass surgery**, the surgeon takes a small blood vessel from the leg or chest and uses it to bypass the section of severely narrowed coronary artery. **Coronary angioplasty** involves insertion of a catheter tipped with a balloon into the narrowed artery. Inflation of the balloon opens the artery, and the surgeon inserts a wire mesh stent to maintain blood flow. Both operations are expensive and they may have complications. Before you get to the point where you require one of the invasive procedures, prevention seems prudent.

False negative results are disturbing because they indicate a failure to diagnose the presence of existing coronary artery disease. A small number of patients who undergo exercise stress tests fall into this category, and most of them do not go on for further evaluation. In such cases, the first indication of a problem may be the last, a myocardial infarction or heart attack. Because of this, the physician cannot rely on the stress test alone, but must employ clinical judgment, the patient's medical history, and other diagnostic tools. For example, patient reports of indigestion or chest pain during exertion may be useful because the gradual **warm-up** of the stress test may allow patients with narrowed arteries to adjust to the increased workload, thus disguising the problem. Research shows that partially occluded vessels, which may not produce symptoms during a stress test, contain unstable plaque, which may rupture and cause a heart attack without warning.

False positive tests are also disturbing because they may cause otherwise healthy people

Nonsurgical Alternative

The United States has just 5 percent of the world's population, but performs nearly half of the angioplasties and bypass surgeries worldwide. Some think that a quarter to a third of all cardiac procedures are unnecessary, and that many people do as well with nonsurgical approaches. How do you know if you need the procedure that your doctor recommends? Dr. Thomas Graboys, a cardiologist at Harvard Medical School, employs three criteria to determine who can follow the nonsurgical route:

1. If the condition of the heart muscle is good
2. If the electrical stability of the heart, especially under stress (treadmill) is good
3. If there is an absence of symptoms such as angina

Those who meet these criteria may want to consider a nonsurgical approach involving drugs and lifestyle changes (Griffin 2004). A 2009 meta-analysis of 61 medical trials suggests that normal care, including medications and exercise, was as effective in reducing mortality and morbidity for heart disease patients as angioplasty (Trikalinos et al. 2009). Once again, the argument can be made for taking responsibility for our own health through physical activity, better diet, and healthy living practices.

to become cardiac neurotics, morbidly obsessed with a heart condition that may not exist. Estimates of the frequency of false positive results range from as little as 10 percent to more than 30 percent, depending on the group studied (Balady et al. 1998). False positive results are more prevalent in highly active subjects and women (who may be more likely to hyperventilate during the test). Endurance athletes often exhibit ECG abnormalities during the stress test, and experienced doctors have learned to disregard the findings in the absence of other signs or symptoms. But what about active nonathletes who receive word that the stress test indicates possible coronary artery disease? What do they do next?

In the past, the coronary angiogram was the only way to confirm or deny the existence of coronary artery disease. If the stress test indicated possible disease, the patient had two choices: have the invasive catheter test or ignore the findings and fret about the possibilities, even giving up an active lifestyle for a heart condition that might not exist. Today the patient has other choices. **Myocardial** scintigraphy involves a less invasive assessment of myocardial blood flow during rest and exercise. In this procedure, radioactive thallium is injected into the circulation, and its uptake in cardiac muscle is observed with a scintillation camera. Cold spots indicate areas where blood flow is inadequate during exercise, allowing confirmation of stress-test results (Froelicher 1984). Recently, drugs have been used to stress the heart and simulate the stress test, and computerized tomography (CT) scans are being used successfully to detect plaques in **coronary arteries**. The ideal will be a simple, noninvasive, low-cost alternative, such as a comparison of blood pressure readings taken from the arm and leg. A difference between the two readings may indicate the presence of circulatory problems or atherosclerosis. These developments may someday make the stress test obsolete as a test for heart disease.

Some experts think that false positive tests occur infrequently. They reason that a coronary artery spasm may occur during the vigorous effort of the stress test. Because the catheterization test is routinely performed at rest, the spasm may not show up. The thallium scan mentioned earlier helps solve this problem, and drugs can indicate the tendency for spasms during catheterization. For more on exercise testing, visit the web pages for the American Heart Association (www.heart.org) and the American College of Sports Medicine (www.acsm.org).

EVALUATING THE RISKS OF ACTIVITY

Anecdotal notes on the dangers of exercise appear often in exercise literature, leading many people to have concerns about the safety of physical activity. Research has confirmed that activity greatly reduces but doesn't eliminate the risks associated with inherited or lifestyle diseases. Habitually active people have a 60 percent lower risk of heart attack than their sedentary counterparts. The risk for the active person rises only 5 times during vigorous exercise, to a level slightly above the risk of sedentary living (Siscovick, LaPorte, and Newman 1985). Meyers (2003) reported that heart attack patients who participated in a formal exercise program reduced their death rate by 20 to 25 percent. When habitually inactive people engage in vigorous exercise, their risk rises 56 times above resting levels when they first start an activity program, but it drops rapidly as the program progresses. Overall risk during nonexercise periods also drops dramatically. The bottom line: Start an exercise program with short duration and low intensity, and gradually increase duration and then intensity. Keep it going, join the active life, and enjoy the lowered risk of heart disease and the improved quality of life for many years to come.

The risks of activity and fitness range from minor musculoskeletal problems to major coronary events. The risks are low for low-intensity and moderate-duration activity. Overuse injuries are more common when a person rapidly increases distance, with more miles (km) per week, with high-intensity training (e.g., **interval training**), and with eccentric exercise (e.g., downhill running). The risk of a coronary event is low for an **asymptomatic** adult, in either training or testing, and the exerciser can cut the risk in half by taking the pre-exercise screening questionnaire (see form 3.1).

When patients take a stress test in a medical setting, the risk is one cardiac episode per 187,000 person-hours of testing. The average test lasts 15 minutes, so the odds of an event are 1 in 748,000, or about 1/100 of the chance of being in a major automobile accident per hour of driving. But when presumably healthy (asymptomatic) people are tested, the risks are much lower. The incident of sudden cardiac death during vigorous exertion in healthy adults is only one death per year in every 15,000 to 18,000 people (ACSM 2005). For patients in a medically supervised cardiac rehabilitation program, the risk of death is one per every 60,000 person-hours of participation. Clearly, the health benefits of physical activity outweigh the risks (Morrey and Hensrud 1999).

Figure 3.5 provides a graphic view of the relationship between the benefits and risks of activity. The figure indicates that benefits increase rapidly at first, but eventually reach a plateau, with little additional reward at higher levels of activity. Risks, on the other hand, rise slowly at first and then more rapidly at higher levels of activity. The prudent approach to maximizing benefits and minimizing risks is to engage in a level of activity associated with enhanced health—regular, moderate activity. Figure 3.6 illustrates warning signs to be aware of when physically active.

For those with special exercise needs or limitations, more specific recommendations are needed. Consult references, the Internet, community services, or your physician for additional information.

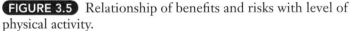

FIGURE 3.5 Relationship of benefits and risks with level of physical activity.

Adapted from K. Powel and R. Paffenbarger, 1985, "Workshop on epidemiologic and public health aspects of physical activity and exercise: A summary," *Public Health Reports* 100 (2):118-126.

• *Older adults.* With age comes increasing need for muscular fitness. Seniors should undertake exercises to develop and maintain muscular strength and endurance. A wise approach is to increase strength to required levels before loss of strength limits self-sufficiency. Chapter 6 explores issues of age, activity, and vitality.

• *Women.* The exercise advice and prescriptions in this book work for both men and women, but women should consider some specific issues. Young women need to know that high-volume vigorous prepubertal training may delay the onset of the menstrual cycle. On the positive side, that delay is associated with lower risk of cancers of the breast and the reproductive system. Long delays in the onset of menstruation or amenorrhea because of excess endurance training in young women can reduce bone mineral content, cause stress fractures, and pose future bone problems (osteoporosis). Conversely, strength training strengthens bones and increases strength and muscle mass.

Pregnant women may continue their exercise habits with physician approval. Most doctors recommend eliminating high-impact aerobics, keeping the exercise heart rate below 140 beats per minute, and avoiding prolonged exposure to high temperature during activity.

Stop Signs

If any of these occur, even once, stop exercising and consult your physician before resuming.

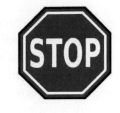

- Abnormal heart action: irregular **pulse**; fluttering, pumping, or palpitations in the chest or throat; a sudden burst of rapid heartbeats; or a very slow pulse that had been beating at a moderate rate a moment earlier (may occur either during or after exercise).
- Pain or pressure in the middle of the chest or in the arm or throat during or after exercise.
- Dizziness, lightheadedness, sudden loss of **coordination**, confusion, cold sweat, glassy stare, pallor, blueness, or fainting. In this case, stop the exercise—don't try to cool down—and lie with your feet elevated or sit and put your head down between your legs until the symptoms pass.

Yield Signs

If any of these occur, try these suggested remedies. If no relief occurs, consult a doctor.

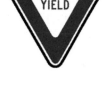

- *Persistent rapid heart action.* Heart rate increases with exercise intensity. High heart rate values may occur when you are exercising vigorously and for 5 to 10 minutes thereafter. To correct the problem, lower exercise intensity (heart rate) to a comfortable level and increase it slowly over a period of weeks. Consult a physician if the action is persistent.
- *Flare-up of bone or joint conditions.* Rest and resume exercise when the condition subsides. If you have no relief with the usual remedies, see your doctor.

Caution Signs

You can usually remedy these signs without medical consultation, although you may wish to report them to your doctor.

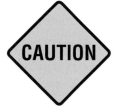

- *Nausea or vomiting after exercise.* Wait at least 2 to 3 hours after eating before you exercise, avoid extreme heat, exercise less vigorously, and take a longer **cool-down** period.
- *Extreme breathlessness lasting more than 10 minutes after stopping exercise.* Exercise less vigorously, at a level at which you can hold a conversation (talk test). If breathlessness persists, see your doctor.
- *Prolonged fatigue.* If you remain tired 24 or more hours after exercising or have insomnia related to physical activity, lower your intensity and increase it gradually over a period of weeks.
- *Side stitch.* Lean forward while sitting and attempt to push the abdominal organs up against the diaphragm.

FIGURE 3.6 Warning Signs in Physical Activity.

Postmenopausal women should participate in activities that put a moderate degree of stress on the muscles and bones of the upper body as well as the legs, to minimize the progress of osteoporosis. And women of all ages need to be aware of their special nutritional needs (e.g., calcium and iron).

• *Children*. Children are not miniature adults; their bones are still forming, and their capacity for exercise in certain circumstances is different from that of adults. Moreover, the value of early (prepubertal) strength or endurance training is still far from established. Therefore, moderation is the best approach. Children should avoid heavy training, prolonged hard work in the heat, and excess competition (if only to prevent later burnout). Give children the freedom to develop their own games, to play, to explore, and to be kids. Don't impose an adult model or adult goals on children, but do encourage an active lifestyle that will last a lifetime.

• *People with disabilities*. Each disability carries its own restrictions, but each has potential as well. People with disabilities participate and compete all the way up to international competitions, but only after establishing control over their conditions. They have learned to ski, to kayak, to do just about anything, and more opportunities are becoming available. Wheelchair athletes compete in marathons, play basketball, and fish at special access sites. People with multiple sclerosis respond better to moderate activity, such as swimming. For more information, contact your recreation department, community service organizations, or the National Center on Physical Activity and Disability, which maintains a wonderful free electronic newsletter and website (www.ncpad.org).

• *Racial considerations*. We've long known about the greater prevalence of hypertension among African-Americans (Lubell 1988). One in every three African-American adults has hypertension, compared with one in four non-African-Americans, and African-Americans are three times more likely to have severe hypertension than whites. All people benefit from aerobic and moderate lifting activities. Those with hypertension may want to avoid extremely heavy lifting or exercises with an isometric (static) component, because straining against a heavy load can elevate blood pressure dramatically. Moderate aerobic exercise and weight loss will help lower blood pressure. People with hypertension should undergo a pre-exercise medical examination, follow dietary recommendations, and take prescribed medications.

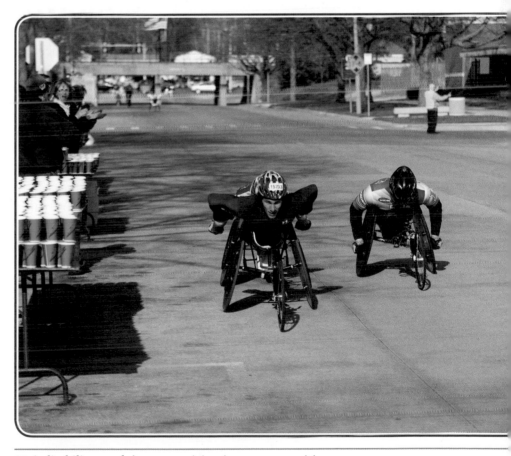

■ A disability needn't stop participation or competition.

INDIVIDUAL HEALTH RISK ANALYSIS

Use the health risk analysis form found in the appendix as a learning tool to identify positive and negative aspects of your health behavior. Although many of the effects are based on real findings from large epidemiological investigations, the estimates are generalized, and you should not take them too literally. Accurately predicting how long you will live or when you will die is impossible.

Plus one (+1) represents a positive effect that could add a year to your life or life to your years, and minus one (–1) indicates a loss in the quantity or quality of life. Complete each section and record the totals in section VIII of the form.

If you find that your risk of heart disease is high, you can take a number of steps to lower the risk, including the following:

- Engage in regular, moderate physical activity, 30 minutes on most days.
- Eat more fresh fruits and vegetables and less saturated and trans fat.
- Eat soy protein and olive oil.
- Keep your body mass index below 25 (see section I).
- Take a low-dose coated aspirin daily or every other day.
- Have one alcoholic drink (red wine or beer) daily or every other day.

SUMMARY

Until recently, the medical community has been cautious concerning exercise, suggesting a visit to the physician and even a stress test before participation. This approach is understandable, given that few medical schools offer more than a few lectures on the established benefits of physical activity. Unless your doctor is active or has special training in physiology or sports medicine, he or she may know little about the benefits of activity and how to prescribe exercise to achieve those benefits. But as the benefits and risks become better understood, physicians are turning to exercise physiologists to design and conduct preventive and rehabilitative exercise programs.

Of course, you don't have to see your physician to participate in moderate activity such as walking. If you feel good and answer no to all the questions in the health-screening questionnaire (page 60), you don't have to spend large sums to confirm what you already know. Start slowly, increase intensity and duration gradually, and continue to read this book. Use health screening, early detection, and periodic medical examinations to help you maintain your health.

Turning Your Life Around

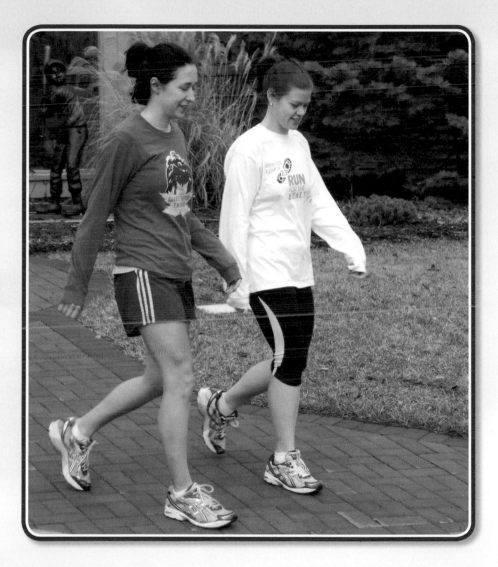

Seventy percent of adult Americans do not meet the physical activity guidelines for health and only 10 percent are active enough to improve fitness. Why have Americans not adapted the active life, even when we know that the benefits include feeling better, a healthier and longer life, better brain function, higher self-esteem and self-efficacy, and even better earning power? Why do most individuals who diet end up weighing the same or more than their starting weight within one to two years? Why are health clubs packed in January with new members fulfilling New Year's resolutions to become more active, only to be sparsely populated by March?

The likely answer is that we do not understand the psychology of behavior change or under-stand the concept of meaningful physical activity. In the first section of this book we covered the benefits of physical activity; all of the reasons why exercise is the truly great universal medicine. Exercise doesn't cure everything, but the benefits with no side effects are so broad in scope, inexpensive, and effective that the non-partisan government accounting office has suggested that if all American adults would meet the guideline of 150 minutes of weekly moderate physical activity, the American health care costs would be cut 50 percent or more.

In the first section we also introduced the idea of purposeful and meaningful physical activity. Bill Morgan developed this idea and has shown that when physical activity is purposeful (such as gardening or biking errands) or meaningful (such as outdoor activities that you enjoy like hiking or cross country skiing—the authors' favorites), we are much more likely to adapt the behaviors into the routine of our lives.

The three chapters in this section should help you understand the psychology of activity, how we can effectively change our behavior using well-documented strategies, and how to incorporate purposeful activity into your life.

Psychology of Activity
Learning to Play

> " In every real man, a child
> is hidden who wants to play. "
>
> *Friedrich Nietzsche*

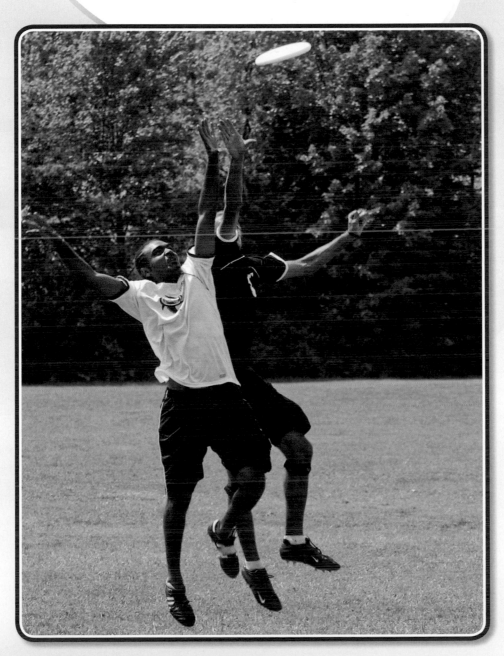

We can safely say that from a health standpoint, the people likely to benefit the most from regular, moderate physical activity seem most resistant to adopting or maintaining the behavior. As teachers and researchers, we have devoted our careers to the proposition that increased knowledge concerning the health benefits of activity and fitness will lead to increased participation. Unfortunately, for the majority, this has not been the case. Indeed, feelings related to well-being, enjoyment, and pleasure seem more important in initiating and maintaining activity than concerns about health or factual knowledge. So, we must journey beyond the comfortable landscape of physiology into the realm of psychology in search of answers to questions of motivation and adherence to regular, moderate physical activity.

This chapter presents ways to help you begin and maintain a healthy, active life. It deals with motivation, the reasons to become involved in regular activity, and adherence, how to sustain that involvement throughout life. Central to the discussion are the concepts of enjoyment, pleasure, satisfaction, and having fun. The active life is not a monastic existence or an exercise in asceticism. Rather, it is a vital, vigorous, and joyful life, replete with satisfactions, healthy pleasures, and even thrills.

This chapter will help you do the following:

- Understand the importance of enjoyment, pleasure, and satisfaction in activity and other life choices
- Appreciate the role of motivation, goal setting, and feedback in the initiation and adherence to the active life
- Identify your current involvement in physical activity
- Plan systematic changes in your activity plan
- Learn to visualize yourself as you would like to be
- Develop a reinforcement schedule to reward new behaviors

MOTIVATION

What motivates people to engage in regular activity? Is it to look or feel good, for weight control, or to improve and maintain health? Far fewer than half of all Americans follow the health recommendation of the Centers for Disease Control and Prevention (CDC) and the American College of Sports Medicine (ACSM) that every adult should accumulate at least 30 minutes of moderate-intensity physical activity on most, preferably all, days of the week (Pate et al. 1995). Fewer still follow the Institute of Medicine recommendation to engage in activity for 60 minutes a day. Among those who do 30 minutes of activity, fewer than 20 percent do so in a way that will bring about improvements in fitness. The rest lack the interest or motivation necessary to ensure regular participation (see form 4.1). Let's examine the psychology of motivation in hopes of finding ways to motivate ourselves, family members, and friends. Motivation involves the arousal, direction, and persistence of behavior.

What reasons have you given for your lack of participation in regular, moderate physical activity?

Interested, but haven't taken action:

- ☐ Can't afford the time; too busy right now
- ☐ Lack of opportunity
- ☐ Not convenient
- ☐ Too expensive
- ☐ Don't know how to start

Not interested:

- ☐ Low priority at this point in my life
- ☐ Concerned about my health
- ☐ Don't want to be embarrassed
- ☐ Bad childhood experiences
- ☐ Have never enjoyed it

What would you say to motivate a family member or friend who expressed one of these reasons for not participating in regular activity?

From B.J. Sharkey and S.E. Gaskill, 2013, *Fitness and health, seventh edition* (Champaign, IL: Human Kinetics).

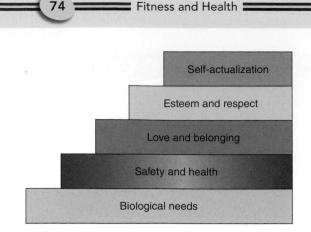

FIGURE 4.1 Hierarchy of needs.

Arousal

Physiological motives or drives are triggered by basic biological needs such as food, water, elimination, and sex. Safety and health needs are next in the hierarchy of human motives or needs—to be safe from threat, to be secure. Then come love and belonging—needs involving genuine affection and a place in one's group. Next in the hierarchy are the esteem needs—to be liked and respected and to respect oneself. At the top of the hierarchy is the need for **self-actualization**, to realize one's potential (Maslow 1954). Any of these needs may serve to arouse a person to action (see figure 4.1).

Directing Behavior

The **direction of behavior**—that is, where and how one behaves when aroused—is a complex study involving a multitude of learned behaviors and their interaction with ever-varying situations. Kenyon (1968) categorized the reasons that people engage in physical activity:

- Social reasons—to meet or be with people or part of a group
- Pursuit of vertigo—the thrill of speed and change of direction while remaining in control
- Aesthetic reasons—the beauty of movement
- Catharsis—relief from stress and tension
- Ascetic reasons—self-denial, discipline, training
- Health and fitness

Many forms of activity can satisfy a person's needs. One could walk, jog, run, swim, or cycle for health and fitness. Or a person could climb, kayak, ski, mountain bike, or windsurf in pursuit of vertigo. The direction chosen depends on several factors, including the level of arousal, previous exercise experiences, opportunity, the physical and social environment, and a bit of chance.

It strikes us that Kenyon's list of reasons that people engage in physical activity needs to be updated. A study of runners indicated additional reasons that people participate, including challenge, centering, afterglow, and because it feels good (Johnsgard 1985). What a surprise—people engage in physical activity because it feels good and brings them enjoyment. Another reason for participation is to improve or enhance appearance. For some, this means losing weight or fat, toning muscles, developing a six-pack set of abdominal muscles, or looking slim and svelte. Wow, exercise not

Finding Your Activity

Before Brian moved to Montana almost 50 years ago, he had never seen a pair of skis, let alone a real mountain. Yet he was motivated to try skiing, in part because friends and coworkers were skiers (social reason). Before long, he realized that skiing was for him. Soon he was skiing not to belong or for esteem, but because it was exciting (pursuit of vertigo), because it felt good, and because he wanted to test himself and find his potential. He became hopelessly hooked, positively addicted to the sport.

only feels good, contributes to vitality, and brings enjoyment, but also improves health and appearance!

Pleasure Principle

In their book *Healthy Pleasures,* Ornstein and Sobel (1989) describe the pleasure principle and its role in the motivation of behavior. Pleasurable sensations reverberate in the nervous system, releasing endorphins and other opiate-like chemicals. These chemicals find their way to receptors and satisfy physiological needs. The authors reason that the human desire for enjoyment evolved to enhance survival. They cite eating, reproductive behavior, and caring for others as examples of pleasures that are good for health and survival of the species. And they suggest that measurable, pleasurable benefits of physical activity may be as close, as easy, and even as enjoyable as a walk in the park. Their advocacy of natural pleasures, of things that feel good, is consistent with the active life. Exercise doesn't have to hurt

■ Participate in activities that are personally meaningful, make you feel good, or help you reach a personal goal.

Type T

Type T (for thrill) is a personality type that describes people who are hooked on excitement, risk, and tempting fate. Jack, a physician friend, is the quintessential type T. Over the years, he has raced motocross, climbed mountains, kayaked rivers, and sailed a catamaran. He mastered downhill skis, moved on to Telemark skis, and is now a board skier. His latest passion, windsurfing, takes him to the Columbia River, the mecca for the sport. Type Ts fit Kenyon's category pursuit of vertigo, defined as the thrill of speed and change in direction while remaining in control. Some find pleasure and satisfaction in pushing the limits, in gaining mastery, in flirting with danger while remaining in control, if just barely. People have said that type Ts get high on their own hormones. Certainly this behavior can become addictive, leading to tougher climbs and more challenging descents. Or it can become somewhat less dangerous, taking the form of in-line skating, scrambling up peaks, or even caving. Following the thrills to an untimely end isn't necessary. A person can channel the addiction into demanding but safer pursuits, compatible with the needs of family and career.

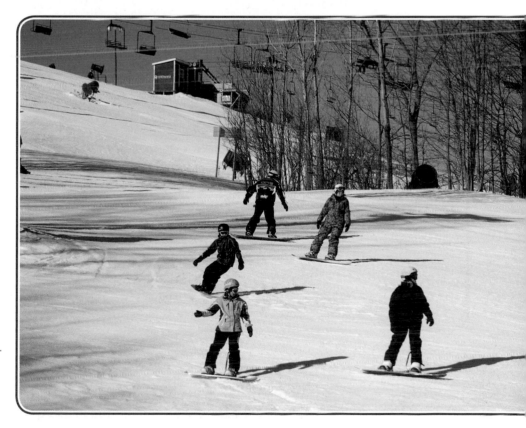

> *Y*ou must be willing and able to delay gratification if you are to experience the pleasure and relief that comes with completion of a difficult task.

to be good; it only has to be regular and moderate to bestow the benefits and healthy pleasures.

Even so, not all healthy pleasures are easy or immediately gratifying. Pleasure is synonymous with enjoyment and satisfaction. Some of the hardest things we have ever done are the most satisfying, such as running or cross-country skiing a marathon, climbing a mountain, or completing a triathlon. The training is always satisfying and usually enjoyable. But you must be willing and able to delay gratification if you are to experience the pleasure and relief that comes with completion of a difficult task.

> *I*t is impossible to live pleasurably without living wisely, well, and justly, and impossible to live wisely, well, and justly without living pleasurably.
>
> **Epicurus**

Intrinsic Motivation

Intrinsic or self-directed goals are more effective in long-term motivation and adherence to exercise. Extrinsic or external sources of motivation may arouse and direct efforts to win a prize, medal, trophy, or scholarship or to gain social acceptance. However, the motivation necessary to persist, to ensure lifelong participation in the active life, must come from within, from the upper reaches of the hierarchy of human needs (self-respect, self-actualization) and from the pleasure principle. Consider the former athletes who lose interest in their sport when the glory fades and the medals tarnish. Then look at your habitually active friends, the hikers, runners, tennis and racquetball players, and skiers. What keeps them going? Do they seek health, a trophy, or a championship? They go out each day because they must, because they are addicted, and because being active feels good. They go out to be themselves, and in the process they come closer to their potential.

Compulsion

An addiction can be nothing more than a habit. Of course, some of us are compulsive, prone to carrying things to extremes. Compulsive exercise behavior shares similarities with anorexia nervosa. Both groups include hard-working achievers who employ an ascetic approach to their problems. Do compulsive runners and those with anorexia nervosa share an obsessive-compulsive disorder? Probably not, but the discussion serves to reinforce the old-fashioned but ever applicable admonition for moderation in all things.

Persistence

Defined as the ability to go on resolutely or stubbornly in spite of difficulties, persistence is the key to success in physical activity and in life. Calvin Coolidge summed up its importance in the following lines:

Nothing in the world can take the place of persistence. Talent will not; nothing is more common than unsuccessful men with talent. Genius will not; unrewarded genius is almost a proverb. Education will not; the world is full of educated derelicts. Persistence and determination alone are omnipotent.

We need persistence to meet fitness, performance, weight-control, or other goals, especially on cold, windy, or rainy days. Persistence implies faith in the eventual outcome, the ability to delay gratification, and confidence in our ability to cope with adversity. Without it, we could never leave our cozy homes and venture forth in cold and snow. Persistence helps us sustain effort over a prolonged period to reach a goal. It is the foundation of adherence.

ADHERENCE

To adhere means to maintain loyalty, to stick fast, to cling. Why do some stick with the active life while others slip away? We define dropouts as those who begin an exercise program and then cease participation. Exercise program dropout rates range from 20 percent to more than 50 percent. People most often cite lack of time as the reason for dropping out, as well as for not starting in the first place. Family, career, or other responsibilities make it difficult for many who say they are just too busy. We think of our recent presidents when we hear this excuse. Even they found time for physical activity in their schedules. Effective time management is one of the hallmarks of success, as is involvement in the active life. Other reasons for dropping out include having no place to exercise, fatigue, inadequate information, inconvenience, and lack of willpower.

Studies have shown that factors associated with dropping out include a sedentary youth and previous unfavorable exercise experience, which underscores the need for enjoyable activity experiences, for having fun in school physical education and youth sports programs. Education and income have also been linked positively with adherence; more education means more income, and both have been associated with adherence. In personality tests, adherers were found to exhibit more self-confidence and emotional stability than dropouts did. Cigarette smoking is usually linked with a higher rate of dropping out of exercise (Willis and Campbell 1992). Family and peer support enhances adherence, and excessive work demands hinder it.

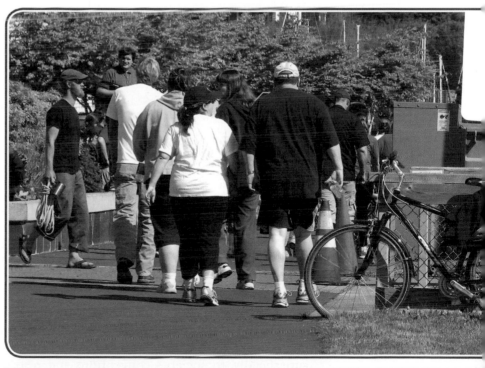

■ Find the environment that will help you stay active. Activities that you enjoy and that are social or purposeful are most likely to be adopted long term.

Programs that are enjoyable and that foster a sense of achievement and satisfaction are more likely to encourage adherence.

A number of factors that influence continued participation have been identified. Some relate to individual participation, and others pertain to exercise programs. Some folks thrive in an individual program, whereas others enjoy group participation and supervision (Greenberg 2011). One local company's wellness program provides for both types, offering both individual time-share programs (in which employees match their personal exercise time with an equal amount of company-paid time), and fitness club memberships that provide group or individual programs. Convenience, good facilities, likable leadership, and social support are factors related to adherence in group programs. Another determinant is how well the program meets participants' needs. The self-regulatory processes of monitoring goal progress and responding to discrepancies has also been shown to be important to adherence (de Bruin et al. 2012).

Finally, we return to the pleasure principle. Programs that are enjoyable and that foster a sense of achievement and satisfaction are more likely to encourage adherence (Petruzzello 2012).

Group cohesion is defined as a dynamic process reflected by the tendency of a group to stick together and remain united in the pursuit of its objectives and for the satisfaction of its members' needs. Increased group cohesion leads to an increase in adherence to an exercise program. Indeed, a summary of research concluded that people who hold strong beliefs about the cohesiveness of their exercise group do the following:

- Attend more classes
- Arrive on time
- Drop out less frequently
- Resist disruptions
- Experience more positive effects
- Improve their attitudes toward exercise
- Achieve confidence in their ability to successfully carry out actions to satisfy situational demands (self-efficacy) (Estabrooks 2000)

Drill Instructors?

Several years ago my old friend Dr. Paul Davis initiated an unusual exercise program in Washington, D.C., called the Sergeant's Program. Former drill instructors staffed the program and led participants through a grueling program of **calisthenics** and running. The instructors used salty speech, derisive comments, and epithets to motivate the group of young male and female lawyers, MBAs, and bureaucrats. To everyone's surprise, the program was a great success.

Climate for Adherence

With maturation comes the satisfaction of lower-order needs and the opportunity to seek self-actualization. Self-actualized people are free to determine their lifestyle and personal goals and to pursue them without anxiety and without the necessity to conform, except superficially, to society's conventions and restraints. Self-actualized people seek to be, not to become. They enjoy their lives as they seek to realize their capacity. They require neither the attention nor the adulation of the crowd, only a personal sense of satisfaction and achievement.

Even self-actualized people sometimes find it difficult to make necessary sacrifices. Pursuing any goal is hard when those around you are not supportive. Fitness studies have shown that the emotional climate created by significant others is highly related to the participant's adherence to the program. When wives, husbands, and loved ones offer encouragement and support, the participant is likely to continue. Why would anyone deprecate a loved one's efforts in a fitness or sports training program? Spouses may complain about the amount of time involved, the cost, and upset schedules and vacations. Of course, some may complain because, secretly, they envy their spouse's dedication and satisfaction, or they fear losing their rejuvenated loved one or the loss of shared experiences.

To avoid emotional conflicts, discuss your interests and goals with loved ones. Realize how your participation may affect them and try to minimize adverse effects. Invent new shared experiences to replace those lost as a result of your personal quest for excellence. A supportive emotional climate is certain to prevail when both husband and wife are happily involved in the active life. Both need not be involved in the same activity, although there are many such cases. If both seek excellence in tennis, they do not necessarily have to play mixed doubles. What matters is that each understands how important participation is to the other and that the emotional climate they create influences enjoyment and adherence.

Climate and geography can enhance or detract from the enjoyment of participation. When young women performed aerobic exercise in a naturalistic environment, the activity was associated with decreases in state anxiety and increases in tranquility, positive engagement, and revitalization (Focht and Hausenblas 2001). In some cases, the environment can preclude certain activities. For example, skiing isn't available in some parts of the country—if you want to participate regularly, you'll have to move or take expensive vacations. The answer, often ignored, is to move to where climate and geography suit your interests. Ridiculous, you say? Perhaps, but we've met hundreds of people who have done just that—left high-paying jobs amid urban sprawl to seek a better way. We've met them by mountain lakes, on ski lifts, running in the desert, and skiing in the wilderness. Do they have any regrets? Perhaps. Decide on your goals, your priorities, and the kind of life you want to live, and then give it your best effort. In time, if you feel the need to change, do it. It's all a part of the process of achieving your potential.

With 85 years at your disposal, you have time to try out several careers and locations. Don't lament time that you must spend away from a favored environment. Enjoy yourself as much as possible and realize that future careers and locations await you. Active, creative lives are available everywhere, not just at distant holiday resorts. Adapt to the environment that you are in and use it to learn new skills, not to regret the ones that don't fit the setting. But never give up on the dream that unites vocation, avocation, and location. One of our dreams has been to live where we can cross-country ski on groomed tracks right outside the backdoor. We haven't quite achieved the dream, but we are close—within a mile.

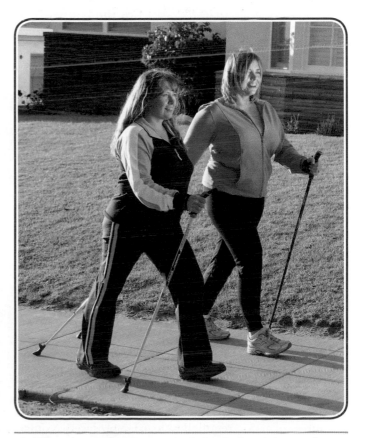

■ Adherence and enjoyment of physical activity can be increased through supportive relationships.

Improving Adherence

We've considered some of the reasons that people drop out and the factors associated with adherence to the active life. We've discussed the emotional climate and the importance of pleasure and having fun. Now let's turn our attention to psychological concepts that shed light on ways to enhance adherence. One concept is the therapeutic use of physical activity as a means of coping with moods, stress, anxiety, depression, and other problems. As part of a daily schedule, the activity becomes preventive, an inoculation against moods that interfere with life satisfaction. For more on adherence, consult Weinberg and Gould's *Foundations of Sport and Exercise Psychology* (2003).

• *Internals versus externals.* The psychological construct called locus of control separates people into internals, those who believe that they can control outcomes in their lives, and externals, who believe that chance or others control their lives. Those with an **internal locus of control** are more likely to adhere to healthy behaviors than those with an **external locus of control** are. Which better fits your view of life? Can you modify your locus of control to enhance adherence to healthy behaviors, such as regular activity? We believe that you can.

*E*xtol your virtues, and you'll boost self-esteem, adherence, and possibly performance.

• *Self-efficacy.* The theory of self-efficacy suggests that coping behaviors such as physical activity are influenced by the perception of acquiring mastery in that area. Perception of mastery influences performance, and theory suggests that positive experience alters this perception. Thus, successful experience may reinforce an activity, leading to continuation of the behavior. Although judgments of efficacy are situation specific, it has even been suggested that enhanced self-efficacy in one behavior may generalize to others. Research indicates that self-efficacy plays a prominent role in the early adoption and adaptation stages of exercise programs, but is less potent in the maintenance stage. Self-efficacy takes on renewed importance when structured programs end and people must rely on their own resources to develop an exercise program (McAuley and Blissmer 2000).

If the perception of mastery reinforces behavior, perhaps we can influence that perception with affirmative statements, or positive reinforcements of progress and performance. Elite athletes use affirmative statements to build confidence and aid performance, part of the

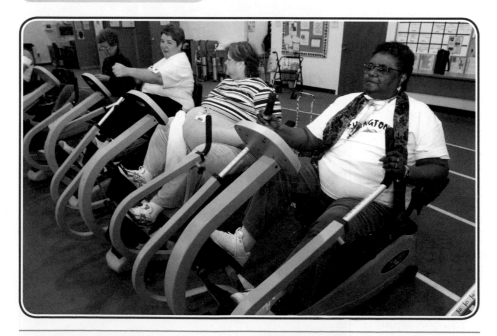

■ "Self-efficacy is the belief in one's capabilities to organize and execute the sources of action required to manage prospective situations" (Bandura 1986).

positive internal dialogue that leads to success, both in sport and in life. If it works for athletes, you too can use positive self-talk to reinforce your sense of success, thereby enhancing adherence. Recognize your sacrifices, your progress, and your achievements. Celebrate your epic adventures. At the same time, you must eliminate negative self-talk. Extol your virtues, and you'll boost self-esteem, adherence, and possibly performance.

Internal Dialogue

The first step toward a positive internal dialogue is to eliminate negatives, irrational thinking, and cognitive distortions from your internal dialogue. Stop blaming yourself, focusing on negatives, overgeneralizing, magnifying, and minimizing. Don't undervalue your accomplishments. Change the negative "I look flabby" into the positive "I need to improve muscle tone." Then select positive affirmations to reinforce your behavior. Add simple statements such as "I can do this," "I'm making progress," "I'm looking good," and "I'm achieving my goals." If you use them regularly, you'll feel better about yourself and your program.

GOAL SETTING

A goal is an aim or a purpose, what a person seeks to accomplish. Goals serve to help focus and regulate behavior, thus affecting both motivation and adherence. Goal setting has a beneficial influence on the performance of a task. Although most folks use goals to a certain extent, few take full advantage of their influence on the motivation for and adherence to physical activity. By using short- and long-term goals, you can devise a strategy to achieve the desired result.

Goal setting works best by using **process-oriented goals**. For instance, a process-oriented goal is to work up gradually to 30 miles (48.2 km) of running per week, or to complete a 10K (6.2 mi) race. An outcome-oriented goal would be to run the 10K race in less than 40 minutes, an outcome that might be very difficult to achieve. **Outcome-oriented goals** have their place, but they need to be reasonable and adaptable. If the day of the 10K race is hot and humid, you'll need to adjust your goal.

We use goals to prepare for upcoming events and adventures, such as our annual winter ski trip in Yellowstone Park. In fall, we engage in muscular fitness training to build strength and endurance in skiing muscles. As soon as the snow flies, we begin training so that we'll be able to keep up with our partners in February. Of course, we thoroughly enjoy every phase of the preparation, particularly the sense of accomplishment at the end of a long, hard trail. Set long-term goals as targets and short-term goals to help attain them. Write down your goals and keep records as you progress. Back when Brian considered himself a serious runner, he set training targets and recorded daily mileage on the calendar. At the end of the week, he'd add the total to see whether he was on target to reach the goal.

Set realistic goals, such as 30 minutes of moderate physical activity most days of the week. When the goal becomes too easy and loses its motivational effect, set a new, more challenging goal. Challenging goals get better results than easy ones. Use specific goals; don't just plan to work hard. Finally, keep the list simple. Don't set too many goals. As you achieve success, you may expand the list. But for now, begin with one or two long-term targets and some short-term steps to guide progress toward the targets (Locke and Latham 1985). When you achieve a significant long-term goal, celebrate!

When Steven was coaching the U.S. Nordic combined team, the team had a sports medicine advisory group that included a sport psychologist, our publisher, Dr. Rainer

The Active Personality

Do activity and improved fitness influence personality, or are some personality types more likely to be active? Personality is a frame of reference that psychologists use in the study of behavior. More than a mask but less than reality, personality is a product of heredity and the environment, usually studied with paper-and-pencil tests or in-depth interviews, but never really defined or measured.

Cattell suggests that our personality indicates what we will do when in a given mood and placed in a given situation. He developed the Cattell 16 Personality Factor Questionnaire, a personality test used widely by researchers (Cattell, Eber, and Tatsuoka 1970). The test, typical of the paper-and-pencil approach, scores the subject on each of 16 factors, or personality traits (aloof–sociable, emotional–calm, timid–adventurous, confident–insecure). Assuming that this approach is valid, let's use it to consider how activity and personality are related.

Studies of the personalities of middle-aged men have shown that highly fit subjects are more unconventional, composed, secure, easygoing, emotionally stable, adventurous, and higher in intelligence than low-fitness subjects are. The most pronounced personality differences were those related to emotional stability and security. The presence of differences between high- and low-fitness groups, however, does not prove that the differences are due to fitness. Emotionally stable and secure men may be more likely to engage in a fitness program. When researchers studied the effects of a 4-month fitness program on these subjects, they noted little personality change in the low-fitness group, in spite of a conspicuous improvement in fitness. The researchers reasoned that it takes years to become fit or unfit, and that a few months of activity is insufficient to bring about significant personality changes (Ismail and Young 1977). Longitudinal studies are necessary to confirm or reject the hypothesis that personality improves with activity or fitness.

Martens. One skill that Rainer taught was the exceptionally helpful tool of **visualization**. After athletes had defined their short- and long-term goals, Rainer helped them visualize themselves accomplishing those goals. Treat yourself as you would like to be and you will become that person. To be a champion, you have to see yourself as a champion and all that it includes. Visualization is a powerful tool to change behavior, self-beliefs, actions, sport technique, and self-image. Change the action in the mind and the mind will control the body.

To begin an exercise program, you need to think of yourself as a person who lives the active life. See yourself achieving the goals that you would like to achieve, and slowly but surely, you will move to the new reality. You can learn more about behavior change in chapter 5.

SETTING YOUR PREFERENCE TO EXERTION

Years ago, we researchers felt that perceptions were too subjective, too prone to error and variation. When an athlete said that he was too tired to go on, we doubted his motivation. But Swedish psychologist Dr. Gunnar Borg changed all that when he developed and validated his **rating of perceived exertion (RPE)** (see table 10.4 on page 197). Borg (1973) realized that the brain integrates sensory stimuli generated during physical effort into a perception of effort. The brain perceives and evaluates stimuli from muscles, respiratory distress, pain, and the sensation of a pounding heart. Subsequent studies have shown that these subjective estimates of effort are highly related to workload, heart rate, oxygen consumption, and even **lactic acid** and hormones. In other words, our subjective estimate of work intensity provides a rather accurate gauge of the load itself, as well as the internal factors affected by the work. Of course, our subjective perception of effort is also closely tied with the pleasure that we derive from participation.

Because we are able to judge our effort accurately in an exercise such as cycling or running, and because the heart rate and metabolic cost of the effort are closely related to those ratings, we should listen to our bodies during exercise. If the exercise feels too difficult, it probably is. In exercise prescription, the heart-rate training zone employs important physiological criteria to determine a safe and effective dose of exercise. You may find that running at your training heart rate feels somewhat hard. Thereafter, you can use that sense of difficulty to guide your exertion. If high temperatures cause your heart rate to rise, your perception of effort will adjust your pace to a more prudent level. Eventually, this sense of effort is all that you need to gauge exercise intensity.

While we're on the subject of perception, let us spend a moment on the concept of

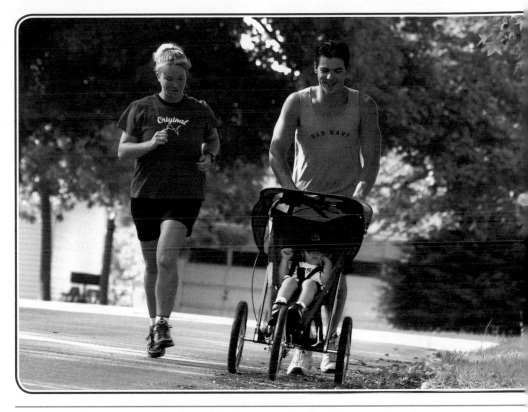

■ Learn to listen to your body and find an exertion level appropriate for your goals and enjoyment.

Finding a Project

To complete her senior project, Steven's youngest daughter decided to take on a formidable challenge. She had read about the Border-to-Border ski across Finland, an event requiring use of traditional cross-country technique to cover 28 to 52 miles (45–84 km) per day for 7 days to traverse the 278-mile (450 km) distance across Finland from Russia to Sweden. Because Steven thought that the trip would be fabulous, he agreed to join her. They began training to develop the technique and endurance that they would need. Having the major goal motivated their training and made it more enjoyable. Because Heidi had never been to Finland, he helped her imagine the rolling landscape near the Arctic Circle. Visualizing the benefits, the sauna at the end of each day, and the feeling of accomplishment helped to sustain the hours of gentle skiing that preceded the trip.

preferred exertion. When subjects participated in a low- or high-preference activity, fatigue and psychological distress were higher in the low-preference condition, and positive well-being was higher and **perceived exertion** lower in the high-preference activity, even though work rate remained constant across conditions (Parfitt and Gledhill 2004).

In another area of preference, experienced exercisers seem to require a certain level of exertion to be satisfied. If the exertion is too easy, their sense of satisfaction diminishes. Training increases the preferred exertion, whereas inactivity lowers it. People who have been involved in highly competitive sports often have learned to prefer a high level of exertion. Some erroneously believe that exercise has to hurt to be good (it does not), or they subscribe to the maxim "No pain, no gain" (also untrue). Therefore, when they resume activity after a prolonged layoff, they overdo it and end up with soreness or injury.

The preference for exertion is learned. For most Americans, the learned preference consists of the minimum, of walking to and from the car. This circumstance could be different. If parents, schools, and community leaders demonstrate and encourage sensible and inexpensive exercise habits, more kids will grow up with a predisposition to regular activity. If parents become involved, the kids will make physical activity a family affair. Elementary, high school, and even college students should be encouraged to participate in healthful activities. Community organizations can sponsor activities for which participation is the major goal. The objective is to raise preferred exertion to the level required to achieve the health benefits of regular, moderate physical activity.

SUMMARY

This chapter examines motivation and adherence to help you initiate and maintain involvement in enjoyable, lifelong physical activity. We've learned that motivation involves the arousal, direction, and persistence of behavior and that **intrinsic motivation** is more persistent than **extrinsic motivation**. We've also learned that internals, those who feel in control of their lives, are more likely to adhere to healthy behaviors than are externals, those who believe that chance or others control their lives. We've seen that success or the perception of mastery reinforces participation and aids adherence. The chapter provides a way to identify current activity patterns, establish realistic goals for new behaviors, and use reinforcement to help ensure attainment of those goals.

Throughout this book, we advocate realistic goals, minor adjustments, and gradual change as a proved approach to improvements in activity and other health behaviors. Research and common sense support this approach. Most people won't need a radical change if they just stick with minor adjustments, such as taking daily walks or substituting low-fat foods for high-fat foods. But one school of thought suggests that moderate changes are hard to measure and easy to ignore, making a slip back into bad habits more likely. Gradual change may not provide the results and positive feedback required to reinforce the behavior, whereas big changes in health behaviors are more likely to yield big results. If you think that you might prefer this second approach, set lofty goals, such as running a marathon or making major changes in diet and body weight. Make a major commitment and see what happens. Use the approach that works for you.

The next chapter explores methods of behavior change. You will determine your attitudes toward physical activity and your willingness to change your physical activity behaviors.

Active people seem better able to cope with the problems of life. These hardy people share several characteristics: a sense of being in control, a sense of involvement and purpose, and the flexibility to adapt to challenges and opportunities (Kobasa 1979). Robust good health and resistance to illness don't absolutely require regular, moderate activity, not if you are blessed with superb genes. But if you are like most of us, activity provides a coping mechanism that contributes to health, adaptability, and resistance to stress. And more important, it's fun.

It's been said, "Begin; the rest is easy." Of course, that isn't true—the rest isn't easy. But unless you begin, you'll never know how easy or hard the road may be. Life is a journey, not a destination.

Behavior Change
Gaining Control

"Two roads diverged in a wood, and I
. . . took the one less traveled by,
and that has made all the difference.

Robert Frost

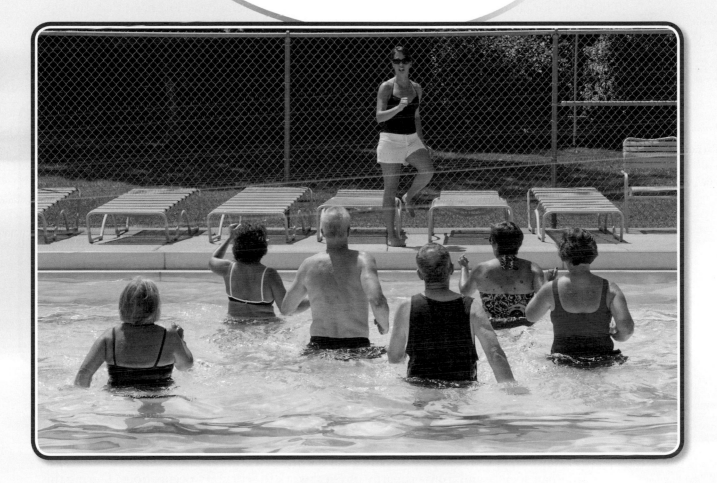

We all have an image of who we are, what we like, and how we will act in most situations. Our physical activity patterns are the combined result of our self-image and our environment. Most of us have developed regular patterns of physical activity or inactivity that define our behavior in this important realm. As authors, one of our primary roles in writing this book is, first, to provide convincing information that the active lifestyle is beneficial and, second, to help you understand how to make desired changes. As noted earlier, from a health standpoint, the people likely to benefit the most from regular, moderate physical activity seem most resistant to adopting or maintaining the behavior. Unfortunately, for Americans and for most people in the developed world, the road of physical fitness is truly the road less traveled.

This chapter discusses why behavior modification is so difficult. We'll help you develop the necessary tools and strategies to get you started down a new pathway of physical adventure. You will truly be taking the pathway less traveled, and it will make all the difference to your health and how you feel and look. It will even help your brain perform better. In some ways, this might be the most important chapter in the book. Since you are reading this, you are either interested in changing your physical activity habits or you are a student required to read this book. While each of you may be in a different stage of behavior change, you are gathering the background (raising consciousness) that can support future actions to become more active or fit. We will discuss the stages of behavior change, help you decide where you fit in the continuum, and provide strategies to start or enhance your journey.

This chapter will help you do the following:

- Learn why it is so difficult to change behaviors such as physical activity and nutrition
- Determine your barriers to physical activity
- Understand how your environment affects your behavior
- Identify your current stage of behavior change
- Plan systematic strategies to help you change
- Learn to visualize yourself as you would like to be
- Develop a reinforcement schedule to reward new behaviors

ACTIVITY IN MODERN SOCIETY

Our ancestors were constantly on the move. Over the last century, Americans and others in industrial and developing societies have witnessed a great migration from a rural to an urban society and from primarily physical work to sedentary occupations. During this same time period, the proliferation of human-energy-saving tools, from cars for personal transport to electric can openers, escalators, and computers, have helped us conserve our personal energy and replace it with external power. This trend is continuing around the world as societies become urbanized. For example, China has seen mass migration to cities and the explosive growth in automobile use. A study by Egger and colleagues (2001) suggests that current Americans walk or jog 5 to 10 miles (8–16 km) less today than we did three or four decades ago.

> **A** difference in activity levels equivalent to walking 8 to 16 kilometers (5–10 mi) per day represents a huge decline in daily energy expenditure. At the upper level, this coincides roughly with previous estimates of reduced activity (James 1995, Cordain et al., 1998). It also accords with the levels of movement required for foraging for survival throughout most of human evolution. Anthropological evidence suggests that early humans, like modern hunter-gatherers, may have transported tools, weapons, and game over a daily range of about 15 kilometers (9 mi). Given their other daily tasks, this would have added up to a substantial daily energy use which was rarely, if ever, exceeded by food intake over an extended period, thus reducing the chances of energy imbalance. As a result, up until the past two or three decades, human populations had not been overweight. The growth of time-saving and time-using technologies, however, means that these activity levels are unlikely to be reached without conscious effort. In the presence of an abundant, energy dense food supply, obesity, at the population level, is an inevitable consequence of modernization.

Adapted from Egger, Vogels, and Westerterp, 2001.

Children watch their parents, other adults, and peers. They imitate the behaviors they see, and without even realizing it, they develop sedentary behaviors that they perceive as the norm. Physical activity has been in a steady decline in the United States for the past half century, with sedentary behavior accelerating during the past two decades. Added to the decrease in human movement is the increased availability of food and a rise in snacking. Restaurant portions have increased, fast food is ubiquitous, and obesity has become an epidemic.

For the two-thirds of American adults now overweight or obese, physical activity becomes even more difficult. Even though most American adults know that physical activity is important for their long-term health and that they will feel better and be more productive if they start exercising, few are able to escape their environment and self-image and begin the regenerative process that physical activity brings. Physical activity is truly the best medicine for the human body. The American College of Sports Medicine promotes a campaign called Exercise is Medicine. The evidence is on their side: Physical activity is the only medicine that offers so many benefits with no negative side effects. Changing behavior to include the medicine of exercise requires more effort than opening a bottle and swallowing a few pills, but it also brings forth many benefits and promotes long-term health.

BARRIERS TO PHYSICAL ACTIVITY

More than 60 percent of adult Americans do not meet the recommended physical activity guidelines for health, and less than 10 percent meet fitness guidelines. A sedentary lifestyle has become the norm as many technological advances and conveniences have made our lives easier and less active. Adults model this behavior to our youth. Over the past decade, sedentary youth behavior has accelerated. Predictably, there has been an associated increase in overweight and obese youth and earlier onset of diabetes and heart disease.

Sallis studied the most common reasons that adults cite for not adopting more physically active lifestyles (Sallis and Hovell 1990, Sallis et al. 1992). His lists include the following:

- Not enough time to exercise
- Find exercise inconvenient
- Lack self-motivation
- Do not find exercise enjoyable
- Find exercise boring
- Lack confidence in ability to be physically active (low self-efficacy)
- Fear of being injured of have been injured recently
- Lack self-management skills such as goal setting, progress monitoring, or a reward process
- Lack encouragement, support, or companionship from family and friends
- Do not have parks, sidewalks, bicycle trails, or safe pleasant paths convenient to the home or office

Each of us can come up with additional reasons as to why we might not be physically active. Understanding the common barriers to physical activity and your personal beliefs and barriers will help you to develop strategies to become more active. You can start by taking the barriers to being physically active quiz (form 5.1). Once you identify your personal barriers, you can use the strategies provided to begin your personal plan toward an active life. What keeps you from being more active?

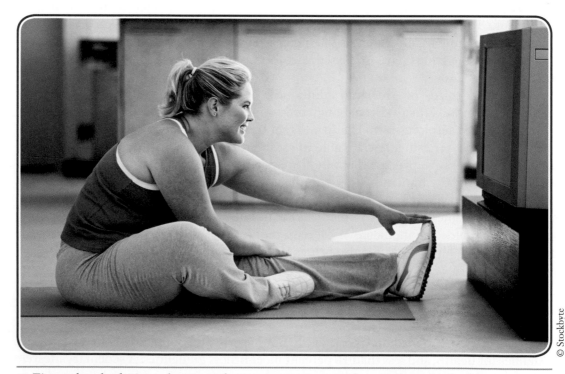

© Stockbyte

■ Fitness breaks during television ads are a great way to reduce sedentary minutes.

Directions: Here are reasons that people give to describe why they do not get as much physical activity as they think they should. Please read each statement and indicate how likely you are to say each of the following statements.

How likely are you to say:	Very likely	Some-what likely	Some-what unlikely	Very unlikely
1. My day is so busy now, I just don't think I can make the time to include physical activity in my regular schedule.	3	2	1	0
2. None of my family members or friends like to do anything active, so I don't have a chance to exercise.	3	2	1	0
3. I'm just too tired after work to get any exercise.	3	2	1	0
4. I've been thinking about getting more exercise, but I just can't seem to get started.	3	2	1	0
5. I'm getting older, so exercise can be risky.	3	2	1	0
6. I don't get enough exercise because I have never learned the skills for any sport.	3	2	1	0
7. I don't have access to jogging trails, swimming pools, bike paths. . .	3	2	1	0
8. Physical activity takes too much time away from other com-mitments—time, work, or family.	3	2	1	0
9. I'm embarrassed about how I will look when I exercise with others.	3	2	1	0
10. I don't get enough sleep as it is. I just couldn't get up early or stay up late to get some exercise.	3	2	1	0
11. It's easier for me to find excuses not to exercise than to go out to do something.	3	2	1	0
12. I know of too many people who have hurt themselves by overdoing it with exercise.	3	2	1	0
13. I really can't see learning a new sport at my age.	3	2	1	0
14. It's just too expensive. You have to take a class or join a club or buy the right equipment.	3	2	1	0
15. My free times during the day are too short to include exercise.	3	2	1	0
16. My usual social activities with family or friends do not include physical activity.	3	2	1	0
17. I'm too tired during the week and I need the weekend to catch up on my rest.	3	2	1	0
18. I want to get more exercise, but I just can't seem to make myself stick to anything.	3	2	1	0
19. I'm afraid I might injure myself or have a heart attack.	3	2	1	0
20. I'm not good enough at any physical activity to make it fun.	3	2	1	0
21. If we had exercise facilities and showers at work, then I would be more likely to exercise.	3	2	1	0

(continued)

Form 5.1 *(continued)*

Follow these instructions to score yourself:

- Enter the circled number in the spaces provided, putting together the number for statement 1 on line 1, statement 2 on line 2, and so on.

Add the three scores on each line. Your barriers to physical activity fall into one or more of seven categories: lack of time, social influences, lack of energy, lack of willpower, fear of injury, lack of skill, and lack of resources. A score of 5 or above in any category shows that this is an important barrier for you to overcome.

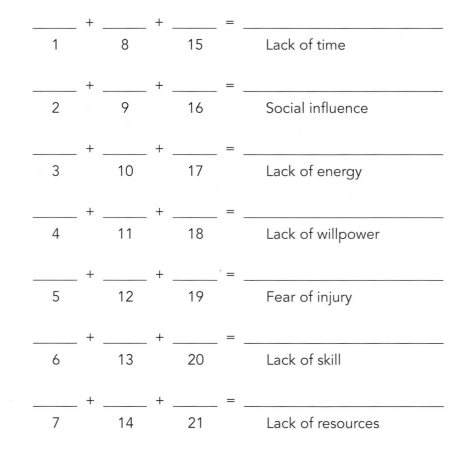

_____ + _____ + _____ =			_____
1	8	15	Lack of time
_____ + _____ + _____ =			_____
2	9	16	Social influence
_____ + _____ + _____ =			_____
3	10	17	Lack of energy
_____ + _____ + _____ =			_____
4	11	18	Lack of willpower
_____ + _____ + _____ =			_____
5	12	19	Fear of injury
_____ + _____ + _____ =			_____
6	13	20	Lack of skill
_____ + _____ + _____ =			_____
7	14	21	Lack of resources

From B.J. Sharkey and S.E. Gaskill, 2013, *Fitness and health, seventh edition* (Champaign, IL: Human Kinetics). Reprinted from Centers for Disease Control and Prevention. Available: http://www.cdc.gov/nccdphp/dnpa/physical/life/barriers_quiz.pdf

Many strategies can help you adapt to an active lifestyle. The remaining portions of this chapter teach you more about behavior change, explain how to identify your stage of change, and provide ideas for moving forward. Before we move on, use the information (adapted from the CDC) in form 5.2 to help you with some ideas to overcome your physical activity barriers. Once you have evaluated your barriers to physical activity, you should have some strategies to begin your journey toward a healthy and energy-filled life. The next section further explores how your environment affects your physical activity. You will need to self-evaluate your environmental factors as you move through the rest of this chapter, looking at stage of change, strategies for change, and how to use visualization to help you change your self-image.

Form 5.2   Suggestions for Overcoming Physical Activity Barriers

Lack of time
- ☐ Identify available time slots. Monitor your daily activities for 1 week. Identify at least three 30 min time slots you could use for physical activity.
- ☐ Add purposeful physical activity to your daily routine. For example, walk or ride your bike to work or to go shopping, organize school activities around physical activity, walk the dog, exercise while you watch TV, or park farther away from your destination.
- ☐ Select activities requiring minimal time, such as walking, jogging, or stair-climbing.

Social influence
- ☐ Explain your interest in physical activity to friends and family. Ask them to support your efforts.
- ☐ Invite friends and family members to exercise with you. Plan social activities involving exercise.
- ☐ Develop new friendships with physically active people. Join a group, such as the YMCA or a hiking club.

Lack of energy
- ☐ Schedule physical activity for times in the day or week when you feel energetic.
- ☐ Convince yourself that if you give it a chance, physical activity will increase your energy level. Next, try it.

Lack of motivation
- ☐ Plan ahead. Make physical activity a regular part of your daily or weekly schedule and write it on your calendar.
- ☐ Invite a friend to exercise with you on a regular basis and write it on both your calendars.
- ☐ Join an exercise group or class.

Fear of injury
- ☐ Learn how to warm up and cool down to prevent injury.
- ☐ Learn how to exercise appropriately considering your age, fitness level, skill level, and health status.
- ☐ Choose activities involving minimum risk.

Lack of skill
- ☐ Select activities requiring no new skills, such as walking, climbing stairs, or jogging.
- ☐ Take a class to develop new skills.

Lack of resources
- ☐ Select activities that require minimal facilities or equipment, such as walking, jogging, jumping rope, or calisthenics.
- ☐ Identify inexpensive, convenient resources available in your community (e.g., community education programs, park and recreation programs, or worksite programs).

Weather conditions
- ☐ Develop a set of regular activities that are always available, regardless of weather (indoor cycling, aerobic dance, indoor swimming, calisthenics, stair-climbing, skipping rope, mall walking, dancing, or gymnasium games).

(continued)

Travel	☐ Put a jump rope in your suitcase and use it.
	☐ Walk the halls and climb the stairs in hotels.
	☐ Stay in places with swimming pools or exercise facilities.
	☐ Join the YMCA or YWCA (ask about reciprocal membership agreement).
	☐ Visit the local shopping mall and walk for half an hour or more.
	☐ Bring your MP3 player with your favorite aerobic exercise music.
Family obligations	☐ Trade babysitting time with a friend, neighbor, or family member who also has small children.
	☐ Exercise with the kids: go for a walk together, play tag or other running games, get an aerobic dance or exercise tape for kids (there are several on the market). You can spend time together and still get your exercise.
	☐ Jump rope, do calisthenics, ride a stationary bicycle, or use other home gymnasium equipment while the kids are busy playing or sleeping.
	☐ Try to exercise when the kids are not around (e.g., during school hours or their nap time).
Retirement years	☐ View your retirement as an opportunity to become more active instead of less. Spend more time gardening, walking the dog, and playing with your grandchildren. Children with short legs and grandparents with slower gaits are often great walking partners.
	☐ Learn a new skill you've always been interested in, such as ballroom dancing, square dancing, or swimming.
	☐ Now that you have the time, make regular physical activity a part of every day. Go for a walk every morning or every evening before dinner. Treat yourself to an exercise bike and ride every day while reading a favorite book or magazine.
Notes	

From B.J. Sharkey and S.E. Gaskill, 2013, *Fitness and health, seventh edition* (Champaign, IL: Human Kinetics). Reprinted, by permission, from Centers for Disease Control and Prevention, 1999, *Promoting physical activity: A guide for community action* (Champaign, IL; Human Kinetics), 31, 72.

ENVIRONMENT AND BEHAVIOR

Our social, economic, built, and even weather environments have changed dramatically over the past three to five decades. Consider that in 1960, nearly 70 percent of adult Americans worked in occupations that required physical labor. Today that number is less than 30 percent. This shift in just the economic environment has resulted in an average daily decrease of 400 to 700 kilocalories of energy expenditure, or the equivalent of walking about 4 to 7 miles (6.5–11 km). It is little wonder that the current guidelines for healthy physical activity levels recommend that we accumulate at least 10,000 steps (about 5 mi, or 8 km) a day to reduce likelihood of chronic disease.

As chapter 12 discusses, simple math suggests that storing only 10 kilocalories a day for a year will result in about a pound of stored fat. This means that the reduction of 400 to 700 kilocalories a day in physical activity would result in weight gains of 40 to 70 pounds (18–32 kg) a year if nutritional intake were constant. Luckily, our physiological systems have some ability to adapt to prevent these great weight shifts. However, too little exercise combined with too much food inevitably results in weight gains.

It is not only our economic environment, but also the built environment that conspires to limit our physical movement. Start to pay attention to the multitude of devices that save you a few kilocalories of effort each time you push a button: your TV remote, automatic car windows, and garage door openers. Consider also the many automatic energy savers that we use without even being aware of it: automatic door openers at many buildings, drive-through windows, escalators, elevators, moving walkways, information obtained by searching the Internet instead of going to the library, and many more. At work, we often use e-mail or the phone to contact colleagues who may be next door or just down the hall rather than walking down to their offices.

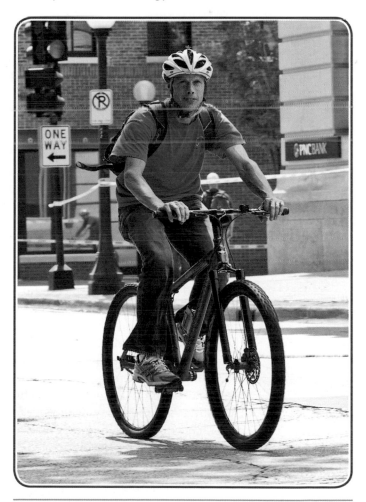

The built environment can also be blamed for much more loss of physical activity. Consider how the automobile has replaced walking or biking for many short trips. In 1970, it was estimated that walking and biking accounted for about 52 percent of trips shorter than 2 miles (3 km) for shopping and visiting. That percentage had dropped to under 10 percent in 1995 (Purcher and Leferve 1996), and it is now estimated to be less than 6 percent (CDC 2009). As the next chapter discusses, adding purposeful activity to your daily life is one of the most effective methods to increase your physical activity. Although both are getting older, the authors of this book continue to walk and use their bikes for most activities around town.

Of course, the built environment can be blamed for much of the reliance on the automobile. Many suburbs do not have nearby stores that are easy to walk to. Sidewalks may not exist, or may be inconsistent, making walking difficult or unsafe. People often live far from work, and mass transit may not be available. We all need to evaluate our

■ Many errands can be done just as, or more, efficiently on a bike than driving.

environment to determine what is possible. You may discover that many opportunities exist. Walking a mile from home to catch a bus that then drops you off a mile from work might be just the purposeful activity to get you going. Walking to a neighborhood store for daily supplies rather than frequently driving to the bigger box store might help you get moving, which will make you feel more energetic. You might consider walking or biking rather than driving to visit friends who live nearby.

The social environment also affects our physical activity. Cultures tend to adapt to social norms. When we see the majority of people driving, sitting, watching television, or using computers, we begin to accept that as normal. As the average waistline gets bigger, our image of normal adapts. Students in our Health and Human Performance class in Missoula conducted a survey, asking other students at the university to view images of people (33% normal weight, 33% overweight, and 33% obese) and rate them as normal, overweight, or obese. The majority of students rated both normal and overweight people as normal and most obese people as either normal or overweight, with few ratings of obese. In our freshman class, where all students complete a body-composition lab, we ask everyone to anonymously self-rate themselves prior to both underwater and **skinfold** measurement and then, again anonymously, to report their percentage of body fat. Eighty percent of overweight students believed they were normal weight, while 24 percent and 43 percent of obese students rated themselves as normal or overweight, respectively. We obviously have a skewed image of a healthy **body composition**.

The social environment goes much further than just image. Someone who associates with sedentary friends is likely to be sedentary. Youth emulate their peers and their parents. In a project to measure physical activity in Missoula schools, we used accelerometers for a week to measure physical activity of more than 800 2nd- through 12th-grade students. Physical activity decreased dramatically from elementary school to middle school. Seniors in high school were doing almost no vigorous physical activity. Only one-third were meeting health guidelines for adult physical activity, and fewer than 15 percent were meeting youth guidelines. They had adopted the American culture by the time they finished high school. Of course, this should be no surprise, since they are only doing what they see their peers and role models doing. In order to break this cycle, it is necessary to understand the stages of behavior change, which the next section discusses.

STAGES OF BEHAVIORAL CHANGE

Understanding that we go through a series of stages in order to modify behavior is important to making any change, such as the initiation and maintenance of regular physical activity. It begins with a sincere intention to change behavior, which is perhaps the best indicator of success. Changing behaviors means altering our self-image. To do that, one really needs a commitment. We then look at the early stages of behavior change, followed by factors associated with program maintenance or adherence. Finally, we review behavior therapy as a strategy to aid the initiation and maintenance of the activity program.

A number of factors influence one's intention to adopt a new behavior, including information, role models, authoritative figures (e.g., physician), previous experience, and social pressure. A person may need time to move from disinterest to readiness to change. The fact that you are reading this book suggests that you are gathering the information and support to make a commitment to the active lifestyle.

The status of exercise behavior model includes six stages of change (Stone and Klein 2004). In the descriptions of each stage, we use examples of physical activity:

1. Precontemplative—Not considering activity. In the **precontemplative stage**, people are either unaware that being sedentary is bad for their health or are in denial. They may

deny that they are sedentary or that changing their behavior to an active lifestyle will improve their lives. In some cases, they may feel that the effort is greater than the reward. Moving from this stage to the next requires education and information. Often, people must be shocked by a significant event in life, such as a heart attack or developing diabetes, to move to the next level.

2. Contemplative—Thinking about it. In the **contemplative stage** of behavior change, people are aware that the active lifestyle will benefit them in terms of health, vitality, energy, or cognition. While they have not yet started to become more active, they are thinking about it and gathering information. During this time, positive support from friends or family and educational material will have great effect. Setting reasonable goals based on good information will also help them get started. Visualizing (see later section) themselves as healthy, able to do activities with friends, having more energy, keeping their brain healthy, and other positive thoughts will help them change their self-image even before they start the activity.

3. Preparation—Exhibiting some activity. In the **preparation stage**, they have begun to take the necessary steps toward a healthy lifestyle. They develop a plan, purchase walking shoes, make plans with friends to be active together, and get started. During this time period, people often **relapse.** Encouragement from peers and others is important. Beginning an exercise program can be difficult. Later, we offer more strategies, including rewards for reaching small goals. The line between preparing and taking the first steps to reach the next level of action is blurry, but once you are moving on a regular basis and have started a program, you have graduated.

4. Action—Fully engaged in the new behavior. During the first several months of starting a physical-activity program, you are considered to be in the **action stage**. During this time, it is vital that you strive to see yourself as you want to be, keeping your eye on your goal of being an active person. These first few months are the hardest. You are still changing your self-image and your body is adapting to the new physical activity. As you gradually increase the duration, variety, and maybe even the intensity of your activities, you will feel better. Eventually, your body will crave the active lifestyle, and you will see yourself as an active person.

5. Maintenance—Active for months. In the **maintenance stage**, you have kept up your new regime for several months, developed an activity routine, and incorporated exercise into your life—you are nearly there. At this point, you may still have to remind yourself of your goals to get out every day. You may have minor relapses, but in general, you are joining the ranks of the physically active. You look forward to those times each day when you can get out and move, get your blood flowing, breathe more deeply, and enjoy the control you have over your health and wellness.

6. Adoption—Activity internalized as part of lifestyle. Finally, you will arrive at the point where you have completely changed your self-image. You *are* an active person. Sure, there may be occasional days when you have to spend long hours at a desk, but even then, you find ways to move. You have adapted a lifestyle that gets you up and around whenever possible. Without thinking, you ride your bike to work rather than drive, or you park farther away from a destination just so you can get in some walking. You smile when you think of getting home so that you can go for a walk with your wife, husband, or dog. At the **adoption stage**, you cannot imagine yourself as anything other than a member of the active life.

You can think of the stages of behavior change as a stairway. We move up the steps to initiate a new behavior. It is also possible to relapse and move back downward. Going backward occasionally is not failure, but reality. We never fail until we quit. We all have

One of the best indicators of future success is a person's readiness to change. If people say they are ready, they probably are.

setbacks, but if you are truly committed, you will persevere and begin your climb again. If you are committed to a goal, and there is no goal more worthwhile than taking control of your health, then the journey will be well worth the struggle. The information in figure 5.1 will help you with strategies appropriate for your stage in behavior change.

One of the best indicators of future success is a person's readiness to change. If people say they are ready, they probably are. Early success is associated with reasonable expectations and goals, gradual change, appropriate reinforcement, social support, and cognitive strategies (relaxation, dissociation).

BEHAVIOR MODIFICATION STRATEGIES

According to the exercise-behavior model, people move through five behavioral strategies as they adopt and maintain a new habit: substituting alternatives, enlisting social support, rewarding themselves, committing themselves, and reminding themselves to persist (Marcus and Forsyth 2003). This section provides a way to identify the desired behavior and make progress toward its acquisition. The essentials are threefold:

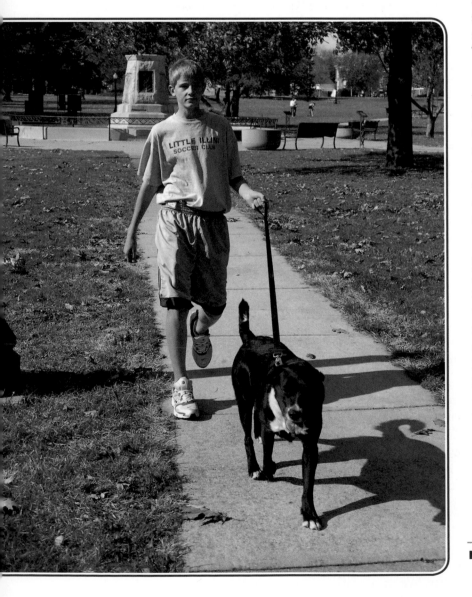

1. Identify the behavior that you wish to modify (e.g., physical activity) and maintain an accurate record of your current behavior. Maintain a weeklong record of all your physical activity (form 5.3). Include the intensity and duration of your involvement, and complete the cognitive question for fitness training and recreational activities.

2. Analyze your current behavior, and then plan needed modifications. Do you need to burn more calories, increase intensity, or do specific training (e.g., muscular fitness)? Plan appropriate modifications to meet your needs and interests. For example, you could increase your activity to meet the activity guideline set by the CDC and ACSM (30 min of physical activity most days of the week).

3. Develop a contract with specific goals and a schedule of rewards to reinforce the new behavior (form 5.4). Use activity benchmarks such as minutes

■ Dogs are effective exercise partners for purposeful activity.

Stage of change	Strategies to enhance change
Precontemplation	In this stage, where you or another person is not yet thinking about change, is helpful to do the following: • Gather or provide information about the benefits of the proposed change. • Understand that you are in control and can change your life. • Obtain information about the consequences of not changing. • Obtain correct information about current health status to overcome feelings of denial. • Get help and information from others who have changed and who can share their positive stories.
Contemplation	In this stage, where you or another person is thinking of change, it is helpful to do the following: • Weigh the benefits and costs of the proposed behavior change. • Evaluate the barriers to change and develop strategies on how to overcome the obstacles. • Start to visualize the benefits of the change and to see yourself, or help another see themselves, living after they have made the positive change.
Preparation	In this stage, where you or another person is beginning to take the necessary steps to begin change, it is helpful to do the following: • Experiment with small changes. • Understand that relapse is a part of change, not a failure. • Develop a plan to gradually incorporate the new behavior into your daily routine. For physical activity, we recommend meaningful activity (see chapter 6). • Develop a support group of people who will give positive feedback and help you move toward your new goal. • Set short- and long-term goals.
Action	In this stage, when you or another person is taking definitive steps toward changing behavior, it is helpful to do the following: • Focus on goals, both short- and long-term. Reset new goals as they are achieved. • Find a support group. • Avoid environments that encourage moving back toward old behaviors. • Understand that relapse is a part of change. It is not failure, but simply a small setback. • Continue to gather supportive information and to visualize positive outcomes. • Continually update strategies to overcome obstacles as they arise. • Understand that it will take up to 6 months for the change to become a part of your normal behavior. • Understand that this stage and the maintenance stage are where the 12-step smoking cessation and weight-loss programs are used. Focus on the specific goals and plan that these programs have developed.
Maintenance	In this stage, where your new behaviors have become a normal part of your life, it is helpful to do the following: • Realize that occasionally old habits return. This is only a temporary setback that is out of character for you. • It remains important to maintain a support group of people who enhance and give positive feedback on your new behaviors. • Continue to evaluate goals, strategies, barriers, and opportunities to help maintain the positive behaviors.

FIGURE 5.1 Stages of Change Model.

Adapted from Prochaska, DiClemente, and Norcross 1992; Miller and Rollnick 1991; Rosenstock 1966.

exercised or miles (or km) walked or run per day or week, weight loss, or other indicators of successful adoption of the new activity. A tangible, universally accepted reward such as money seems to work for most of us. Spend the reward immediately or save it for something that you really want but might not otherwise buy. Don't worry about the expense. The new behavior will save more than the cost of the reward in medical and other expenses. In time, the behavior will become a healthy habit, and you will be able to focus on new goals or new behaviors (e.g., weight control, time management).

POSITIVE BEHAVIOR MAINTENANCE

Adherence to a newly adopted behavior can be difficult; 50 percent of participants drop out of exercise programs within the first year. Certain strategies help improve the odds of success (Taylor and Miller 1993). People continue activity in the following scenarios:

- The activity meets a need.
- The activity is purposeful (see chapter 6) and fun.
- They have social support.
- They see evidence of change.

To ensure lifelong participation, the person must move from extrinsic to intrinsic motivation, become self-sufficient (independent of the instructor and the setting), and develop strategies to deal with factors that threaten continued participation. Work, illness, or family crises may interrupt participation in regular, moderate activity, but must never terminate it.

Develop a network of support systems to ensure your adherence. Support is available from family and friends, interest groups, professionals, clubs, programs, publications, and organizations.

- *Family.* Spouses provide support by taking a sincere interest in each other's activity, and when possible, by participating together. Family members often select gifts to encourage or enhance participation. Trips may revolve around a shared experience, such as hiking, canoeing, skiing, or golf.

- *Friends.* Most of our longtime friends share our interests. The shared interests are the foundation of the relationship, the glue that holds it together. Their presence gets us out and keeps us going. Together, we do more than any of us would do alone.

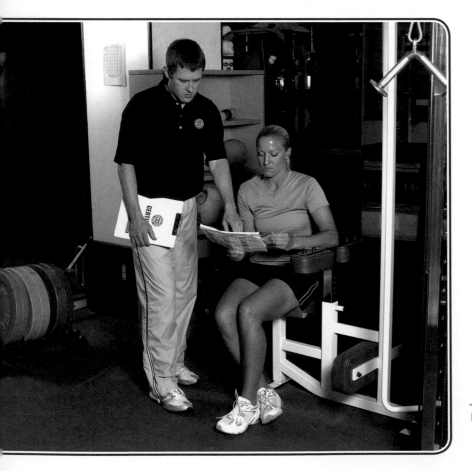

■ Keep a log of your activities and reward yourself when you reach specific goals.

Date _____

Time	Place	Exercise	Intensity	Duration

What were your thoughts during exercise?

_____

_____

Intensity scoring		Duration scoring	
Score	Intensity	Score	Duration
5	Sustained heavy breathing and perspiration	4	Over 30 min
4	Intermittent heavy breathing and perspiration—as in tennis	3	20–30 min
3	Moderately heavy—as in recreational sports and cycling	2	10–20 min
2	Moderate—as in volleyball, softball	1	Under 10 min
1	Light—as in fishing, walking	—	

Note: Include all forms of physical activity, including work, walking, and household chores.

From B.J. Sharkey and S.E. Gaskill, 2013, *Fitness and health, seventh edition* (Champaign, IL: Human Kinetics).

Form 5.4   Activity Reinforcement Schedule

Date	Activity	Distance or time	Reward*
	Weekly total		
	Weekly total		
	Weekly total		
	Weekly total		
	Total for month		

Note: Daily reward—for meeting activity goal (e.g., 2 mi, or 3 km); weekly reward—for meeting activity goal (e.g., 12 mi, or 19 km); monthly reward—for meeting activity goal (e.g., 50 mi, or 80 km; improved fitness score). Adjust goals as fitness improves.

*Rewards: daily—a small monetary award (e.g., $1) or a cool drink; weekly—a larger monetary reward (e.g., $5) or a special favor (e.g., movie); monthly—a substantial monetary reward (e.g., $20) or a very special favor (e.g., concert, dinner out). Rewards can be saved for a special purpose (e.g., new warm-up outfit, tennis racket).

From B.J. Sharkey and S.E. Gaskill, 2013, *Fitness and health, seventh edition* (Champaign, IL: Human Kinetics).

• *Interest groups.* We all have access to hiking, skiing, running clubs, and more. Our local canoe-racing group welcomes neophytes to join their Wednesday evening training sessions. If you can't find a group with your interests, start one.

• *Professionals.* From personal trainers to fitness and sport instructors, a wide array of help is available. Seek out experts for advice and motivation. Get professional instruction to improve your performance and enjoyment of tennis, skiing, or other recreational sports.

• *Clubs.* By joining a health and fitness club, you'll gain access to equipment, instruction, and an added bonus, the social support of fellow members. Club-based programs often succeed when home-based programs fail because of the social and psychological support. Joining an organization or a recreational league can help you maintain a fitness routine.

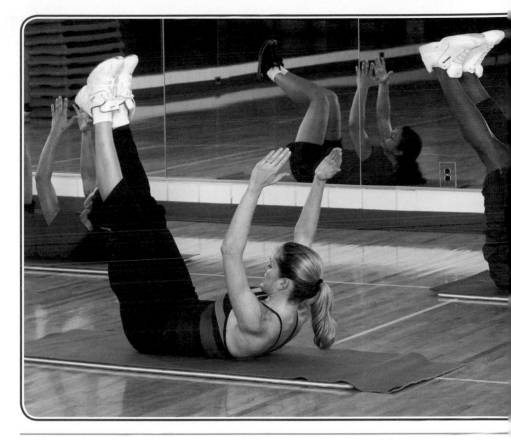

■ Social physical activity can promote enjoyment and meaningfulness.

• *Programs.* Take advantage of your workplace wellness program and become involved in new activities. The wellness program at our university has provided us with weightlifting, swimming, inline skating, ski clinics, and many other classes. Our campus recreation program has welcomed us on winter ski trips and in canoe and kayak classes.

• *Publications.* Many books are available to help you maintain or expand your interests. Magazines cater to general *(Outside)* or specific interests *(Backpacker).* Videos and computer programs provide instruction in everything from golf to mountain biking.

• *Organizations.* The American College of Sports Medicine (ACSM) provides information and publications on fitness, exercise science, and sports medicine. ACSM also publishes position papers on a wide range of topics (www.acsm.org). Sport organizations such as the United States Tennis Association provide sport-specific pamphlets, instruction, and tournaments.

Sometimes a new piece of equipment will generate or revive interest in an activity. For example, adjustable ski poles increase interest in and enjoyment of backcountry hiking. The poles aid uphill travel, relieve aging knees on the downhills, and provide balance in crossing logs and streams. Sporting goods stores and equipment catalogs provide ways to make activity more pleasurable. Take advantage of these and other support systems to ensure lifelong involvement in physical activity.

RELAPSE SOLUTIONS

Participants often relapse, slipping back to inactivity after an initial change for the better. Relapse occurs for many reasons, ranging from emotional and social to physical. Because the event is so common, if it happens, you should not let it bother you. Relapse is part of the process of change, for athletes as well as for newcomers. In dieting, relapse is par for the course. What can you do to prevent or recover from relapse? One approach calls for a planned relapse, just to test the reaction when instructor support is still available. To date, most relapse prevention programs have been labor intensive, teaching how to anticipate and cope with relapse using strategies that we have already discussed, such as behavior therapy and goal setting. Most have yielded modest results.

Our suggestion is to search for intrinsic motivation and to strive for internal control. Free yourself from the need for external validation from fitness instructors. Their responsibility is to lead you to a level of independence so that you will no longer rely on them for information or encouragement. Wean yourself from dependence on their motivation and control. Then develop your own approach to relapse prevention. Build the social support and emotional climate you need to keep going. Don't depend on one activity; be ready to adapt in the event of injury or chronic illness. When relapse comes, and it will, return to your goals, to behavior therapy, and to your support systems. Study your schedule and find opportunities for activity. Set new goals, avoid negative messages, and focus on your strengths (Blair, LaMonte, and Nichaman 2004). People who develop behavioral or cognitive strategies, such as positive self-talk, are more successful at coping with relapse (Willis and Campbell 1992). By devising your own solution, you'll be better prepared for the future.

Get a Dog

What are the secrets of long-term participation in physical activity? Studies of lifelong participants show that a number of factors are associated with their persistence. These people are higher in self-motivation and self-efficacy and lower in negative barriers than those less persistent. They cite fitness, well-being, and energy as reasons to continue. They enjoy activity and make it a priority (Stone and Klein 2004). Morgan (2001) argues for the importance of purposeful or meaningful physical activity (see chapter 6). In his study of long-term adherents, he found two meaningful categories of activity—transportation and dog walking. Those of us with dogs understand how much they enjoy their time out and that this walk is as good for us as it is for them.

VISUALIZATION STRATEGIES

Visualization, or imaging yourself as you would like to be, can be a very powerful tool to help change behavior. Visualization includes imagining your goals. It is also helpful to be careful with the use of words, thoughts, and feelings, since they greatly influence your self-beliefs and self-image. Thus, visualization really involves the process of beginning to see yourself as the new person that you are moving to become. By using words, thoughts, and emotions that support your new behaviors, those new actions will become a permanent part of who you are.

Studies with athletes and others working to change behavior have shown that the more senses you add to your imagery, the more likely that you will be able to change. Even if you have trouble seeing images with your eyes closed, it is possible to use words that influence thoughts and emotions. Simply stating that you enjoy walking will help change your belief about physical activity.

People who are in the contemplative, preparation, or action stages of behavior change can enhance their ability to adapt by spending a few minutes every day visualizing themselves accomplishing something meaningful—seeing, feeling, hearing, and thinking as clearly as possible to see yourself attaining your goals. This may be a self-image of feeling much better, being able to participate in activities that you have had to give up, or living with vitality and vigor. Bring every aspect of the positive new behaviors into your image so that you feel positive emotions. See yourself demonstrating the behavior, reaching your goals, and benefiting from your action. Work to develop a vision that makes you feel motivated, passionate, and enthusiastic.

How do you do this? Imagine that your goal is to end your sedentary lifestyle and become more active. In your mind, you would imagine yourself as a slimmer person full of vitality. You might see yourself playing tennis, walking down the beach in the surf, fitting into your clothes well. Additionally, you want to imagine feeling whole and healthy. You have no aches and pains, and you are able to smile at life as you take it by the horns. You might even imagine your medical check-up with normal blood pressure and cholesterol, where the provider tells you how well you are doing.

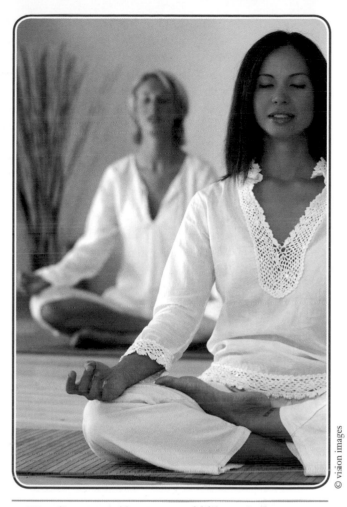

© vision images

■ Visualize yourself as you would like to become.

Relaxation

Sit in a comfortable chair in a quiet room and repeat a simple sound (mantra) such as *Easy* each time you exhale. Concentration on the breathing and the mantra masks disturbing thoughts, and the body begins to relax. As you become more proficient with the technique, you may achieve a transcendent state of relaxation, clear thought, imagery, well-being, and openness. In time, you'll be able to use the skill during activity and sport. Meditation is not a substitute for exercise; it will not induce the many physiological changes that result from regular activity. On the other hand, some find activity to be as effective as meditation in the achievement of relaxation. While relaxed, it is often the best time to do visualization and to begin to see the new you.

Dissociation involves diverting attention from how you feel during exercise by focusing on other topics or conversation with a partner. For some people, the first 20 minutes of activity before pain-killing endorphins kick in are the hardest. Similarly, the first few weeks of a new program are the toughest. So, it helps to have ways to cope until appreciable changes become evident or until you become addicted. Behavior therapy seems to work for difficult cases.

Image achieving your goals; make that the picture you see. Change your self-image from what you are to what you want to become. Once you have changed the internal image, you will begin to demonstrate the actions to become that new person. After all, the brain controls actions. Once you have changed your self-image, you will naturally begin to act as that new person. So, when you visualize it, feel it, touch it, smell it, taste it, hear it, see it, and generate the emotions that go with the healthy behaviors. If you use visualization at least once a day and take consistent action, your success will be greatly enhanced.

SUMMARY

This chapter shows why it is so difficult to change behaviors such as physical activity and nutrition. The good thing is that you can now identify your personal stages of change and barriers to physical activity. You should also be more aware of how your environment affects your nutritional and physical activity patterns. Based on your stage of change, you should be able to develop strategies to move toward a more active life. Remember to visualize your goals, see yourself as you would like to be, and consider personal rewards as you meet milestones along the way.

In the next chapter, we will help you shift to an active lifestyle by including meaningful physical activity in your personal routine, leading to vitality and health in all stages of life.

Meaningful Activity
Lifetime Vitality

> " Time is really the only capital that any human being has, and the one thing that he can't afford to lose. "
>
> *Thomas Alva Edison*

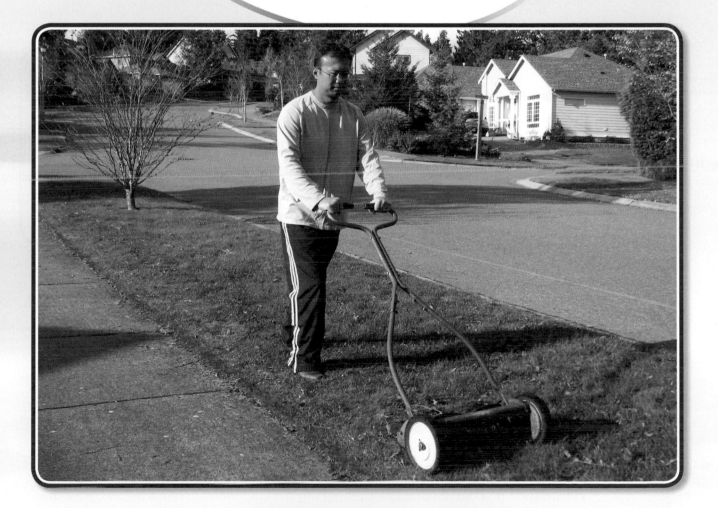

One of the most common excuses for physical inactivity is the lack of available time. In today's busy world, this is a valid concern and a major barrier to the active life. In truth, this says more about one's priorities than it does about the inability to incorporate activity into a busy life, which can be done by replacing sedentary pursuits, such as driving, with physical activities, such as walking or biking. Many small behavior changes can lead to major health benefits. Finding ways to move muscles as a part of your daily routine can be done at any age. When incorporated into everyday life, this will start you on a path to lifelong vitality.

Age tells little about your health, your appearance, your fitness, or your ability to perform. Although aging inevitably leads to death, it does so at different rates for different people, depending on heredity and on personal decisions about how you choose to age.

Sometime after the peak reproductive years, when the direct evolutionary advantage has passed, virtually all tissues and organs begin to age. Parents remain important, at least until the child becomes a young adult, and grandparents serve to pass on wisdom or assist the parents. But when a person reaches the 70s, biological justification to continue life diminishes, and indeed, life expectancies range from 83.3 for women and 73 to 75.5 for men. But life expectancies, which have risen throughout the past century, tell only part of the story.

This chapter will help you do the following:

- Incorporate purposeful physical activity into your life
- Differentiate life expectancy from life span
- Understand how activity and other habits influence longevity
- Appreciate how fitness influences your **physiological age**
- Understand how activity and fitness extend the prime of life

MEANINGFUL PHYSICAL ACTIVITY

Purposeful or meaningful physical activity is activity that is done in the normal course of daily living that accomplishes a necessary, meaningful, or enjoyable task. Purposeful physical activity provides meaning or purpose beyond the simple movements and results in an immediate outcome, such as walking to the store, biking to work, or walking your dog. Other purposeful activities include gardening, mowing or raking the lawn, shoveling snow, playing with kids and grandkids, exercising with friends, or hiking, running, or biking outside on a beautiful day (versus exercising indoors). People who engage in purposeful and enjoyable activities are more likely to remain active throughout life.

Our remote-control lifestyles have evolved along with the combustion engine and the introduction of electricity to our homes. During the last 75 years, we have changed from a civilization that did physical labor during our working hours to one where we have the option of moving very little during the day. By the 1950s, automobiles and farm machinery had, for the most part, replaced physical labor. A gallon of gasoline could do more work in an hour than man and animal could do in a day.

We celebrate the luxury of modern conveniences that make our lives easier. The thermostat automatically controls the furnace or air conditioner. Not long ago, it required a lot of physical activity to keep one's house warm. We now program the thermostat and take the climate-controlled environment of home or work for granted.

With each passing year, technology advances with new tools, toys, and apps that reduce the need for muscular movement. Cars, which keep us from walking and running, now have automatic transmissions, power steering, and electric window openers. Manual typewriters became electric, and then were replaced by the computer. We no longer turn pages on a book, but read from a screen. We no longer walk through a library; instead, we surf the Internet. Fruits and vegetables, which once required extensive labor, are now found year-round in supermarkets.

Each small step toward reduced human movement brings with it unintended consequences. Terms such as *couch potato*, *obesity*, and *sedentary lifestyle* have become commonplace. Along with the energy-saving lifestyle come previously rare chronic diseases, which now top the list of the causes of morbidity and mortality.

It is now possible to order nearly everything we need to live at home, including groceries, by sitting at the computer, ordering it, and having it delivered. Instead of preparing meals, we eat packaged foods or drive to a restaurant. It has been proposed that modern man expends about 600 to 1000 fewer calories per day during activities of daily living (purposeful exercise), than did our ancestors who hunted, farmed, and did physical labor for nearly every task of living. At the same time, we are eating as much or more than our active ancestors. It is no wonder that we are becoming an obese society with all of the associated chronic diseases.

Finding Meaning in Your Activity

John, an exercise science student at the University of Montana, was diligently working to help his girlfriend Mira become more physically active. He persuaded her to meet at 6:45 a.m. at the student recreation center for a cup of coffee. Afterwards, they could do a workout on the treadmill or other exercise machines. John prevailed for four mornings, but Mira continued to complain about getting up early, driving to the gym, and running aimlessly on the treadmill, with news blaring from the TV at the front of the room. She suggested that they ride their bikes to a local trailhead, go for an easy run, and enjoy the beauty of the morning and the chance to talk. The first outing was a great success that ended with both enjoying a cup of coffee and looking forward to the next run. Mira explained to John that she needs to feel some meaning or purpose in her exercise. Getting outside and the chance to talk were both valuable to her. They continued the tradition through the next three years, when they graduated and were married.

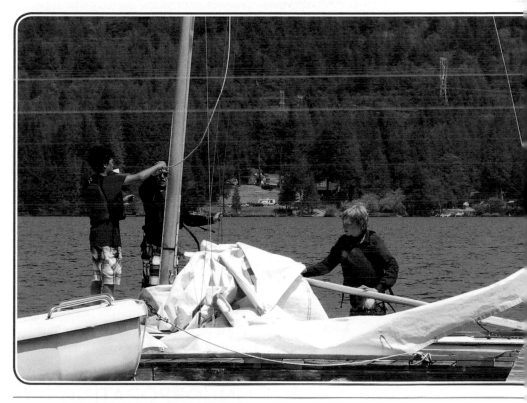

■ The family that plays together stays together.

To compensate, the modern exercise gym has evolved. We drive miles to exercise at the health club in order to become more fit and meet recommended guidelines of physical activity for health. Others choose home treadmills or stationary bikes where they run or bike to nowhere. Some people elect to walk or run around town or in the country to become fit. Research shows that most people who start exercise programs soon give up for lack of time or interest. This seemingly purposeless physical activity has a lower priority than other tasks that need to be done. Thus, we drop out and go back to driving from one sedentary activity to another.

Maybe it is time to build meaningful physical activity into our lives. Walking and biking are making a comeback in some communities. Growing our own food is gaining in popularity. Participatory rather than passive spectator sports are gaining a foothold. It is time to start finding ingenious ways of putting exercise back into our daily routines. The more we do, the more our bodies and our environment will thank us.

We know that people who regularly meet health guidelines for physical activity do so by incorporating purposeful physical activity into their daily living. The first part of this chapter discusses how to do this through small changes in your daily routine.

In order to clarify different terms used in this chapter, we will adhere to the following definitions from the American Heart Association and American College of Sports Medicine (Thompson et al. 2003).

• *Physical activity* is defined as any bodily movement produced by skeletal muscles that results in energy expenditure beyond resting expenditure.

• *Exercise* is a subset of physical activity that is planned, structured, repetitive, and purposeful in the sense that improvement or maintenance of physical fitness is the objective.

• *Physical fitness* includes **cardiorespiratory fitness**, muscle strength, body composition, and flexibility, comprising a set of attributes that people have or achieve that relates to the ability to perform physical activity. When defining the amount of physical activity or exercise, an important interrelationship exists between the total dose of activity and the intensity at which the activity is performed.

• *Dose* refers to the total amount of energy expended in physical activity.

• *Intensity* reflects the rate of energy expenditure during activity (Pate et al. 1995). Intensity can be defined in absolute or relative terms. **Absolute intensity** reflects the rate of energy expenditure during exercise and is usually expressed in **metabolic equivalents**, or **METs**, where 1 MET equals the resting metabolic rate of ≈ 3.5 ml $O_2 \cdot kg^{-1} \cdot min^{-1}$. **Relative intensity** refers to the percent of aerobic power utilized during exercise. It is expressed as percent of maximal heart rate or percent of $\dot{V}O_2max$. **Moderate-intensity activities** are those performed at a relative intensity of 40 to 60 percent of $\dot{V}O_2max$ (or absolute intensity of 3 to 6 METs). **Vigorous-intensity activities** are those performed at a relative intensity of >60 percent of $\dot{V}O_2max$ (or absolute intensity of >6 METs). For example, brisk walking at 4.8 kilometers per hour (3 mi/hr) has an absolute intensity of ≈ 4 METs. In relative terms, this intensity is considered light for a 20-year-old healthy person, but represents a vigorous intensity for an 80-year-old person (Fletcher et al. 2001).

INCORPORATING PURPOSEFUL ACTIVITY INTO DAILY LIVING

How we adjust our lifestyles to incorporate purposeful physical activity depends on environment and the ability and willingness to change. As noted in the box ahead, Steve and Kathy, who are both about 60 years of age, have found ways to include purposeful activity into their lives. Your environment may be different, but each of us can find ways to integrate meaningful activity into our lives.

Modern conveniences have allowed us to pack more into each day. Incorporating purposeful physical activity may take a little more time (biking or walking to the store rather than driving), but it will take less time than driving to the gym for a workout.

Research and empirical data have demonstrated that people are most successful meeting physical activity health guidelines that require only moderate-intensity physical movement through purposeful activity. However, in today's culture, in order to meet fitness standards (see Physical Activity Guidelines box), it may be necessary to plan specific exercise time, as reported by O'Dougherty and colleagues (2010). In a study of women, the quarter of participants who met fitness standards did so largely through planned exercise such as jogging, biking, or similar vigorous activities, while their moderate physical activity to meet health recommendations was met through purposeful activities of daily living such as shopping, housework, social activities, and dog walking. Thus, becoming physically fit requires going beyond purposeful physical activity. It is possible to incorporate vigorous physical activity into purposeful tasks by simply increasing your intensity, such as running or vigorous cycling to work. While this works for some people, it may require a change of clothes and access to a shower at work. But your fitness sessions should also be meaningful and enjoyable.

Training to improve performance in a sport or activity is meaningful for adults of all

It's Easy Being Green and Healthy

Author Steve and his wife Kathy both work at the University of Montana, about 3 miles (5 km) from their home. They commute to work daily by walking or riding their bikes, occasionally cross-country skiing or taking the bus when the weather is particularly bad. Walking to work takes about 90 minutes for the full round trip, while biking requires about 30 minutes. Riding the bus requires a half-mile walk on each end or 1 mile (1.6 km; 30 minutes) a day. The 30-minute bike ride or walk to catch the bus fulfills their recommended physical activity for health. Biking to work is faster than driving (including finding a parking space and walking to their building). Both log their self-powered commute miles with the Missoula Way to Go Club. Each has accumulated more than 18,000 miles (29,000 km) in the past 11 years. They estimate that they have saved more than 1,200 gallons (4,500 L) of gas and many dollars of related car and parking expenses. They also feel good about their small carbon footprint (greenhouse gas production). Additionally, Kathy typically does 30 minutes of bike errands during her lunch break around town, and both Steve and Kathy do errands on their way home to pick up groceries and other home items. They have incorporated other purposeful activities into their lives. They mow their large lawn with a manual push mower every few days. When they get behind, they have a small gas mower they use to catch up. They walk for most social trips or go by bike for longer trips. Their large garden provides more reason for meaningful physical activity. Of course, they still own a car and use it for out of town trips, and use their TV remote, but they limit TV to less than 1 hour a day.

ages. We do aerobic and **muscular training** to improve performance in tennis, skiing, and other sports. We train to improve performance in running, swimming, cycling, and cross-country skiing. And some train to improve enjoyment and performance in hiking, cycling, paddling, backcountry skiing, and other outdoor adventures. The training has purpose and the performance goals serve as strong motivation to continue on a regular basis. Sometimes training for one activity, such as mountain biking, improves performance in another (hiking) or in a coming season (alpine skiing). Many continue to pursue performance goals into their 70s or even their 80s. That is exercise with a purpose.

There are many ways, from small to large, that purposeful physical activity can be incorporated into your life. It is often helpful to think about physical activity guidelines for health in terms of energy expenditure. We tend to measure energy in **nutritional calories**. Each nutritional calorie listed on a food package is the amount of energy necessary to raise 1 liter of water (1.057 qt) 1 degree centigrade (1.8 °F). The physical activity guidelines require metabolizing about 150 to 400 calories during moderate physical activity most days of the week. Additional calories expended doing light activities, such as standing, fidgeting, and slow walking also burn calories. These activities can have a positive effect on weight loss, but they are not counted in the calorie expenditure needed to meet the physical activity guidelines.

Physical Activity Guidelines

Physical activity guidelines for adults include accumulation of 30 minutes or more of moderate intensity physical activity—at least 10 minutes at a time—most days of the week. Guidelines for youths up to age 18 recommend accumulating 60 minutes of moderate and vigorous physical activity most days, including some muscle-strengthening activities. A higher physical fitness standard requires at least 30 to 50 minutes of vigorous exercise at least 3 days a week. Meeting the physical fitness standard and meeting health guidelines on the other days of the week also qualifies for meeting physical activity health recommendations. For both adults and youths, with planning and purpose, you will find that these guidelines are easy to accomplish.

To determine calories expended during walking, multiply miles × weight (pounds) × .667 (km × weight [kg] × .908). Thus, a 150-pound (68 kg) person will expend about 100 calories each mile and a 200-pound (90 kg) person will burn about 133 calories. If you walk at pace of 3 miles (5 km) per hour (brisk walk) for 10 minutes at a time, three times a day, you will have accumulated 1.5 miles (2.4 km). For a 200-pound person, this would be 200 nutritional calories, which meets the guidelines both by total activity time and energy expenditure. Optimally, 400 calories a day of physical activity are recommended. With some thought and planning, you will discover that it isn't hard to incorporate activity into your daily life, even without an exercise program. Form 6.1 looks at how people can add purposeful physical activity into their daily routines.

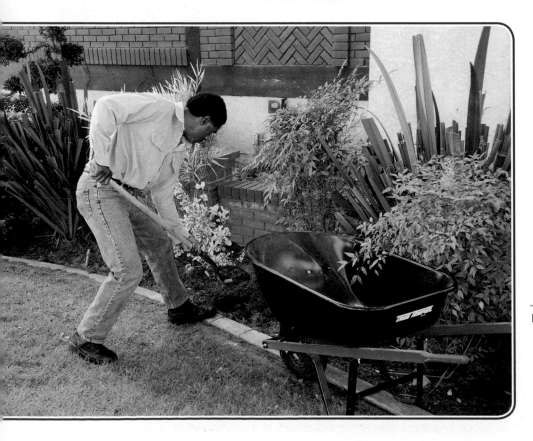

■ Gardening is a purposeful activity that can burn 3 to 6 calories per minute. At a modest intensity, one can meet the physical activity health guidelines with 30 to 40 minutes of enjoyable activity.

In order to meet health guidelines, the physical activity needs to be at an intensity equivalent to or higher than a brisk walk. Which of these activities can you work into your lifestyle?

- ☐ Walk or bike instead of driving to and from work or school.
- ☐ Walk or bike instead of driving to the bus stop on the way to and from work or school.
- ☐ Walk or bike with your child to and from school rather than driving them.
- ☐ Use public transportation whenever possible, since it generally requires more human-power movement than driving alone.
- ☐ Walk up and down stairs instead of taking an elevator or escalator.
- ☐ Get off the bus a few stops early and walk the remaining distance to your destination.
- ☐ Park at a more distant parking lot from work or school and walk the final mile.
- ☐ Mow the lawn with a push mower rather than a riding mower. For small yards, consider a hand mower.
- ☐ Rake leaves by hand rather than by using power tools.
- ☐ Work in the garden.
- ☐ Push a stroller.
- ☐ Clean the house.
- ☐ Walk, bike, or run with your dog to give you both exercise.
- ☐ Make frequent trips to the store by foot or bike rather than making major shopping trips with your automobile.
- ☐ Golf socially, being sure to carry your clubs.
- ☐ Do traditional sports for social fun or competition.
- ☐ Dance for both purposeful activity and social fun.
- ☐ Have walking rather than sit-down meetings at work when possible.
- ☐ At the office, get up and walk to other offices to talk, rather than calling or sending e-mails.
- ☐ What can you come up with? _____

_____

_____

_____

_____

_____

ENVIRONMENT AND PURPOSEFUL ACTIVITY

Unfortunately, many communities have been developed for automobile transport, with limited infrastructure to promote purposeful physical activity. Lack of sidewalks, bike paths, bike racks, neighborhood stores, street lights, parks, and playgrounds all reduce your access to physical activity in your neighborhood. While there may be many local barriers to physical activity, if you recognize the barriers, you will be able to develop strategies that allow you to achieve purposeful physical activity that meets the health guidelines. Remember, health starts at 30 minutes a day and improves as you do more, working up to 60 minutes or more every day or adding intensity to your 30 minutes. Even better, you can do the activity in bouts as short as 10 minutes at a time.

Chapter 5 helps you identify your personal barriers to physical activity and strategies for overcoming those barriers. Form 6.2 lists common neighborhood barriers to physical

Form 6.2　Common Neighborhood Barriers to Physical Activity

How would you rate your neighborhood for the following?

	None (major problem)	Poor (problem)	Good (not a problem)
Sidewalks	☐	☐	☐
Walking paths	☐	☐	☐
Bike paths and bike racks	☐	☐	☐
Safe routes for youths to walk or bike to school	☐	☐	☐
Local stores that you can walk or bike to	☐	☐	☐
Bus system	☐	☐	☐
Unleashed or uncontrolled dogs make physical activity unsafe	☐	☐	☐
Traffic makes physical activity unsafe	☐	☐	☐
Crime	☐	☐	☐
Physical activity is socially unacceptable	☐	☐	☐
Adequate parks and playgrounds	☐	☐	☐
Local recreation center (and safety of the recreation center)	☐	☐	☐
Local swimming pool	☐	☐	☐
Local sport fields	☐	☐	☐
School facilities with times for open public recreation	☐	☐	☐
Nearby shopping mall with a walking program	☐	☐	☐

From B.J. Sharkey and S.E. Gaskill, 2013, *Fitness and health, seventh edition* (Champaign, IL: Human Kinetics).

activity. Go through the checklist, noting barriers and possibilities. Once you have identified your local barriers to physical activity, you can make a difference by becoming locally involved. Become an activist for building the infrastructure needed for a healthier neighborhood. Bike paths and sidewalks get built when community members put pressure on local governments. Businesses will put in bike racks when they are made aware that there is a demand. Schools will develop safe walking routes to school when parents speak out.

You can find many stories of people who have made incredible differences by increasing access to physical activity in their neighborhoods. If you do an Internet search for "physical activity community action," you will be amazed at the wide variety of stories and support material online. The U.S. Centers for Disease Control (CDC) and many other organizations have written plans and ideas for how to become an advocate for physical activity in your community. The CDC has a number of great tools along with many success stories. Their website is www.cdc.gov/healthycommunitiesprogram/tools.

The remainder of this chapter discusses growing older with vitality. While this may seem unrelated to purposeful physical activity, people who develop an active lifestyle are more likely to live longer. More importantly, they will live independently for longer. They remain healthier as they age and can better enjoy their golden years. Purposeful activity built into your daily routine is one of the best ways to invest in your future health.

AGING AND ACTIVITY

Life expectancy has gone up in proportion to declines in infant mortality and infectious diseases. But the attainable life span, the highest possible age in a life free of serious accident or illness, has not changed noticeably in the past 200 years. In other words, we are not living longer, we are simply avoiding premature death. Survival curves point to a theoretically attainable life span of about 85 years, with a standard deviation of 4 years (figure 6.1). Thus, 68 percent of the population have the potential to live between 81 and 89 years (85 plus or minus 4 years), and 95 percent of deaths from natural causes would fall between 77 and 93 years (85 plus or minus 2 standard deviations, or 8 years). Rare indeed are people who live beyond 97 years, more than 3 standard deviations above the mean. The oldest documented life spans are in the neighborhood of 120 years (Fries and Crapo 1981).

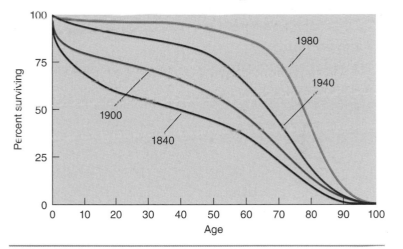

FIGURE 6.1 Survival curves. With less infant mortality and trauma (accidental death), more people survive to the attainable life expectancy, 85 years. With good health habits, more are able to postpone chronic debilitating illness, remaining vigorous until the last years or months of life.

Adapted from *Vital statistics of the United States, 1977, Volume II, Section 5*, DHEW Publication PHS 80-1104, National Center for Health Statistics.

The decline of chronic illness has extended the period of adult vigor, so life remains physically, emotionally, and intellectually vigorous until shortly before its close (figure 6.2). Appropriate behaviors can modify many of the factors believed to be associated with age, including heart and lung function, bone density, blood pressure, and cholesterol. People who choose not to age rapidly can reduce morbidity and extend the vigorous years by living an active, healthy life (Fries and Crapo 1981). On the other hand, those who decide to age rapidly are destined to become a burden on family, health care, and community support systems.

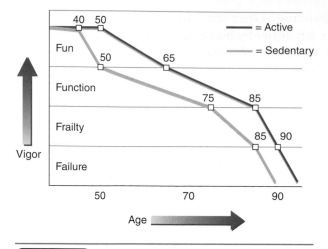

FIGURE 6.2 Vigor and the active life. Active living extends the periods of fun and function and shortens the time of frailty and failure.

> **A**ctivity adds life to your years as well as years to your life! Unfortunately, as some have said, the years you add all come at the end.

Earlier, we quoted studies that indicate an increase in longevity for those who lead the active life. Activity adds life to your years as well as years to your life! Unfortunately, as some have said, the years that you add all come at the end. And some have suggested that the years you add are about equal to the time that you spent in exercise. Can that be true? One study found at least a 2-year increase in life expectancy associated with activity. If you exercise 1 hour every day for 40 years, you'll spend 14,560 hours engaged in exercise. Divide that number by 24 hours per day, and you get 607 days, or 1.67 years, somewhat less than the 2 years or more that you'll earn. Of course, you will enjoy the time you spend in exercise, recreation, and sport, and you will extend the years of fun and function, the prime of life.

Theories of aging are many, including those dealing with gene defects or chromosomal damage, errors in protein synthesis, and limits to the number of cell divisions (the Hayflick limit). Other factors associated with aging include caloric intake, inherited factors, **free radicals**, stress, and lifestyle.

• *Caloric restriction.* Animal studies have shown that eating fewer calories (up to 40 percent less) can extend survival time dramatically (28 percent in one study) when adult animals were put on a low-protein diet (Miller and Payne 1968). Some researchers have felt that the most important factors determining life span were those that influenced body fatness. Animals fed fewer calories also had a lower tumor incidence and less chronic disease (Comfort 1979). When Alexander Leaf studied healthy elderly people in three remote parts of the world, he found their diets low in calories and fat (1973). Leaf believed that the low-calorie diet, combined with regular activity and a productive and respected role in society, contributed to good health and long life.

• *Inherited factors.* People with exceptional longevity and their offspring have significantly larger particles of low-density lipoprotein (LDL) cholesterol, which are associated with lower prevalence of hypertension, cardiovascular disease, and metabolic syndrome. This genetic variation is favorable because the larger LDL is less likely to adhere to artery walls. Although genes probably determine this favorable particle size, studies suggest that exercise can enlarge the LDL particles (Barzalai et al. 2003).

• *Free radicals.* One theory of aging holds that so-called free radicals (reactive molecules with one or more unpaired electrons) prove toxic to vulnerable tissues. In the biological world, life span is inversely related to metabolic rate. Exercise produces free radicals that can harm the body. But moderate activity enhances antioxidant protection and the immune system. Chronic heavy exertion may produce an excess of free radicals, raise the risk of heart disease, and depress the immune response (Demopoulos et al. 1986). The role of free radicals in exercise and aging requires more study. In the meantime, vitamins C and E and other antioxidants are believed to provide some protection against these potentially toxic by-products of oxidative metabolism, especially when consumed in food rather than in pills.

• *Stress.* Working in a stressful job is associated with a doubling of the risk of death from cardiovascular disease. Workers with the greatest disparity between effort and reward and those with high job strain and perceived lack of control over their jobs were more than twice as likely to die from heart disease compared with those with a better balance among these factors (Kivimaki et al. 2002).

In terms of aging, studies of women caring for the chronically ill or children suggest that stress or the perception of stress is linked to aging. Researchers studied telomeres, DNA protein complexes that cap the ends of chromosomes and promote genetic stability. As cells divide, a portion of the telomere is lost, and after considerable loss, the cell stops dividing. The oxidative stress of continuous care was linked with shortening of the telomeres of the cells, equivalent to a decade of additional aging when compared with women under low stress (Epel et al. 2004).

At present, no single theory explains the decline that occurs with age. What is surprising is the realization that the rate of decline, or senescence, is not fixed. It is variable, subject to considerable modification.

A list of changeable aspects of aging has emerged, markers that are subject to changes brought about by one's personal decisions and behaviors (Fries and Crapo 1981) (table 6.1).

A definite pattern emerges from a consideration of the changeable aspects of aging, pointing to the importance of daily habits as the way to improve your health span, or your active life expectancy.

> **W**hat is surprising is the realization that the rate of decline (senescence) is not fixed, but is variable, subject to considerable modification.

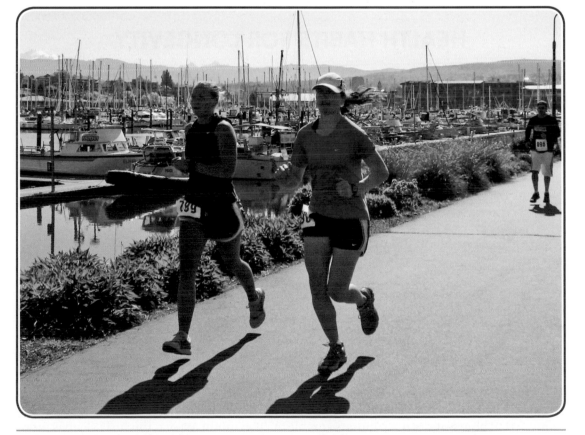

■ Activity helps you extend the physically and mentally vigorous years of your life.

Table 6.1　Changeable Aspects of Aging

Aging marker	Personal decision or behavior
Cardiac output	Exercise
Glucose tolerance	Exercise, diet, weight control
Osteoporosis	Weight-bearing exercise, diet
Pulmonary function	Exercise, nonsmoking
Blood pressure	Exercise, diet, weight control
Endurance and strength	Exercise
Reaction time	Training, practice
Cholesterol	Diet, weight control, exercise
Arterial wall rigidity	Diet, exercise
Intelligence and memory	Training, practice
Skin aging	Avoid sun

Several factors affected by aging appear to be nonmodifiable. These include graying and thinning of hair, elasticity of skin, kidney reserve, and degeneration of the eyes including cataracts and macular degeneration.

Adapted from J. Fries and L. Crapo, 1981, *Vitality and aging* (New York, NY: W.H. Freeman & Company), 125. By permission of James Fries.

HEALTH HABITS FOR LONGEVITY

In 1962, researchers at the Human Population Laboratory of the California Department of Health began a study of the relationship of health to various behaviors or habits. Health and longevity are associated with the following:

- Adequate sleep (7 to 8 hr/day)
- A good breakfast
- Regular meals (avoid snacks)
- Weight control
- Not smoking cigarettes
- Moderate alcohol consumption
- Regular exercise

The study found that men could add 11 years to their lives and women 7 years, just by following six of these habits (Breslow and Enstrom 1980). Let's examine each practice to see whether it fits your current lifestyle. Then you can decide if changes are in order.

Adequate Sleep

When men or women sleep 6 hours or less per night, they are not as healthy as when they sleep 7 or 8 hours. Those who sleep 9 hours or more are slightly below average in health. Thus, 7 to 8 hours of sleep are most favorable. As you might expect, too little sleep is more of a problem than too much.

Sleep is characterized by alternating stages. One stage involves **rapid eye movements (REM)** and changes in heart rate, blood pressure, and muscle tone. This stage may serve as a rest period for the inhibitory nerve cells of the brain. It usually is accompanied by dreams. If it is interrupted, we become anxious and irritable. This REM sleep constitutes about 20 percent of the total for the night. Deeper or quieter periods provide the rest necessary for recovery from fatigue. If you miss some sleep one night, the body will not make any serious attempt to recover the sleep deprivation.

However, if a substantial amount of the loss is REM sleep, more REM sleep will occur on subsequent nights (figure 6.3). Going without sleep seems to impair creative capabilities, which suggests that another function of sleep is to restore a cerebral cortex fatigued by consciousness.

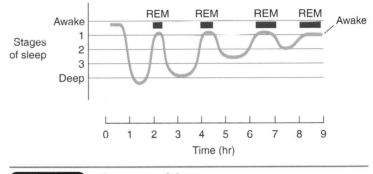

FIGURE 6.3 The stages of sleep.

Moderate physical activity seems to enhance the ability to fall into deep sleep without altering the time spent in REM sleep. Too little or too much exercise appears to result in sleep disturbance, and significant sleep loss seems to suppress the immune system.

Nutritious Breakfast

In the California study, those who ate breakfast almost every day experienced better health than those who ate breakfast some of the time (Breslow and Enstrom 1980). Furthermore, a good breakfast may be a prerequisite to good performance in work and sport. Breakfast often comes 12 hours after the evening meal, so you can see why it is important for energy and cellular metabolism. A few researchers suggest that breakfast should be the largest and most important meal of the day, and everyone agrees that it should include more than a cup of coffee and a doughnut.

Regular Meals

Erratic eaters have poorer health than those who eat regular meals. Those who seldom or never eat between meals have better health than those who regularly eat between meals. Unfortunately, this study did not compare the health status of those who eat smaller but more numerous nutritious meals, but it does indicate the effects of erratic eating behavior and snacking. We can only guess at the content of the between-meal snacks, but chances are that they were toxic foods, high in simple sugars and saturated fat and low in nutrients (Breslow and Enstrom 1980).

Weight Control

When weight is more than 20 percent above or more than 10 percent below the desirable weight, health status declines. For example, if your desirable weight is 150 pounds (68 kg), your health status is most favorable when you maintain your weight between 135 pounds (61.2 kg; minus 10%) and 180 pounds (81.6 kg; plus 20%), a broad margin of error indeed. An interesting study would be to compare the effects on health of low body weight (more than 10% below desirable) because of malnutrition, illness, or smoking with the effects of low body weight resulting from habitual, vigorous exercise. Personal observation indicates that low body weight associated with vigorous exercise and good nutrition is at least as healthy as being at or above the desirable weight.

Avoid Smoking

Smoking remains the leading modifiable cause of death in the United States (435,000 deaths in 2000). But factors associated with overweight and obesity—poor diet and physical inactivity—may soon overtake tobacco as the leading cause of death (400,000 deaths) (Mokdad et al. 2004). If you don't smoke, don't start. If you do smoke, stop. Quitting could be the best thing that you ever do for yourself. If you can't stop for your own health, think of loved ones, especially children, who are exposed to your habit.

Secondhand tobacco smoke is responsible for asthma and respiratory problems, not to mention lung cancers, for many thousands of children. Is quitting worth the trouble? Data from numerous studies show that quitting has many benefits, including better oxygen-carrying capacity, lower blood pressure, improved night vision, and increased effectiveness of prescription drugs. Although some tobacco-related diseases, such as emphysema, cannot be reversed, others seem to repair with time. Repair time for smoking-induced illnesses include 10 years for heart disease and 10 to 15 years for cancer. Quit today and help make the nation smoke free.

Moderate Alcohol

Poor health is associated with heavy alcohol consumption (five or more drinks at one sitting). Those who never drink and those who drink moderately (one to two drinks a day for men, one to three per week for women) enjoy the same level of good health. Believers in the French paradox ponder why the French seem to tolerate rich foods without an increase in heart disease. The answer may lie in regular consumption of wine. Some studies show that those who drink one or two alcoholic drinks daily have a lower risk of heart disease, perhaps because alcohol is associated with higher levels of HDL cholesterol (Gaziano et al. 1993). You should not construe this finding as a broad endorsement of alcohol consumption. Some level of alcohol consumption, if continued for a sufficient period, may lead to degenerative effects on the liver, even when nutrition is adequate. The best advice is to drink moderately (one to two drinks per day for men, one every other day for women) or to avoid drinking altogether. And no, you cannot save your daily drinks for a weekend binge.

Regular Activity

Researchers in the California study compared the health benefits of five types of activity: active sports, swimming or long walks, garden work, physical exercises, and hunting and fishing. Only hunting and fishing (seasonal and infrequent) were not associated with improved health. For all the other activities, those who participated most often experienced the best physical health. The best health was associated with active sports, followed by swimming or walking, physical exercise, and gardening. The lowest death rates occurred among those who were often active in sports, and the highest death rates were for those who chose not to engage in any exercise.

Take up one good health habit (the authors recommend sitting less each day) and others will follow.

In summary, physical health, longevity, and the rate of aging are associated with your daily health habits and your lifestyle. These health habits have more to do with your health and longevity than all the influences of medicine. The California study indicated that a man 55 years old who follows all seven health habits has the same health status as a person 25 to 30 years younger who follows fewer than two. Moreover, the researchers found a positive relationship between physical and mental health (Breslow and Enstrom 1980). A new research review confirms that Breslow had it correct back in 1980. Staying active, eating right, utilizing social and environmental resources, employing coping skills developed across the life span, and developing new strategies can enhance longevity and the quality of life as we get older (Wessell and Edwards 2012). In their review, Wessell and Edwards note many of the health habits identified by Breslow. You know that an association or relationship between variables does not imply cause and effect, that good physical health doesn't necessarily cause good mental health. However, you are probably familiar with psychosomatic illnesses, so you should realize that the opposite effects are possible. A healthy body is an important aid to good mental health, and you can help maintain physical health by following the recommended health habits.

> **Y**our daily health habits and your lifestyle have more to do with your health and longevity than all the influences of medicine.

ATTRIBUTES FOR LONGEVITY

One key to longevity, what it takes to live well beyond normal life expectancy, is your lifestyle. Observations of healthy older people (aged 75 years and over) provide intriguing insights into the personality traits and living habits associated with long-term survival. The following characteristics are associated with longevity:

- *Moderation*. Moderation is a common denominator in all phases of life, including diet, vices, work, and physical activity. Long-term survival in a footrace or the human race depends on pacing.

- *Flexibility*. Psychological flexibility implies the ability to bend but not break, to accept change, to avoid rigid habits.

- *Challenge*. Accept challenges. Create them if necessary. Don't allow life to become too easy. But when a challenge becomes too great, say so, and seek an alternative.

- *Health habits*. A relaxed attitude toward health characterizes long-term survival. Older survivors are not obsessive about health habits. They eat a variety of foods and are not terribly concerned about avoiding items such as cholesterol. They are moderate in their use of alcohol, and some even smoke now and then. These people demonstrate the need for balance and moderation. In general, they lead healthy lifestyles.

- *Relationships*. Older citizens enjoy other people. They maintain an interest in and continuous contact with friends and family. They enjoy their marriages.

- *Outlook*. Healthy elders maintain a positive outlook. They recognize the effects of advancing age and plan to enjoy each phase of life. They realize that long life means growing old, and they are prepared to enjoy both.

- *Active life*. Of course, those who age successfully are engaged in daily routines that require activity. They find reasons to be socially and physically active. Involvement in daily chores provides the purpose, rhythm, and activity that everyone needs. The active life can benefit you in a number of ways, including the following:

  - *Health*. Regular activity enhances both physical and mental health.
  - *Mobility*. Regular aerobic activity, supplemented with resistance exercises, retains or restores mobility and the capacity for a free and independent life.

- *Economy.* To save money, walk, jog, or ride a bike. Cross-country skis are cheaper than a snowmobile and better for you.
- *Ecology.* The active life, with emphasis on muscle-powered sport and recreation, helps conserve limited energy supplies. Physically active people have less effect on the environment than do their sedentary counterparts, who use energy-consuming recreational vehicles and leaf blowers.
- *Adaptability.* The active person retains the ability to adapt to changes in life, the economy, or the environment.
- *Survival.* Older people are survivors. Along the way, they accumulate wisdom and insights that have value to coming generations. The axiom in nature applies to the human race as well: The fittest survive. When fitness is measured and subjects are followed for years, the data supporting the concept of survival of the fittest are strong and compelling (Balady 2002).

Active people view each moment as one to be lived. They avoid people who depress them. When they feel moody or depressed, they do something. They take risks, engage in life, and enjoy it. They don't waste the present with moods, worry, or immobilizing thoughts about the future. Depression, worry, guilt, and anger can lead to (or be caused by) subtle changes in brain chemistry and hormone levels. Physical activity can directly affect moods and the chemistry of behavior, and it can divert attention and provide enjoyment and a sense of self-satisfaction that minimizes or eliminates self-defeating behavior.

You are free to think, feel, and act as you desire. Circumstances, biorhythms, behavior traits, genetics, or deep-seated psychological problems do not control you. You can create

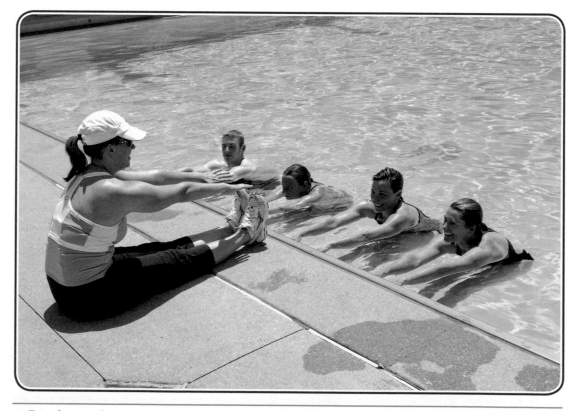

■ Regular involvement in activity is one key to longevity.

the life that you desire if you really want to. Don't fall back on excuses like "I haven't got the time," "I'll start next week (month, year)," "I'm too busy right now, but when the kids are a little older . . ."

Finally, consider the factors that characterize the happy–well group in a longitudinal study (Vaillant 2001). Six factors, measured at age 50, predicted the most successful group at age 80: a stable marriage, a mature adaptive style, no smoking, little alcohol, maintenance of normal weight, and regular exercise.

AGE AND PERFORMANCE

As we've said, chronological age is a poor predictor of health or performance. Health is a function of your habits, heredity, environment, and previous illness. Performance in work or sport is a function of physiological age, not chronological age.

Physiological age (also called biological or functional age) is a composite of health, physiological capacity, and performance measures. The best single measure of physiological age is probably your level of aerobic fitness. That number tells you about the health and capacity of the respiratory, circulatory, and muscular systems. Moreover, a considerable body of evidence shows an inverse relationship between aerobic fitness and a number of risk factors. Thus, an active 55-year-old may have higher health and performance capabilities with fewer heart disease risk factors than a sedentary 20 year-old. This fact has considerable relevance when it comes to changing our

What is Aerobic Fitness?

Aerobic fitness is our ability to use oxygen for aerobic (with oxygen) exercise. The most common unit of measurement is how much oxygen we consume per kilogram of body weight each minute during maximal intensity exercise, which is called our maximal oxygen utilization ($\dot{V}O_2$max). Average $\dot{V}O_2$max values for moderately active young men and women are respectively about 38 and 42 milliliters of oxygen consumption per kilogram of body weight each minute ($ml \cdot kg^{-1} \cdot min^{-1}$). Less-active people tend to have lower values, and endurance athletes may have values of 70 to 90 milliliters per kilogram per minute ($ml \cdot kg^{-1} \cdot min^{-1}$). You will learn a lot more about aerobic fitness in chapters 8 and 10.

society's view of aging and its consequences, such as age discrimination in hiring. Age does not ensure a rapid decline in performance, and when physical performance is important, physiological age is a more accurate predictor of performance potential than chronological age (Sharkey 1987).

Other indicators of physiological age include your family history, health habits, measures such as blood pressure and cholesterol (see the health risk form in the appendix), and measures of strength, **reaction time**, vision, hearing, and other variables.

Aerobic Fitness and Age

Cross-sectional studies show that aerobic fitness declines at the rate of 8 to 10 percent per decade. But among moderately active people, the decline is 4 to 5 percent, and among trained people, the rate of decline can be 2 percent or less.

Figure 6.4 depicts the decline of people who begin with an aerobic fitness of 50 ($ml \cdot kg^{-1} \cdot min^{-1}$). Imagine the differences that occur with a very fit athlete (70 $ml \cdot kg^{-1} \cdot min^{-1}$) who continues to train versus an unfit person (30 $ml \cdot kg^{-1} \cdot min^{-1}$) who remains sedentary. In 10 years, the athlete drops 2 percent to 68.6, whereas the inactive person declines 10 percent to

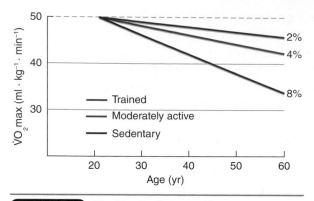

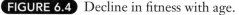

FIGURE 6.4 Decline in fitness with age.

Vicious Cycle

Excess fat restricts exercise capacity, causing a decline in fitness, which further reduces activity, resulting in additional fat accumulation—a vicious cycle indeed. Additionally, sedentary behavior decreases lean body mass, further reducing resting metabolism, thus pushing the **energy balance** toward ever-increasing fat storage. As caloric intake greatly exceeds expenditure, a person's ability to internally adjust resting metabolism to maintain a constant weight is overcome. Internal set-points for weight appear to increase, making future weight loss more difficult. Compounding the problem, aerobic fitness is calculated per kilogram of body weight. Thus, even if a person is able to maintain muscle mass, a rise in weight and fat equates to a decline in fitness and functional capacity.

27. Avoiding gains in body weight and fat minimizes the rate of decline in fitness. Increased body fat, less training, and reduced muscle mass accounts for a significant portion of the decline in fitness and performance that occurs with age.

Eventually, most highly active people cut back on training. Some gain weight, thereby increasing the rate of decline in fitness. The rate of decline in $\dot{V}O_2$max after 50 years of age in endurance-trained individuals was related to a decline in training volume (Pimentel et al. 2003). If you increase your level of activity and maintain the higher level, you can slow the rate of decline until the sixth or seventh decade of life.

The beneficial effects of exercise and weight control on fitness, performance, and health are clear. The quality of life depends on the ability to pursue a variety of activities. Negative factors that affect this capacity for activity, such as excess body fat, should receive attention before irreversible physiological deterioration occurs. A reduction in body fat allows and promotes a more active life and minimizes the decrease in fitness and performance previously blamed on increasing age.

Strength

Strength declines rather slowly with age until the fifth decade, when the rate of decline increases. This loss of muscle mass has been called **sarcopenia**, or vanishing flesh. Sarcopenia is an important component of frailty in older people, contributing to a loss of strength, increased falls, and fractures (Welle 2002). It has been linked to other afflictions of aging, osteoporosis, insulin resistance, and arthritis. Sarcopenia results from loss of **muscle fibers** and fiber **atrophy**, because of lack of use, decreased muscle-building hormones (**testosterone**), and possibly an increase in catabolic hormones and other agents that accelerate the rate of muscle wasting in older people (Deschenes 2005). People who use their strength regularly retain muscle function much longer. Evidence suggests that very old men and women (average age 87 years) can counter muscle weakness and frailty with resistance training (Fiatarone et al. 1994). Activities of daily living such as gait **velocity**, stair-climbing power, and spontaneous physical activity all improved in the resistance-training group. Muscle mass increased as well, in contrast to a decline for the inactive control group. Indeed, this study, along with others, suggests that maintenance of strength throughout the life span may reduce the prevalence of functional limitations (Brill et al. 2000).

SUMMARY

We're all concerned about saving enough and investing wisely during our working years to ensure financial security in retirement. Fiscal fitness is important, but that is only part of the story. To ensure a vigorous and independent retirement, you need to invest in physical fitness as well. In personal finance, the sooner you start to invest the better, so that you can enjoy the fruits of compound interest. The same is true with fitness. You'll achieve maximum gains with an early start. The best time to begin the active life is when you are young. The second best time to start is now.

Incorporating physical activity in a purposeful manner into your daily routine is the best way to ensure that you will continue to bank your investment. Purposeful physical activity accomplishes a necessary or enjoyable task, providing meaning beyond the simple movements, and results in an immediate outcome such as walking to the store, biking to work, or walking your dog. Purposeful and meaningful activities allow you to accomplish necessary or pleasurable tasks while also gaining the health and many other benefits of the active life.

In many ways, the active life and fitness represent money in the bank by reducing future medical costs, minimizing the need for long-term care, and eliminating future burdens on family, friends, and society. The active life represents an investment in vitality and vigor that will pay off many times over in your retirement years. In crass financial terms, the several years of extended life are like a greater starting balance in your retirement fund, giving you an extended return on your annuities and social security. But the greatest return is having the vigor and independence to pursue life to the fullest, all the days of your life.

Activity and training maintain fitness and other measures of performance that normally decline with age. Tennis players and other avid sports participants maintain reaction and movement times, which typically slow with age. The body doesn't wear out, it rusts out. So the old adage "Use it or lose it" is worth noting. Humans were not designed for a sedentary life. For early humans, living required physical activity. Now, we need to build purposeful activity into our lives.

With good genetics and a sensible diet, you may live a long life. Would you rather spend the final years of your life in a nursing home or living independently, traveling, and enjoying the active life? It is never too late to start saving for the future or investing in physical vitality.

Understanding Fitness

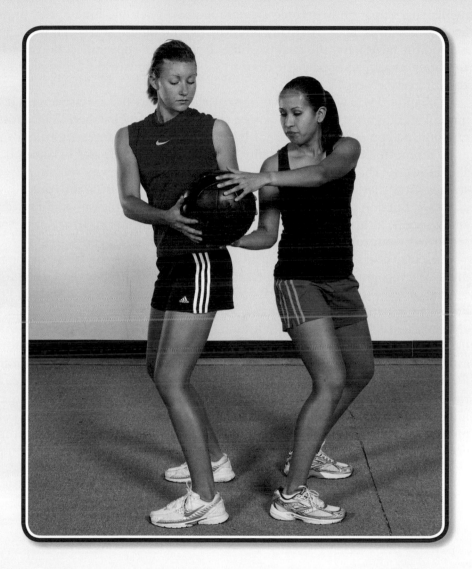

Fitness consists of two parts, energy and muscular. Energy fitness, covered in chapter 7, is how we produce the energy needed for muscular movement, and includes both aerobic (with oxygen) and anaerobic (without oxygen) means. Somewhere above the pace of your normal daily activities but well below maximal effort, you will find aerobic exercise. If you do aerobic exercise often enough you will improve your aerobic fitness, and as fitness improves you'll enhance your health, appearance, vitality, and quality of life. As intensity increases, the ability to produce all the necessary energy using only aerobic means becomes overwhelmed, and an increasing proportion of energy is produced anaerobically.

Aerobic fitness, covered in chapter 8, describes how well you are able to take oxygen from the atmosphere into your lungs and then into your blood and pump it through the heart and circulatory system to working muscles, where it is used to oxidize carbohydrate and fat to produce energy. No other measure says more about the health and capacity of your lungs, heart, circulatory system, and, most important, your skeletal muscles. Rhythmic large-muscle activities such as brisk walking, jogging, cycling, swimming, cross-country skiing, and rowing are aerobic exercises. They demand sustained increases in respiration, circulation, and, most importantly, muscle metabolism, and lead to adaptations in the systems and muscles involved. Aerobic exercise is associated with health and longevity; regular participation in aerobic exercise improves aerobic fitness, and improved fitness further enhances health. In many physical, psychological, and social ways, aerobic fitness is good for health and the quality of life. It improves appearance, boosts self-confidence and body image, and opens the door to a challenging world filled with new experiences and interesting people.

In chapter 9 you will learn that muscular fitness is more than strength; it also includes muscular endurance, flexibility, power, speed, agility, and balance. With most physiologic capabilities, you either use them or lose them, and that is certainly true for muscular fitness. Strength, endurance, flexibility, power, speed, agility, and balance all decline with age. However, the rate of decline is much slower for those who remain active. Numerous studies show that we have the capability to build strength even into our 90s (Fiatarone et al. 1994)! But don't wait until you are 90 to experience the pleasures and rewards of aerobic and muscular fitness. Begin now. You will soon notice that tasks are easier, your muscles are firmer, your tummy is flatter, and you feel better about yourself and life in general.

Muscular fitness once occupied an awkward position on the fringe of the fitness movement. We recognized its contributions to performance in sport and some forms of work, but we lacked conclusive evidence linking muscular fitness with health and the quality of life. That situation has changed and we can now say with confidence that both aerobic and muscular fitness contribute substantially to health. Muscular fitness training increases muscle mass, the furnace that burns fat. Exercises that improve muscular fitness help you avoid the crippling bone demineralization known as osteoporosis. Attention to muscular fitness is essential if you are to avoid the low-back problems and repetitive motion injuries that plague millions of Americans. Continued participation ensures the capacity for independence and mobility in your postretirement years. The essential components of muscular fitness are strength, muscular endurance, and flexibility. Other important components include power, speed, agility, and balance.

Physiology of Fitness

Muscles, Oxygen, and Energy

> "To understand is hard. Once one understands, action is easy."
>
> *Sun Yat-sen*

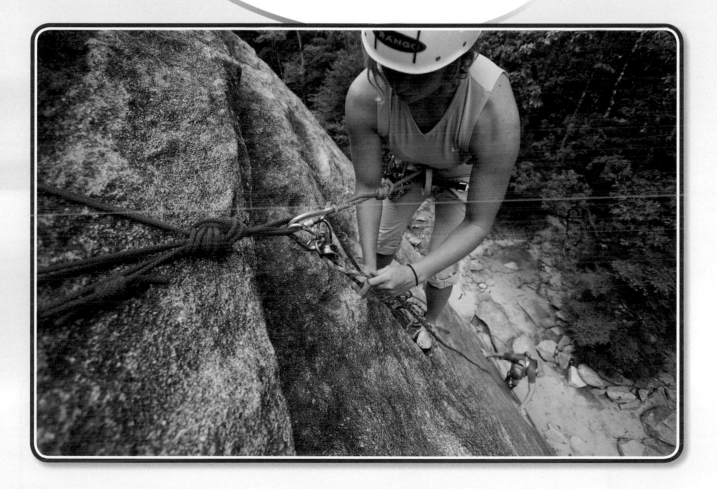

Physiology is the study of how organisms function. The **physiology of fitness** shows how muscular contractions move the body to participate in exercise, sport, and strenuous work. How do these muscles function? What makes them move, and what causes fatigue? What is the energy for muscular contractions, and how is oxygen central to movement and performance? And why is physical activity good for your health? This introduction to the physiology of aerobic and muscular fitness provides the answers to these and other questions.

The brain tells the muscles when and how to contract. When the cerebral cortex makes the decision to move, the action is initiated by the motor cortex. Nervous impulses from the **motor area** of the cortex are routed via neurons that descend the spinal cord and **synapse** with **motor neurons**, which leave the cord and pass the message to muscle fibers (figure 7.1). As they descend, many neurons cross to the other side of the cord, which explains why an injury or stroke on one side of the head affects movements on the other side of the body. The motor neuron and the muscle fibers it controls are called a **motor unit**. Each motor unit includes from a few to many hundreds of muscle fibers.

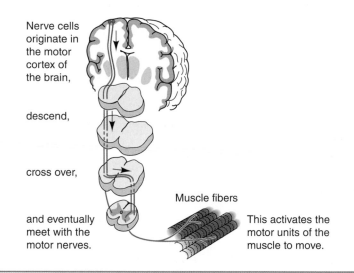

Nerve cells originate in the motor cortex of the brain,

descend,

cross over,

and eventually meet with the motor nerves.

Muscle fibers

This activates the motor units of the muscle to move.

FIGURE 7.1　The motor cortex and the control of muscles.

This chapter will help you do the following:

- Understand the structure and function of muscle fibers
- Determine the energy sources for contractions
- Outline the role of oxygen in metabolic pathways
- Identify the roles of the respiratory, cardiovascular, and **endocrine systems**
- Understand how activity and training improve the function of muscles and support systems, thereby enhancing performance and health

This chapter presents an overview of exercise physiology, explaining how muscles contract, the sources of energy, metabolic pathways, and the role of oxygen. It also identifies supply and support mechanisms of the respiratory, cardiovascular, and hormonal systems that supply and augment the working muscles.

MUSCLE CONTRACTIONS

Each muscle contains thousands of spaghetti-like muscle fibers that range from less than 1 centimeter to more than 35 centimeters (14 in.) in length. The fibers contain the contractile proteins **actin** and **myosin**. Muscle fibers shorten and produce movement when the muscle is stimulated by its neuron. The actin and myosin filaments creep along each other via the tiny crossbridges that reach out from the thicker myosin, attach to the actin, and pull like oars. The barely perceptible movement produced in one segment of the muscle is added to the shortening produced along the length of the fiber, resulting in visible motion (figure 7.2). Because muscles attach to bony lever systems, their movement is multiplied to produce useful work.

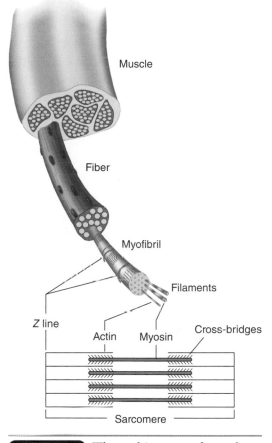

Force

Since each muscle fiber contracts to the best of its ability (all or none), force is dependent on the number of motor units and fibers involved in the contraction. The brain recruits slow-twitch fibers for low force output and larger fast-twitch fibers when more force is required (see box on muscle fibers). More frequent nerve impulses can lead to increases in force. Force output declines with fatigue, so more motor units are required to produce the same force.

Fatigue

A fatigued muscle fiber still attempts to contract all or none of its contractile proteins, but its force declines. Power output declines as intramuscular stores of energy are used (**glycogen** and fat) and substances involved in contractions (calcium) are depleted, and as acid metabolites increase (lactic acid) and energy production drops. These factors are not unrelated. Increased

FIGURE 7.2 The architecture of muscle.

lactic acid brought on by intense effort alters the cell's acid–base balance and reduces the rate of energy production, thereby increasing the rate of energy depletion. This is called **peripheral fatigue**. Proper training can increase energy stores, improve energy production, and reduce the appearance of lactic acid.

Central fatigue occurs after muscle glycogen, the storage form of glucose, becomes depleted after prolonged exertion. The muscle turns to glycogen stored in the liver to supply blood glucose for energy. Eventually, as liver glycogen is depleted, blood glucose levels begin to fall. Since the brain and nervous system rely on glucose for energy, the drop in blood glucose (**hypoglycemia**) is accompanied by impaired nervous system and brain function, confusion, poor coordination, and extreme fatigue. Fortunately, central fatigue can be delayed by consuming carbohydrate supplements in solid and liquid form. Carbohydrate supplements have improved work output of wildland firefighters by 20 percent or more during the latter hours of a 14-hour work shift (Ruby et al. 2004).

Muscle Fibers

Humans have three types of muscle fibers: slow-twitch (slow, oxidative, or SO) fibers and two types of fast-twitch fibers (fast, oxidative-glycolytic, or FOG, and fast, glycolytic, or FG). Most people average around 50 percent slow- and 50 fast-twitch fibers, with 35 percent FOG and 15 percent FG. Endurance athletes have a higher percentage of slow fibers and power athletes usually have more fast fibers. Interestingly, each muscle fiber in a single motor unit is of the same fiber type, slow or fast. In fact, the motor neuron dictates the characteristics of the muscle fiber. If the fiber is consistently recruited for slow work, it takes on the characteristics of a **slow-twitch muscle fiber**. If it is recruited for fast contractions, it develops the characteristics of fast-twitch fibers (table 7.1).

Slow-twitch fibers contract and relax slowly, but they are very resistant to fatigue. They have energy sources and metabolic pathways needed for endurance. **Fast-twitch muscle fibers** contract twice as fast as the slow ones and produce more force, but they fatigue quickly. FOG fibers have a bit less endurance than slow fibers, but far more than FG fibers, which are usually reserved for short, intense bursts of effort. Endurance training enhances the oxidative capacity of fast-twitch fibers, leading to greater stamina. Strength training improves the strength of both fiber types.

Table 7.1 Characteristics of Muscle Fibers

Characteristics	Slow, oxidative (SO)	Fast, oxidative-glycolytic (FOG)	Fast, glycolytic (FG)
Average fiber percentage	50%	35%	15%
Speed of contraction	Slow	Fast	Fast
Force of contraction	Low	High	High
Size	Smaller	Large	Large
Fatigability	Fatigue resistant	Less resistant	Easily fatigued
Aerobic capacity	High	Medium	Low
Capillary density	High	High	Low
Anaerobic capacity	Low	Medium	High

ENERGY SOURCES

Energy, the ability to do work, comes from the sun. It is converted into chemical compounds by plants and animals and is eventually consumed as food in the form of carbohydrate, fat, and protein molecules. The chemical breakdown of these molecules, oxidation, releases the stored energy and uses it to power human muscles.

Carbohydrate

Throughout the world, carbohydrate provides the major source of energy. It is available in simple and complex forms. Simple sugars, such as glucose, fructose, and sucrose (refined sugar, composed of molecules of glucose and fructose), contain energy but few nutrients (i.e., vitamins and minerals). Complex carbohydrate found in beans, brown rice, whole-grain products (bread and pasta), potatoes, and corn comes with important nutrients and fiber. Unfortunately, average Americans get half their dietary carbohydrate from concentrated or refined simple sugar, packed with so-called empty calories (empty because they lack nutrients). Fresh fruits contain simple sugar, but they also provide important nutrients.

Digestion of complex starch molecules begins in the mouth, where an enzyme reduces complex carbohydrate to simple sugar. It is temporarily halted in the stomach, then continued in the small intestine, where starches are further digested. Final breakdown to glucose is completed by **enzymes** secreted by the wall of the intestine. The glucose is then absorbed into the bloodstream. The absorption is rather complete; most of the carbohydrate you eat gets into the blood. The absorbed molecules travel to the liver and muscles to restore glycogen stores. Remaining carbohydrate is stored as fat. We recommend that 60 percent of calories come from complex carbohydrate (beans, brown rice, whole-grain bread and pasta, potatoes, and corn). Simple sugars can be used to supplement carbohydrate during long hours of physical activity.

Fat

Fat is the most efficient way to store energy, with 9.3 calories per gram versus the 4.1 and 4.3 calories for carbohydrate and protein, respectively. Dietary fat is broken down and absorbed in the small intestine. It then travels via the **lymphatic system** (tiny vessels and nodes that transport and filter cellular drainage). The fat clumps (**chylomicrons**) are eventually dumped into the circulation for transport to cells for energy, or to adipose tissue for storage. However, dietary fat intake isn't the only way to acquire this source of energy. Excess carbohydrate or protein can be converted to fat and stored in adipose tissue. Humans have many ways to acquire fat, but only one good way to remove it: physical activity. We recommend that you limit fat intake to one-fourth (25%) of your total calories and limit saturated fat to one-third of fat intake. Avoid trans fat, since it contributes to atherosclerosis and heart disease.

Protein

When we ingest animal or plant protein, the large molecules are cleaved into amino acids and absorbed. The amino acids are building blocks used to construct cell walls, muscle tissue, hormones, enzymes, and a variety of other molecules. Training builds proteins: Aerobic training builds aerobic enzyme protein for energy production and strength training builds contractile proteins (actin and myosin) to exert force. So, it should be no surprise to learn the importance of protein to the active life. We recommend 15 percent of daily caloric intake in the form of protein. While sedentary people need about .8 grams of protein per kilogram of body weight, those who engage in physically demanding activities need 1.2 to 1.6 grams per kilogram (e.g., 1.4×80 kg, or 176 lb, equals 112 g of protein per day. There are 454 g in 1 lb).

More important than quantity, however, is the quality of protein. High-quality protein is high in **essential amino acids**, those that cannot be synthesized in the body. These essential amino acids are **macronutrients**, major food sources that must be available for optimal function. When essential amino acids are missing from the diet, the body is unable to construct proteins that require them. Although animal protein is a better source of essential amino acids (as well as iron and vitamin B_{12}), proper combinations of plant protein can meet nutritional needs. You may be surprised to learn that protein isn't a major source of energy at rest or during exercise—it seldom amounts to more than 10 percent of energy needs. When one trains hard while dieting to lose weight, the body senses starvation and begins to utilize tissue protein for energy. To avoid the loss of muscle tissue and achieve the benefits of training, ensure adequate protein and **energy intake** (see chapter 13 for more on protein and energy).

ENERGY FOR CONTRACTIONS

Muscles cannot directly use carbohydrate and fat. These nutrients are processed by cellular enzymes to produce high-energy compounds that fuel muscle contractions, **adenosine triphosphate (ATP)** and phosphocreatine (PCr). When the motor nerve tells the muscle to contract, ATP is split into adenosine diphosphate to provide immediate energy for contractions (ATP → ADP + P + energy). Because the amount of stored ATP is small, it must be replenished with the splitting of PCr (ADP + PCr → ATP + Cr). Oxidation of carbohydrate and fat replenishes the limited stores of ATP and PCr.

1. Nerve impulse triggers contraction, requiring ATP to provide energy.
2. PCr splits to provide energy to resynthesize ATP.
3. Glucose (or glycogen) is broken down (glycolysis) to pyruvic acid and two ATP molecules are formed.
4. Pyruvic acid or fat is oxidized in muscle **mitochondria** to form CO_2, H_2O and energy to form 36 ATP molecules.

Steps 1, 2, and 3 are nonoxidative, or anaerobic; they do not require the presence of oxygen. Step 4 requires oxygen, so it is called aerobic. Anaerobic metabolism of glucose leads to the formation of 2 molecules of ATP, whereas the aerobic or oxidative metabolism of glucose yields 36 molecules of ATP. Aerobic metabolism is a far more efficient use of fuel.

Think of muscles as a controlled combustion chamber where the energy stored in carbohydrate and fat is slowly transferred to ATP (see figure 7.3). The key to the process are

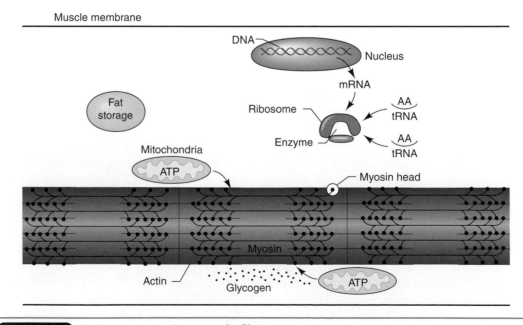

FIGURE 7.3 Basic structures in a muscle fiber.

enzymes, organic catalysts that release and transfer energy. The 6-carbon glucose molecule is systematically cleaved to form 3-carbon pyruvic acid in the pathway called glycolysis. The 3-carbon pyruvic acid molecule enters the mitochondria, where it is oxidized along with fat.

Short-Term Energy Sources

Stored ATP and PCr are good for 3 to 4 calories of energy, and can be exhausted in a few seconds of maximal effort, such as running uphill. As it is depleted, anaerobic glycolysis kicks in to produce more ATP from nonoxidative breakdown of glucose. But the anaerobic pathway is not efficient, and muscle glycogen stores are limited. The aerobic or oxidative breakdown of carbohydrate and fat provide a long-term supply of ATP. After an hour or more of vigorous effort, the muscle glycogen supply begins to decline. The muscle then gets its glucose from the blood. Blood glucose is supplied by liver glycogen stores. When that supply is depleted, the blood glucose declines, and fatigue is imminent. Muscle cannot work as hard without carbohydrate, and the brain and nervous system require carbohydrate for energy (figure 7.4).

Long-Term Energy Sources

For prolonged activity, we must use aerobic pathways. They are more efficient than anaerobic pathways, and the fuels are more abundant. Table 7.2 portrays the supply of available energy. Fat is, by far, the most abundant source of available energy, enough to run hundreds of miles. Carbohydrate stores are more limited, but they can be raised with training and diet (**carbohydrate loading**), or supplemented with solid and liquid sources during exercise.

The contribution of fat and carbohydrate varies during work. For light work, muscle uses mostly fat, supplied with muscle triglyceride and plasma free fatty acids (FFA) that are mobilized from adipose tissue and transported via the circulation. As exercise intensity

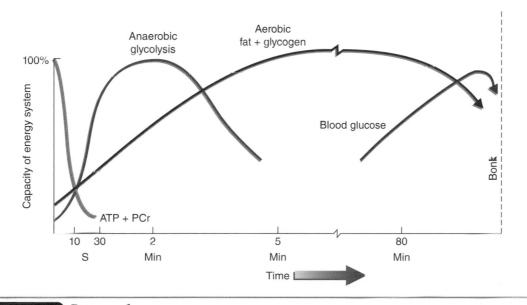

FIGURE 7.4 Pattern of energy use.

Table 7.2 Available Energy Sources

Source	Supply	Energy (kcal)	Miles*
ATP and PCr	Small amount in muscles	4–5 kcal	.045
CARBOHYDRATE			
Muscle glycogen	20 g per kg muscle	1,600	16
Liver glycogen	80 g	320	3.2
Blood glucose	4 g	16	0.16
FAT			
Muscles	Limited, varies with training	1,500	15
Adipose tissue	Variable**	30,000–70,000	300–700

*Assume 100 kcal/mile and all energy in working muscles.

**Depends on body weight and % body fat: 10% fat × 150 lb = 15 lb fat × 3,500 kcal/lb = 52,500 kcal.

PCr = phosphocreatine

Adapted, by permission, from B.J. Sharkey and S.E. Gaskill, 2006, *Sport physiology for coaches* (Champaign, IL: Human Kinetics), 126.

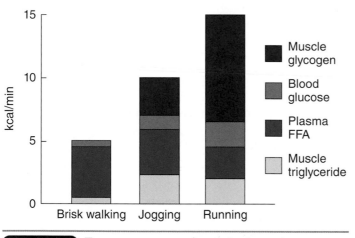

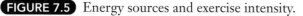

FIGURE 7.5 Energy sources and exercise intensity.

increases, carbohydrate use also increases, becoming predominant at high levels of effort (figure 7.5).

A small amount of fat is stored in muscle. This muscle triglyceride may be increased with endurance training. During long-duration effort, fat utilization increases with time. Fat mobilization from adipose tissue is delayed in the first half hour of exercise. But as the activity continues, fat use increases. Training increases fat utilization, with early supplies coming from muscle triglyceride (Holloszy et al. 1986). As training improves fat utilization, it spares utilization of limited muscle and liver glycogen, an important factor in work or sport.

Long-Term Energy Sources Require Oxygen

Oxygen is the key to aerobic exercise. When you can't supply sufficient oxygen to the muscles, you are forced to use inefficient anaerobic pathways and limited sources of energy, such as ATP, PCr, and glycogen. When you begin to exercise, **oxygen intake** does not immediately meet the demand. An **oxygen deficit** results as you rely on ATP, PCr, and anaerobic glycolysis (leading to the formation of lactic acid). When oxygen intake begins to meet the demand, a steady state is achieved. Exercise can continue so long as you are able to meet the fuel and oxygen requirements. After exercise, oxygen intake returns slowly to resting levels. Recovery oxygen intake in excess of resting needs is called the **oxygen debt**. The debt, or **excess post-exercise oxygen consumption (EPOC)**, is used to repay the oxygen deficit, to replace ATP and PCr, to remove lactic acid, and to replace some of the energy used during the exercise (figure 7.6).

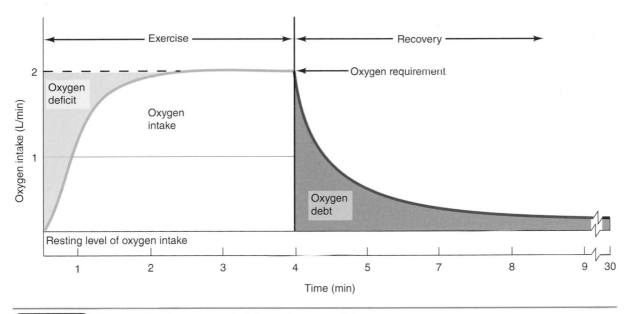

FIGURE 7.6 Oxygen intake, oxygen deficit, and oxygen debt.

Oxygen is the key to prolonged activity. The ability to take in, transport, and utilize oxygen in muscles, or aerobic fitness, is essential for the performance of physically demanding tasks. Let's see how the respiratory and cardiovascular systems carry oxygen and energy to working muscles.

SUPPLY AND SUPPORT SYSTEMS

The respiratory and cardiovascular systems and, to a degree, the hormonal (endocrine) system function as supply and support systems for working muscles. The respiratory system takes air into the lungs and allows the transport of oxygen to red blood cells in the circulation. The cardiovascular system transports blood to the heart and then to the muscles, where oxygen and energy are utilized. The muscles produce by-products such as carbon dioxide, lactic acid, and heat, which are transported from the muscle by the circulation. Carbon dioxide is eliminated during exhalation, lactic acid is buffered or used as a fuel by other muscle fibers, and heat is dissipated through the **evaporation** of sweat.

Respiratory System

Respiration has two main functions: getting oxygen into the body and getting rid of carbon dioxide. **Ventilation (V)**, the amount of air you breathe per minute, is the product of respiratory rate (or frequency: f) and the volume of air per breath (**tidal volume**, or TV), so $V = f \times TV$. The ventilation during prolonged hard work ranges from 40 to 60 liters per minute (40 L = 20 × 2 L), well below the ventilation of maximal effort ($V = 120$ L/min = 40 × 3 L). Fit workers have a lower frequency and larger tidal volume, so their respiration is more efficient. The ventilation during a maximal oxygen intake test is well below the maximal ventilatory volume (MVV = 180 L/min). The healthy respiratory system is overbuilt for its job. Unfortunately, age reduces that margin, especially in those who elect to remain sedentary.

When the diaphragm contracts, it creates an area of lower pressure, causing air to rush into the lungs. When air reaches the tiny air sacs called **alveoli**, oxygen crosses the alveolar and capillary membranes and hitches a ride on **hemoglobin (Hb)** attached to red blood cells (figure 7.7). Under favorable conditions, **hemoglobin saturation** with oxygen is about 97 percent of the available space. As one goes up in altitude and the oxygen concentration and barometric pressure falls, the hemoglobin saturation declines. The respiratory system joins with the kidneys and **buffers** in the blood to control the acid–base balance, which can be disturbed with acid by-products during very vigorous effort, especially in untrained workers.

Cardiovascular System

We have followed oxygen from the atmosphere to the blood. Now let us see how it gets to the muscles. The blood serves to transport oxygen and carbon dioxide as well as fuels, waste products, hormones, antibodies, and heat. Blood buffers (hemoglobin, buffer systems, and protein molecules) help to regulate the acid–base balance. Your 5 liters of blood contains about 5 million red cells per cubic millimeter! The hemoglobin on red cells uses iron to carry oxygen, and the healthy diet must include sufficient iron to avoid anemia. One important outcome of endurance training is a 10 to 15 percent increase in blood volume, which aids oxygen delivery, endurance performance, and the ability to tolerate hot working conditions. The increase in blood volume also aids the efficiency of the cardiac pump (see figure 7.8).

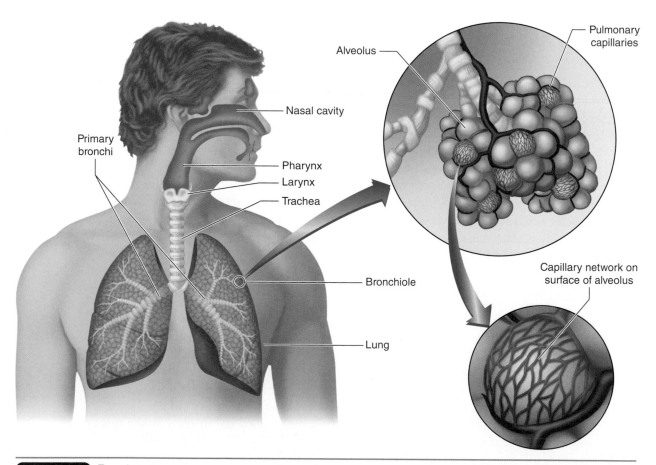

FIGURE 7.7 Respiratory system.

Reprinted, by permission, from W.L. Kenney, J.H. Wilmore, and D.L. Costill, 2012, *Physiology of sport and exercise*, 5th ed. (Champaign, IL; Human Kinetics), 165.

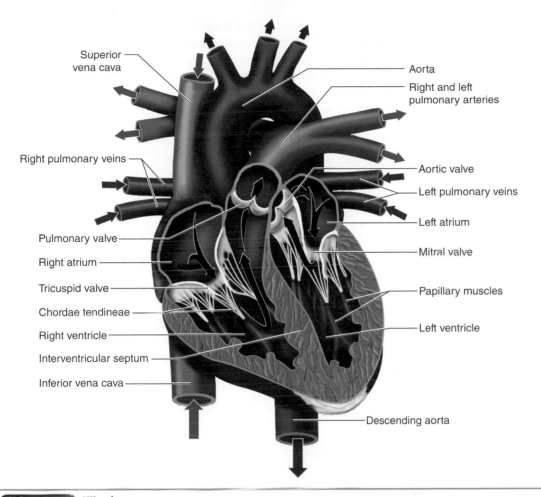

Superior vena cava

Aorta

Right and left pulmonary arteries

Right pulmonary veins

Aortic valve

Left pulmonary veins

Left atrium

Pulmonary valve

Mitral valve

Right atrium

Tricuspid valve

Papillary muscles

Chordae tendineae

Left ventricle

Right ventricle

Interventricular septum

Inferior vena cava

Descending aorta

FIGURE 7.8 The heart.

Reprinted, by permission, from W.L. Kenney, J.H. Wilmore, and D.L. Costill, 2012, *Physiology of sport and exercise*, 5th ed. (Champaign, IL; Human Kinetics), 141.

The heart is the ultimate endurance muscle, amply supplied with mitochondria for oxygen utilization. It has a well-developed system of blood vessels (coronary arteries) for delivery of oxygen and fuel to cardiac muscle. The heart consists of two pumps: the right side, which sends blood to the lungs, and the left side, which pumps blood through the rest of the body (figure 7.8).

The output of the cardiac pump depends on two factors: the beating rate of the pump (heart rate, HR) and the volume per stroke (stroke volume, SV).

$$\text{Cardiac output} = \text{HR} \times \text{SV}$$

With a resting HR of 72 beats per minute (bpm) and a stroke volume of 70 milliliters, the **cardiac output (Q)** is about 5 liters of blood per minute. Heart rate increases with work rate ($\dot{V}O_2$). Figure 7.9*a* illustrates the rise in heart rate for untrained and trained people. Figure 7.9*b* shows how stroke volume responds for the untrained and trained. It is clear that the trained worker has a larger stroke volume, allowing a much larger cardiac output and a much greater supply of oxygen to the muscles during exertion.

The coronary arteries receive blood when it is pumped from the left side of the heart (figure 7.10). When the arteries are narrowed with atherosclerosis, the heart is compromised and is at risk for a heart attack (myocardial infarction). For sedentary people, the risk rises more than 50 times during exertion. Aerobic fitness training lowers the risk of heart disease from 30 to 70 percent, depending on the degree of activity. Those who acquire as many as 3,500 kilocalories of exercise per week achieve the greatest reduction. For example, if you burn 100 calories walking or running a mile (1.6 km), you would have to do 5 miles (8 km) a day, 7 days a week to achieve the maximum reduction in cardiovascular risk.

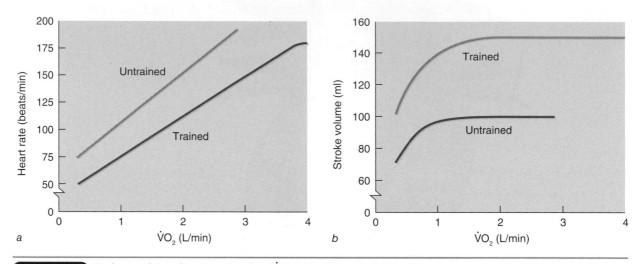

FIGURE 7.9 Relationship of oxygen intake ($\dot{V}O_2$) to HR and SV: (*a*) Rise in heart rate for trained and untrained people, (*b*) stroke volume response for trained and untrained people.

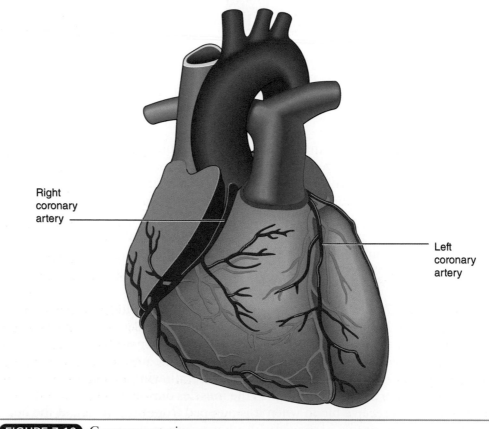

FIGURE 7.10 Coronary arteries.

Endocrine System

The hormones of the endocrine system can be viewed as part of the support system for muscles. Several hormones can increase blood glucose levels (glucagon, epinephrine, norepinephrine, and cortisol), but insulin is the only one that can move glucose into the muscle. Fortunately, glucose is able to enter muscle during physical activity, even in the absence of insulin. That is one reason why physical activity and diet are important components of treatment for diabetes. Physical training improves insulin sensitivity, requiring less insulin to do its work. Hormones are also involved in mobilization of fat from adipose tissue during exercise and the conservation of body water during exercise in the heat. Growth hormone promotes growth of bone and muscle and the use of fat for energy (thereby sparing glycogen and glucose).

GENETIC RESPONSES TO EXERCISE

When you engage in an exercise, such as jogging or lifting weights, at a level above your normal daily activity (load), you **overload** the muscles and their support systems, including the heart and lungs. If you repeat the exercise regularly (e.g., every other day), your body begins to adapt to the overload imposed by the exercise. We call the adaptations *the training effect*. How does exercise signal muscle fibers and support systems to undergo changes that will permit more exercise in the future? The answer lies in the genes and DNA.

Genes influence potential, but they don't assure it. The 30,000 genes that form the blueprint of the human body are subject to the influence of the environment and behavior. Your **genotype** is your genetic constitution, while the **phenotype** is the observable appearance resulting from the interaction of the genotype and the environment. In sport, genetic potential can only be realized when genes are switched on through the process of training. Genes carry the code for the formation of proteins. When a specific type of training is performed, it turns on a promoter that activates specific genes. Through a process called *transcription*, an RNA strand is formed on the template made up of the gene's DNA. The RNA becomes the messenger (mRNA) that exits the nucleus, enters the cytoplasm, and binds to a **ribosome**, whose function is to synthesize protein. The mRNA translates the genetic code into a sequence of amino acids to form a specific protein. Transfer RNA (tRNA) reads the mRNA blueprint and then captures appropriate amino acids for use in the synthesis of the desired protein. Without training, genetically gifted people cannot achieve success in sport. But heredity is much more complicated than genes, DNA, and RNA.

The genetic response to a specific form of training resides in a cluster of genes, and each can be influenced by the presence or absence of so-called enhancers, regulatory elements that influence the degree of response. That helps to explain why the individual response to identical training is so variable. Factors that may influence the response to training could include maturation (hormones), nutrition (energy, amino acids), adequate rest, and even chemically related emotional factors such as stress (other hormones).

Endurance training leads to an increase in the concentration of oxidative enzymes and to a rise in the size, quality, and number of mitochondria, the cellular power plants where all oxidative metabolism takes place (Hood et al. 2000). These particular adaptations are specific to endurance training, and they take place only in the muscles used in training. Endurance training also improves the function of respiratory muscles and the heart, and it increases the blood volume, which improves the **stroke volume** and cardiac output. The rise in blood volume helps explain why the resting and exercise heart rates decline with training.

With a greater blood volume and blood redistributed from other regions (e.g., the digestive system), more blood enters the heart and is pumped out with each beat. So, you can do the same work with a lower heart rate (and larger stroke volume). A large portion of the enhanced cardiovascular function of endurance athletes is due to the training-induced increase in blood volume and its effect on cardiac function, increased hemoglobin and stroke volume, and decreased heart rate and blood viscosity (Gledhill, Warburton, and Jamnik 1999). Training-induced changes in blood volume account for almost half of the improvements in $\dot{V}O_2$max with training: The results are similar for continuous or interval training (Warburton et al. 2004).

Strength training leads to the production of contractile proteins, actin and myosin. Other specific effects of strength training include an increase in muscle mass and a toughening of connective tissue (see figure 7.11). With training, we learn to exert force more effectively. Core training to strengthen back and abdominal muscles contributes to performance and a lower risk of musculoskeletal injury (see chapter 11). Since aerobic and muscular fitness training lead to the production of proteins, both forms depend on a diet adequate in energy and protein.

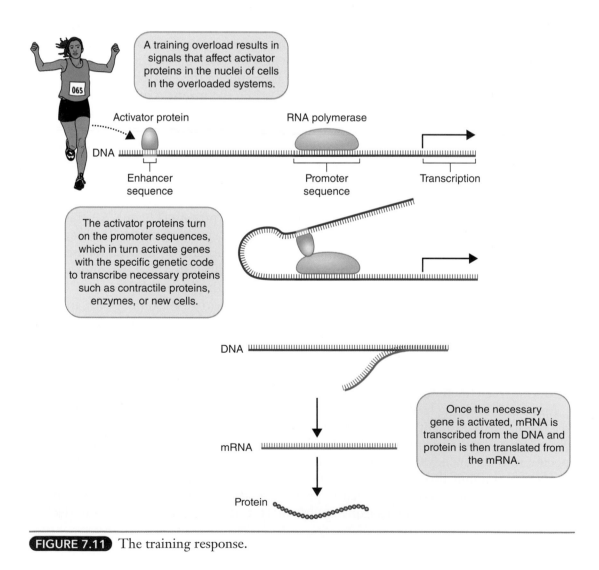

FIGURE 7.11 The training response.

SUMMARY

This chapter provides a brief understanding of the structure and function of muscle fibers and the energy sources used for contractions. Understanding is the key to knowledge. A basic knowledge of exercise physiology should help you understand the complex interactions between training and fitness. Individualized fitness programs require an understanding of the physiology of fitness.

This chapter also explains the essential roles of fat and carbohydrate as the primary sources of energy for prolonged exertion. The reason why we burn more fat at a lower intensity and turn to carbohydrate for vigorous effort should now be clear. Ultimately, oxygen is needed for all energy metabolism, even to metabolize the by-products of **anaerobic** (nonoxidative) metabolism. The respiratory, cardiovascular, and endocrine systems all work together to deliver oxygen to working muscle and to control energy utilization and movement. Finally, this chapter describes the important mechanisms by which training improves the function of muscles and support systems.

You need to understand that training is specific. If you train for aerobic fitness, you synthesize enzyme protein that improves your ability to use oxygen. If you train for strength, you synthesize contractile proteins that improve your ability to exert muscle force. Training-induced adaptations take place in the muscles utilized in training. You cannot train arm muscles to improve leg endurance, or vice versa. Train the muscles you will need for the activity or sport. Now it is time to learn more about aerobic fitness (chapter 8) and muscular fitness (chapter 9).

Aerobic Fitness

Stamina and Efficiency

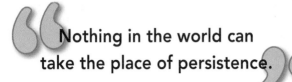

" Nothing in the world can take the place of persistence. "

Calvin Coolidge

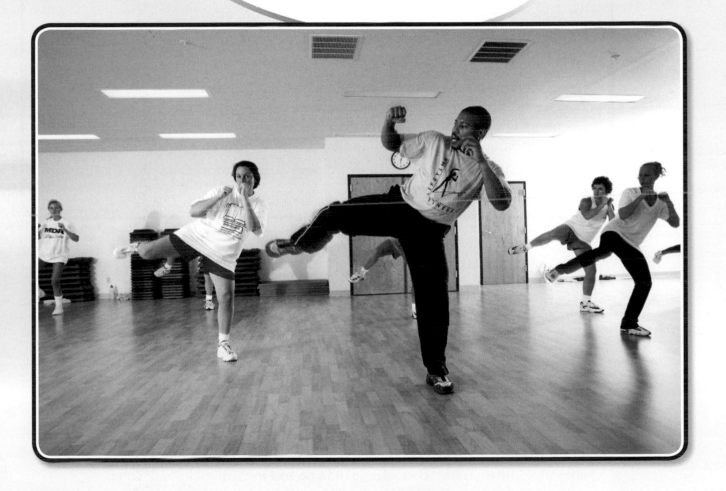

Aerobic fitness is synonymous with endurance, or stamina. It describes the ability, part inherited and part trained, to persevere or persist in prolonged endeavors. Those who pursue fitness earn far more than enhanced health and performance. For many, the process becomes more important than the goal, providing discipline, challenge, and time for reflection. For the moment, we'll consider the physiology of fitness; later, we'll ponder how fitness affects performance in work and sport.

This chapter will help you do the following:

- Understand the terms *aerobic* and *anaerobic*
- Determine the meaning of aerobic exercise and aerobic fitness
- Experience the concept of exercise intensity and the **lactate thresholds**
- Differentiate between aerobic and anaerobic effort
- Understand the factors that influence aerobic fitness
- Define the effects of aerobic training
- Understand how systematic exercise (training) stimulates changes in muscle fibers, respiration and oxygen transport, blood volume, the heart and circulation, the endocrine system, fat metabolism and body composition, and bones, ligaments, and **tendons**
- Understand the **specificity** of training and its importance for the design of effective programs

---

AEROBIC EXERCISE

To learn about **aerobic exercise**, dress for exercise, warm up, and head out at a walking pace. Increase the pace a little as each minute passes, going from a slow to a fast walk. As you approach 5 miles (8 km) per hour (12 min/mi, or 7.5 min/km), you'll feel the need to jog. Continue to increase your speed gradually until the effort becomes uncomfortable and breathing becomes labored, and you doubt your ability to continue. As you increase your intensity from easy to hard, you have moved from aerobic exercise, which means exercise in the presence of oxygen, to exercise that relies increasingly on anaerobic, or nonoxidative, energy production. During aerobic exercise, energy comes from the oxidation of fat and carbohydrate. If you continue to increase the intensity of exercise, the muscles gradually make a transition to anaerobic energy production, which involves intense effort of necessarily short duration and accumulation of lactic acid in the muscles and blood.

Lactic acid is both an energy carrier and a metabolic by-product of intense effort. Its accumulation is a sign that you are using energy faster than your body can produce it aerobically. Too much lactic acid interferes with the contractile and metabolic capabilities of the muscles. Lactic acid and the high levels of carbon dioxide produced in vigorous effort are associated with labored breathing, fatigue, and discomfort. Aerobic exercise can be defined as exercise below the point at which blood–lactic acid levels rise—the lactate

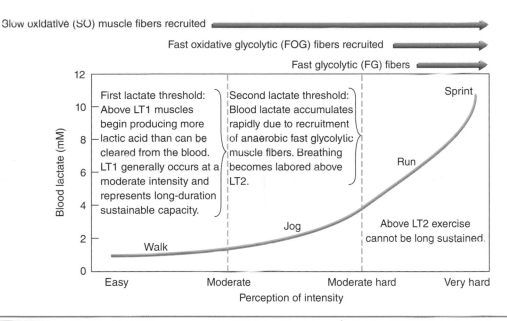

FIGURE 8.1 Lactate thresholds. As exercise intensity (percent $\dot{V}O_2max$) increases, we continually recruit additional slow, oxidative (SO) fibers, fast, oxidative-glycolytic (FOG) fibers, and, finally, fast, glycolytic (FG) fibers. Above LT1, and especially above LT2, more blood lactate accumulates because FG fibers produce more lactic acid and because most muscle fibers are active and therefore unable to remove (take up) lactate.

threshold (see figure 8.1). In simple terms, aerobic exercise includes all large-muscle activities that you can comfortably sustain for 15 minutes or more.

Aerobic metabolism is far more efficient than anaerobic metabolism, yielding 38 molecules of adenosine triphosphate (ATP), the high-energy compound that fuels muscular contractions, per molecule of glucose, versus only 2 molecules of ATP through anaerobic metabolism. Because it produces little lactic acid, aerobic exercise is relatively pleasant and relaxing, not painful. The oxidation of abundant fat reserves during aerobic exercise ensures an adequate supply of energy for extended periods of effort. You can sustain aerobic exercise for several minutes to many hours, and you can carry on a conversation during moderate aerobic exercise.

Stored fat (triglycerides) and carbohydrate are the fuels for aerobic exercise. As exercise intensity increases, we move from reliance on fat during low-intensity exercise to increasing use of carbohydrate at higher intensities of effort. Carbohydrate produces 50 percent of ATP during easy effort. At the **first lactate threshold**, carbohydrate produces 75 percent of ATP, and at the second lactate threshold, 100 percent of ATP comes from carbohydrate oxidation (see figure 8.1).

Aerobic and **anaerobic exercises** differ in intensity; light to moderate activity is aerobic, whereas extremely vigorous or intense effort is anaerobic. Table 8.1 illustrates how heart rate and breathing increase with exercise intensity, and how we switch from burning fat to carbohydrate as exercise becomes more vigorous. The table also shows how the nervous system recruits different **muscle-fiber types** as the effort becomes more intense.

Humans have three main types of muscle fibers: slow-twitch (slow, oxidative, or SO) fibers that are efficient in the use of oxygen; a faster-contracting type that can work with oxygen or without (fast, oxidative-glycolytic, or FOG); and a fast-twitch fiber that uses

The oxidation of abundant fat reserves during aerobic exercise ensures an adequate supply of energy for extended periods of effort.

muscle glycogen for short, intense contractions (fast, glycolytic, or FG) without oxygen. As we go from a walk to a jog to a run, we sequentially recruit SO, FOG, and then FG fibers to help us go faster. If we recruit too many FG fibers, the effort becomes anaerobic. The fibers produce lactic acid, and we are forced to slow down or stop.

Table 8.1 Levels of Exercise Intensity

Component	EXERCISE INTENSITY		
	Light	Moderate	Intense
Example exercise	Walking	Jogging	Running
Metabolism*	Aerobic	Aerobic	Aerobic and anaerobic
Energy source*	Fat > CHO	CHO > fat	Mostly CHO
Heart rate**	<120	120–150	>150
Breathing*	Easy	Can talk easily	Hard to talk
Muscle fiber recruited	SO	SO + FOG	SO + FOG + FG

CHO = carbohydrate
SO = slow oxidative fibers
FG = fast glycolytic fibers
FOG = fast oxidative glycolytic fibers
*Depends on fitness
**Depends on age and fitness

Endurance

A biologist friend who has studied locomotion throughout the animal kingdom has noted that when it comes to running short distances, humans are inferior to other species. Cheetahs, gazelles, antelopes, horses, camels, and even grizzly bears are much faster than humans. But as the distance increases, the human becomes more competitive, and at long distances, human endurance qualities stand out. Unfortunately, this superiority emerges only at distances few are willing to negotiate. When a proud Montana horseman bragged about the endurance and speed of his Arabian, a local physician wagered that he could outrun the horse over a mountainous marathon course (26.2 mi, or 42.2 km). Perhaps the distance wasn't long enough, because the horse finished 16 minutes ahead of the physician. Another factor may have been that however fit, the 49-year-old physician was slightly past his prime, whereas the horse was not.

We have ample evidence that humans are able to run extremely long distances. The Tarahumara Indians of Mexico run more than 100 miles (161 km) on mountain trails while kicking a small ball, and runners throughout the world do 100-mile footraces, sometimes over difficult mountain terrain. Early in the 20th century, crowds flocked to big cities to watch 6-day races in which athletes ran as far as they could. Today, the 6-day record is well over 635 miles (1,022 km), for an average of 106 miles (171 km) per day! In spite of the publicity given to short races and sports that emphasize bursts of speed, the human body has evolved with the capacity to accomplish prodigious feats of endurance.

AEROBIC FITNESS

Aerobic fitness, defined as the maximal capacity to take in, transport, and use oxygen, is best measured in a laboratory test called the **maximal oxygen intake** (or **$\dot{V}O_2$max**) **test**. This test defines the highest intensity of effort. Calculation requires a treadmill or other exercise device (e.g., bicycle **ergometer**), a computer, and a metabolic measurement system to measure oxygen, carbon dioxide, and the volume of expired air. After a health risk assessment, the person being tested signs an informed consent form and is fitted with ECG electrodes to monitor the heart and measure heart rate.

After a brief warm-up, the person begins the test wearing a mask or mouthpiece to direct the expired air into the analyzer. The test involves increasing intensity of exercise, starting at an easy rate and grade, with increases every minute or two. Oxygen intake is computed each minute as the test proceeds toward maximal effort. The test ends when oxygen intake levels off in spite of increased treadmill rate or grade, or when the person can no longer keep up with the treadmill. The highest level of oxygen used is called the **maximal oxygen intake ($\dot{V}O_2$max)**, or peak aerobic fitness.

The $\dot{V}O_2$max test signifies the maximum volume (V) of oxygen (O_2) used. The test takes between 8 and 12 minutes, and uses either metabolic measurements to measure oxygen intake or a table to estimate the value. The protocol should allow the test to be tailored to the subject's level of fitness and previous training. The test should be specific to the person's activity—a treadmill for runners and a bicycle ergometer for cyclists. The test can be conducted on any **mode** of aerobic exercise. Our example focuses on the treadmill.

Measure oxygen intake or use the final rate and grade on the treadmill to estimate $\dot{V}O_2$max (see table 8.2). For example, if the last minute of the test was at 6 miles (9.7 km) per hour and 10 percent grade, the aerobic fitness estimate is 50 milliliters of oxygen per kilogram of body weight per minute. The person being tested should not hold on to the railing of the treadmill if the intention is to estimate the maximal value. Holding on to the railing reduces the workload and overestimates the estimation of oxygen uptake.

Scores in the range of 3 to 4 liters of oxygen per minute are typical, and values of 5 to 6 liters have been reported for endurance athletes. When reported in liters per minute (called **aerobic capacity**), the score provides information about the total capacity of the cardiorespiratory systems and is a predictor of endurance performance in non-weight-bearing sports (e.g., cycling, rowing). But because this value is related to body size, larger people tend to have higher scores.

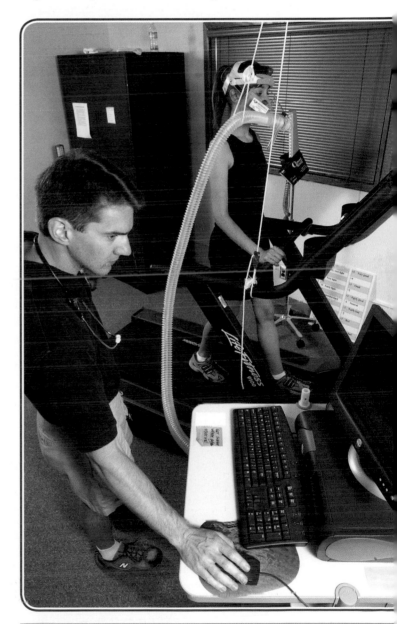

■ The $\dot{V}O_2$max test measures the maximal capacity to take in, transport, and use oxygen.

Table 8.2　Estimating V̇O₂max From Treadmill Test: Approximate Oxygen Intake Required for Final Rate and Grade Combinations*

Miles (km) per hour	GRADE				
	8%	10%	12%	14%	15%
WALK					
3.0 (4.8 km)	22	26	30	34	37
3.5 (5.6 km)	24	29	34	39	43
4.0 (6.4 km)	26	32	38	44	48
RUN					
6.0 (9.7 km)	47	50	53	56	59
7.0 (11.3 km)	54	58	61	65	69
8.0 (12.9 km)	62	66	70	74	78

*ml · kg⁻¹ · min⁻¹, varies with efficiency

To eliminate the influence of body size, the maximal oxygen intake score in liters (1 L = 1,000 ml) is divided by the body weight in kilograms (1 kg = 2.2 lb). In this example, maximal oxygen intake score is 3 liters (3,000 ml), and body weight is 60 kilograms (132 lb):

$$3 \text{ L/min} \div 60 \text{ kg} = 50 \text{ ml} \cdot \text{kg}^{-1} \cdot \text{min}^{-1}$$

The resulting value allows direct comparison of different people regardless of body size. This measure, also known as **aerobic power**, is more related to endurance performance in running and other weight-bearing sports, and it is the preferred way to express **maximal aerobic fitness**. If two people have the same score in liters, which one is more fit, the one who weighs 60 kilograms (132 lb) or the other who weighs 100 kilograms (220 lb)? Divide the score for the latter by the respective body weight:

$$3 \text{ L/min} \div 100 \text{ kg} = 30 \text{ ml} \cdot \text{kg}^{-1} \cdot \text{min}^{-1}$$

In a footrace, the one with a score of 50 would be better able to take in, transport, and use oxygen in the working muscles than the one with the score of 30. The average young male (18 to 25 years old) scores 42 to 45 milliliters per kilogram of body weight per minute, and the average young female scores 39 to 41. Active men score in the 50s and 60s, and similarly active women in the 40s and 50s. Male endurance athletes achieve measurements in the 80s, and top female athletes are not far behind with scores in the 70s (see table 8.3). Although average values decline with age, as much as 8 to 10 percent per decade in sedentary populations, regular activity cuts the rate of decline in half (4%–5% per decade), and aerobic training can cut that rate in half again (2%–3% per decade).

Historically, the aerobic fitness score (V̇O₂max) was viewed as the best measure of fitness and was believed to be correlated to health. As more has been learned about aerobic fitness, other aerobic fitness measures such as the lactate thresholds have emerged as better correlates to endurance and performance in work and sport. The maximal oxygen intake test, or V̇O₂max test, which uses the highest score attained, is a test of **exercise intensity**, best correlated to events lasting 5 to 15 minutes.

Table 8.3 Aerobic Fitness Comparison

Subjects	Age	Men (ml · kg^{-1} · min^{-1})	Women (ml · kg^{-1} · min^{-1})
Untrained	18–22	43	38
Active	18–22	50	43
Trained	18–22	57	53
Elite	18–22	70	63
World class	18–22	≥80	≥70
Untrained	40–50	36	27
Active	40–50	46	39
Trained	40–50	52	44
Elite	40–50	≥60	≥50

As exercise intensity increases from easy to moderately hard, aerobic metabolism shifts from primarily using fat to a greater reliance on carbohydrate to provide the energy for metabolism. The first lactate threshold (LT1) is defined as the intensity of aerobic exercise at which blood lactate begins to increase. The intensity at which this occurs is generally defined as moderate. It is associated with the highest intensity that a person can comfortably sustain for an hour or more. This threshold defines the point at which lactic acid begins to accumulate in the blood more rapidly than it can be removed. The first lactate threshold is an excellent indicator of performance in aerobic events lasting more than 3 hours. This threshold also defines what we call *sustainable aerobic fitness*—the intensity that people can sustain for long periods. The first lactate threshold is an important measure of aerobic fitness (see figure 8.1).

Laboratory tests can identify LT1 by drawing blood samples during each stage of an incremental exercise test and then analyzing the blood for lactate levels. During easy to moderate intensities, blood lactate will remain level, since the blood clears the lactate as quickly as it is produced. After LT1 is reached, blood-lactate concentrations begin to increase gradually until the second lactate threshold is reached, where blood lactate increases more rapidly. Ventilatory measurements during the exercise test permit a less invasive measure of LT1. Several methods can be used to select LT1 through respiratory measurements. Most exercise laboratories or clinical centers are able to perform these measurements.

The second lactate threshold can also be estimated using respiratory data. The **respiratory compensation point**, defined as the point at which ventilation (air in L/min) rises disproportionably to increasing work, corresponds to LT2. This point is also referred to as breakaway ventilation. This rapid rise in ventilation (respiratory rate and depth) provides a perceptible signal, indicating that the person is flirting with excess anaerobic effort and exhaustion, and should ease off. Perceptive people learn to listen to the information that their bodies provide during exertion.

The second lactate threshold is a better indicator of endurance performance than aerobic fitness ($\dot{V}O_2$max) in events such as a 10K road race. The threshold indicates the oxygen-using capabilities of the muscles. Chapter 10 shows you how to use the thresholds

Dimensions of Aerobic Fitness

Aerobic fitness has three important dimensions. Each has its own value, and a single treadmill test can determine all of them (see table 8.4).

The first lactate threshold defines the level of effort that a person can sustain for prolonged periods. Expressed as a percentage of $\dot{V}O_2$max, it may be low or high, depending on the person's level of activity and training. People can increase all dimensions of aerobic fitness by training according to the principles presented in chapters 10 and 14.

Table 8.4   Dimensions of Aerobic Fitness

Measurement	Value	Predicted event duration
$\dot{V}O_2$max	Maximal aerobic power	Events lasting 5 to 15 min (1 to 3 mi, or 1.6 to 4.8 km)
Second lactate threshold (LT2)	Medium duration aerobic power	Events lasting 30 min to 3 hr (10K to marathon)
First lactate threshold (LT1)	Sustainable aerobic fitness	Prolonged work or sport (4 hr or longer)

in an aerobic training program, and chapter 14 shows you how to use the thresholds in training for competition.

Is a high aerobic fitness score the product of heredity or training? How much can training influence fitness? How do other factors such as sex, age, and body fat influence your attainable level of fitness? The following sections cover factors that positively and negatively influence aerobic fitness.

Heredity

Achieving high-level endurance performances requires tremendous natural endowment and years of systematic training. Researchers who studied differences in aerobic fitness among fraternal (dizygotic) and identical (monozygotic) twins found that intrapair differences were far greater among fraternal twins than among identical twins. The largest difference between identical twins was smaller than the smallest difference between fraternal pairs (Klissouras 1976). Bouchard and colleagues (1999) estimated that heredity accounts for 47 percent or more of the variance in $\dot{V}O_2$max values, and Sundet, Magnus, and Tambs (1994) contend that more than half of the variance in maximal aerobic power is due to genotypic differences, with the remainder accounted for by environmental factors (nutrition, training). This finding supports the notion that one way to become a world-class endurance athlete is to pick your parents carefully, especially your mother, because maternal transmission accounts for almost 60 percent of the inherited component (Bouchard et al. 1999)!

One way to become a world-class endurance athlete is to pick your parents carefully.

Having talented parents may help you achieve elite athlete status, but training will dictate how close you get to your potential. In a training study, 80 percent of the improvements in ventilatory threshold (LT1) were due to training, with the remaining 20 percent related to familial or genetic influences (Gaskill et al. 2001). Genes play an important role in how sustainable fitness responds to training, but the majority of the effects are due to training.

We inherit many factors that are important to aerobic fitness, including the capacity of the respiratory and cardiovascular systems, the size of the heart, the number of red blood cells and hemoglobin, and the percentage of oxidative (SO and FOG) muscle fibers. Mitochondria, the energy-producing units of muscle and other cells, are inherited from the maternal side. Studies indicate that the capacity of muscle to respond to training is also inherited, with improvements in aerobic fitness ranging from 5 percent to more than 30 percent (Bouchard et al. 1988). Other inherited factors, such as physique and body composition, also influence the potential to perform at a high level.

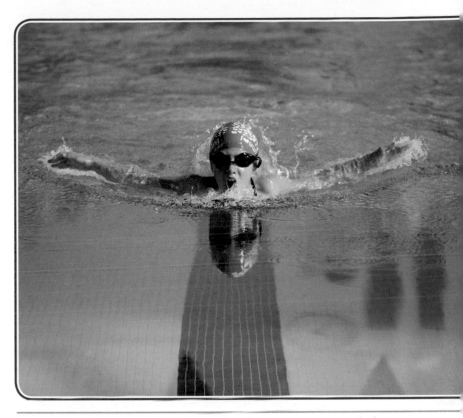

■ Although heredity influences aerobic fitness, training can help you reach your potential.

Training

The potential to improve aerobic fitness ($\dot{V}O_2$max) with training is limited. While most studies confirm the potential to improve 20 to 25 percent (more with loss of body fat), only adolescents can hope to improve much more than 30 percent. Consider two people, one with an untrained $\dot{V}O_2$max of 40 milliliters per kilogram per minute and the other with a score of 60. Let us assume that heredity accounts for the difference in scores. What happens if each trains and gains a 25 percent improvement in $\dot{V}O_2$max?

$$40 \text{ ml} \cdot \text{kg}^{-1} \cdot \text{min}^{-1} \text{ increased } 25\% = 40 + 10 = 50 \text{ ml} \cdot \text{kg}^{-1} \cdot \text{min}^{-1}$$

$$60 \text{ ml} \cdot \text{kg}^{-1} \cdot \text{min}^{-1} \text{ increased } 25\% = 60 + 15 = 75 \text{ ml} \cdot \text{kg}^{-1} \cdot \text{min}^{-1}$$

Training raises the first person above the average for young men, whereas the second person rises to the level of elite endurance athletes. Even in an untrained state, the second person has a higher $\dot{V}O_2$max than the first person does when trained. Whoever said that life was fair?

Training improves the function and capacity of the respiratory and cardiovascular systems and boosts blood volume. However, the most important changes take place in the muscle fibers used in the training. Aerobic training improves the ability of the muscles to produce energy aerobically and metabolize fat. Training makes muscle an efficient furnace for the combustion of fat, producing perhaps the single most important health benefit of regular exercise. Burning fat reduces fat storage, blood fat levels, and cardiovascular risk, and it improves insulin sensitivity and reduces the risk of diabetes. This fat metabolism may

Training makes muscle an efficient furnace for the combustion of fat, producing perhaps the single most important health benefit of regular exercise.

also contribute to a lower risk of some cancers. Of course, training enhances the ability to perform, but the improvement is limited to the activity used in training. Long-duration training will increase LT1, and higher-intensity effort will raise LT2. We'll say more about the specificity of training in later chapters.

Sex

Before puberty, boys and girls differ little in aerobic fitness, but from then on, girls fall behind. Young women average 10 to 20 percent less in aerobic fitness compared with young men, depending on their level of activity. But highly trained young female endurance athletes are only 10 percent below elite males in $\dot{V}O_2$max and performance times. One reason for the difference between sexes may be hemoglobin, the oxygen-carrying compound found in red blood cells. Men average about 2 grams more hemoglobin per 100 milliliters of blood (15 g versus 13 g/dl), and total hemoglobin is correlated to $\dot{V}O_2$max and endurance. On the other hand, some women have higher values than male endurance athletes do (Sharkey 1986).

Other reasons may be that women are smaller and have less muscle mass, or that women have more body fat than men on average (25%–30% versus 12.5%–17.5% for college-age women and men, respectively). Because aerobic fitness is usually reported per unit of body weight, those with more fat and less lean tissue (muscle) will have some disadvantage. Of course, a portion of the difference is sex-specific fat that is essential for reproductive function and health. For those and other reasons (e.g., osteoporosis), women shouldn't try to become too thin. We raise the issue only to explain why the average male has some advantage over the average female in aerobic fitness.

Until the 1970s, women were discouraged or even banned from competing in races longer than .5 mile (.8 km). Overprotective or prejudiced officials worried that frail females couldn't stand the strain. Today women run marathons and 100-mile (160 km) races, compete in the Ironman triathlon, and swim, ski, and cycle prodigious distances. A woman led much of the 1994 high-altitude Leadville 100-Mile Trail Run until a male Tarahumara Indian from Mexico passed her. We've learned that women are well suited for fat-burning endurance events and that some tolerate heat, cold, and other indignities as well as or better than men. Yet at the highest level, women's endurance performances remain about 10 percent behind those of the best males.

Age

Earlier we alluded to the effects of age on aerobic fitness, with a decline approaching 8 to 10 percent per decade for inactive people, regardless of their initial level of fitness (see figure 8.2). Those who decide to remain active can cut the decline in half (4%–5% per decade), and those who engage in fitness training can cut that rate in half again (2%–3% per decade).

A friend who served as a subject in many of our studies had a $\dot{V}O_2$max of 46 milliliters per kilogram per minute when he started aerobic training at age 30. His score rose to 54 in a few months and then declined slowly for three decades as he continued his active lifestyle. When retirement allowed him time for even more activity, his fitness score was 52, well above his starting point at age

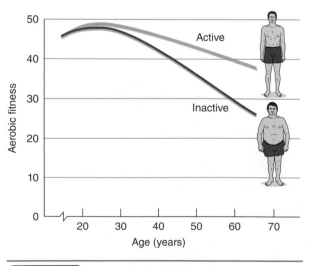

FIGURE 8.2 Age and aerobic fitness.

Adapted from B.J. Sharkey, 1997, *Fitness and work capacity*, 2nd ed. (Missoula, MT: USDA Forest Service).

30. Although trainability may decline somewhat with age, exercise gerontologist Dr. Herb deVries has shown that people can improve their fitness even after age 70 (deVries and Housh 1994). It is never too late to start. At age 81, Eula Weaver had a heart attack to add to her problems of congestive heart failure and poor circulation. Unable to walk even 100 feet (30 m) at first, she worked up to jogging a mile (1.6 km) each day and riding her stationary bicycle for several more. She even lifted weights several days a week. At age 85, she won the gold medal for the mile run in her age group at the Senior Olympics. We say more about age and performance in chapter 6.

Body Fat

Remember that fitness is calculated per unit of body weight, so if fat increases, aerobic fitness declines. About half the decline in fitness with age can be attributed to an increase in body fat. So the easiest way to maintain or even improve fitness is to get rid of excess fat. For example, if Bob, at 100 kilograms (220 lb) and 20 percent fat, loses 10 kilograms (22 lb), or half his body fat, his aerobic fitness score will go from this:

$$4 \text{ L} / 100 \text{ kg} = 40 \text{ ml} \cdot \text{kg}^{-1} \cdot \text{min}^{-1}$$

to this:

$$4 \text{ L} / 90 \text{ kg} = 44.4 \text{ ml} \cdot \text{kg}^{-1} \cdot \text{min}^{-1}$$

Without any exercise, just weight loss, his fitness, both maximal and submaximal, has improved 10 percent! Now, if he earns an additional 20 percent improvement from training, his fitness could rise above 53 milliliters per kilogram per minute ($44.4 \times 20\% = 8.88$ ml $\cdot$ kg^{-1} $\cdot$ min^{-1} + $44.4 = 53.3$). Unlikely? Not at all. Our old friend Ernie smoked two

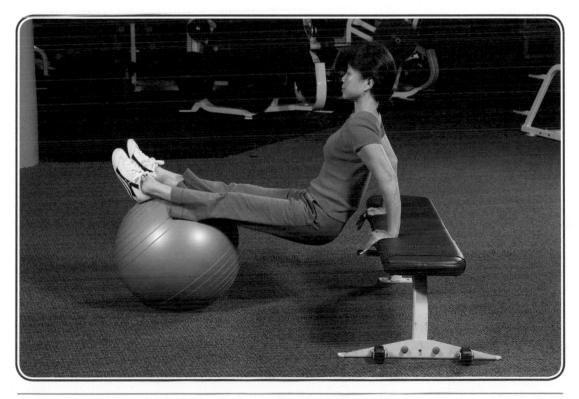

■ What you do day after day shapes your health and vitality.

Relative Fitness Comparison

Aerobic training is the process of doing the best we can with what we are given. One way to monitor progress is to use a concept called **relative fitness**—the percentage of maximal aerobic capacity that you can sustain. As people become more fit, they can sustain a higher percentage of their maximal capacity. Relative fitness shows what percentage of $\dot{V}O_2$max people can sustain for events of different duration. This can be defined using either LT1 or LT2 in comparison with $\dot{V}O_2$max. As you train, both $\dot{V}O_2$max and your thresholds tend to increase. As your training program continues past several months, $\dot{V}O_2$max will plateau, while improvements in submaximal fitness (LT1 and LT2) will continue. The closer your threshold values are to your maximal value, the more effective your training has been. Table 8.5 shows typical values for relative fitness. Over the course of training, the intensity gradually increased from 50 percent to 85 percent of $\dot{V}O_2$max.

A surprising finding in a large study of sedentary people was that many of the older participants had high relative fitness values, whereas some of the younger participants, including a number with $\dot{V}O_2$max values greater than 50 milliliters per kilogram per minute, had low relative fitness (Gaskill et al. 2001). Because all these people had low levels of activity, they had similar relative fitness scores. Relative fitness is calculated by dividing $\dot{V}O_2$ at the first lactate threshold by $\dot{V}O_2$max. For example, a genetically gifted but sedentary 21-year-old male with a $\dot{V}O_2$max of 54.5 milliliters per kilogram per minute and LT1 of 19.8 milliliters per kilogram per minute has a low relative fitness of 36 percent, whereas a 60-year-old sedentary female with a $\dot{V}O_2$max of 25.8 milliliters per kilogram per minute and a LT1 of 18.6 milliliters per kilogram per minute has a high relative fitness of 72 percent.

Relative fitness tells us what percentage of maximal capacity we can sustain. Because sedentary people require about 18 milliliters per kilogram per minute of oxygen to do tasks of daily living, they are essentially training at that level. By performing tasks of daily living, the older woman maintains her sustainable fitness at a relatively high percentage of her maximal capacity, whereas the young man is using but a low percentage of his capacity. Training will help these people increase both $\dot{V}O_2$max and sustainable fitness (LT1). Of course, the young male has much more room for improvement.

Training and genetics influence $\dot{V}O_2$max, while submaximal fitness seems to be related to what we do with our potential. Of course, to be successful at the elite level, an athlete must have both a high maximal capacity and high relative fitness.

Table 8.5 Relative Fitness

Relative fitness level	LT1 as a % of $\dot{V}O_2$max	LT2 as a % of $\dot{V}O_2$max
Low	35–50%	45–60%
Medium	50–60%	60–70%
High	60–70%	70–80%
Very high	70–80%	80–90%

packs a day, weighed more than 250 pounds (113 kg), and bragged about his sedentary lifestyle. When he took a fitness test, it was all he could do to finish with a score in the low 30s. Ernie got the message. He stopped smoking, started training, and paid attention to his diet. Years later, you wouldn't recognize him. Under the fat, he discovered a trim, handsome body. He now weighs around 170 pounds (77 kg), has a fitness score of 58, and thoroughly enjoys the active life.

Activity

Finally, let us comment on the most obvious influence on fitness: your regular level of activity. What you do, day by day, year after year, shapes your health, vitality, and quality of life. You can lose the effect of years of training in a mere 12 weeks with the cessation of activity (Coyle, Hemmert, and Coggan 1986). Three weeks of complete bed rest, for example, may cause a fitness decline of 29 percent, or almost 10 percent per week, but you can easily restore the loss with regular activity (Saltin et al. 1968). Moderate activity leads to improved fitness and substantial health benefits, training leads to a higher level of fitness and extra health benefits, and prolonged, systematic training helps you achieve your potential. The choice is yours, but remember: Health has more to do with regular, moderate activity than with your level of fitness.

AEROBIC TRAINING EFFECTS

Fifty years ago, the term *cardiovascular* was used to define fitness. Next came the term *cardiorespiratory*, and today we speak of *aerobic fitness*. The changes in terminology reflect insights derived from decades of research, based on a clearer view of the effects of training. We used *cardiovascular* when the best-documented effects of training were about the heart and circulation, measures of transport. *Cardiorespiratory* became popular when we began to understand the importance of oxygen intake as well as transport. And *aerobic* was adopted to indicate that oxygen intake, transport, and utilization all improved with training. Since 1967, when research first documented the effects of endurance training on the ability of the muscles to use oxygen, we have become increasingly aware that some of the most important effects of training involve skeletal muscles and their ability to carry out oxidative, or aerobic, energy production. To emphasize that point, we like to say that skeletal muscle is the target of aerobic training.

You've heard that fitness is good for the heart and the lungs, and that is true. But training requires the use of muscles, and the major effects of training take place in the muscles that are used in training. Of course, important secondary adaptations take place in the cardiovascular, respiratory, and neuroendocrine systems and other tissues (fat, bone, ligaments, tendons). But it is impossible to improve the health or function of organs such as the heart without involving the skeletal muscles. All the beneficial changes begin with muscular activity. If you train the muscles properly, the secondary benefits follow. If you fail to train the muscles, the other changes are unlikely to occur.

When you engage in an exercise such as walking or jogging at a level above your normal daily activity (load), you overload the muscles and their support systems, including the heart and lungs. If you repeat the exercise regularly (e.g., every other day) your body begins to adapt to the overload imposed by the exercise. We call the many adaptations the training effect. The exercise somehow signals muscle fibers and support systems to undergo changes that will permit more exercise in the future. How does it work? Let's look at a muscle fiber.

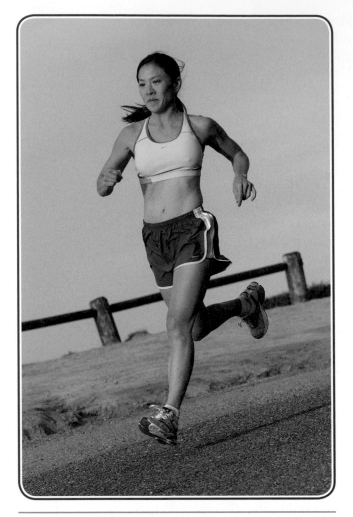

■ The major effects of training take place in the muscles that are used in training.

Figure 7.3 illustrates the basic structure of a muscle fiber. Something associated with training (metabolic by-products, chemical messenger, hormone) tells the **deoxyribonucleic acid (DNA)** in the nuclei of the muscle fiber to produce specific messengers in the form of **ribonucleic acid (RNA)**. The messenger RNA (mRNA) travels to structures within the fiber called ribosomes to direct the synthesis of specific proteins, like aerobic enzymes. Transfer RNA (tRNA) reads the mRNA blueprint and then captures appropriate **amino acids** for use in the synthesis of the desired protein. Endurance training leads to an increase in the concentration of oxidative enzymes and to a rise in the size and number of mitochondria, the cellular power plants where all oxidative metabolism takes place (Hood et al. 2000). These particular adaptations are specific to endurance training, and they take place only in the muscles used in training.

The effects of training have been determined in experimental studies. A typical study involves pretesting of volunteer subjects for aerobic fitness, lactate thresholds, and other measures; random assignment to experimental or control groups; weeks or even months of systematic and progressive training; and posttesting to measure the adaptations resulting from training. Studies have ranged from low to high intensity, using low- to high-fit subjects. We'll review the effects of aerobic training and then differentiate specific effects of long-duration, low-intensity training versus high-intensity training.

A variation of the training study involves **detraining** already fit subjects. Researchers convince habitual exercisers to forgo training for a period while they observe the decline of important measures and performance. Although this approach has limits, it eliminates the need for prolonged training. We'll look at both types of studies as well as animal research to help you understand the training effect.

AEROBIC TRAINING AND MUSCLE FUNCTION

Muscle, the motive force and source of many of the benefits associated with exercise, is the primary target of training. The effects of aerobic training on muscle relate to the utilization of oxygen. Oxidative metabolism, the enzymatic breakdown of carbohydrate and fat to produce energy for muscular contractions, takes place in cellular powerhouses called mitochondria (Coggan and Williams 1995). Long, slow training improves the oxidative capabilities of slow, oxidative (SO) fibers, whereas high-intensity training enhances the capabilities of fast, oxidative-glycolytic (FOG) fibers. Aerobic training has the following effects on muscle:

• Increases the concentration of aerobic enzymes (protein compounds that catalyze metabolic reactions) needed for the metabolic breakdown of carbohydrate and fat to produce energy in the form of ATP (adenosine triphosphate, the cellular energy supply).

- Increases the size and number (volume) of mitochondria, which produce energy aerobically (with oxygen).
- Increases the ability of the muscle to use fat as a source of energy.
- Increases the size of the fibers used in training.
- Long–slow training improves the oxidative capabilities of SO fibers.
- High-intensity training enhances the capabilities of FOG fibers.
- Increases the storage of muscle glycogen.
- Increases the supply of intramuscular fat.
- Increases the **myoglobin** (a compound that carries oxygen from the cell membrane to the mitochondria) in muscle fibers.
- Increases the number of capillaries serving muscle fibers.

> *The effects of aerobic training on muscle relate to the utilization of oxygen.*

Cellular Effects

Before 1967, research had failed to demonstrate the effects of training on muscle fibers. Dr. John Holloszy reasoned that previous studies failed to overload aerobic pathways, so he subjected laboratory rats to a strenuous treadmill program. Trained rats were eventually able to continue exercise for 4 to 8 hours, whereas untrained animals were exhausted within 30 minutes. Following the 12-week program, the animals were sacrificed to allow study of the muscle tissue. Holloszy found a 50 to 60 percent increase in mitochondrial protein, a twofold rise in the oxygen consumption of trained muscle, and enhanced ability to use (oxidize) carbohydrate and fat (1967). Other researchers have replicated these findings and confirmed them in humans, using a **muscle biopsy** technique.

Muscle biopsy technique: A hollow needle is inserted through an incision in the skin and fascia into the muscle. By removing a small piece of muscle about the size of a popcorn kernel, it is possible to measure aerobic and anaerobic enzymes, muscle glycogen stores, and gene expression as well as the study of an ever-increasing list of muscle functions.

Today we know that the increase in mitochondrial mass is due to branching of existing mitochondria, and that the increase provides greater capacity for oxidation of energy sources, especially our abundant supply of fat (we store 50 times more fat energy than we do carbohydrate energy, and training makes that supply more available).

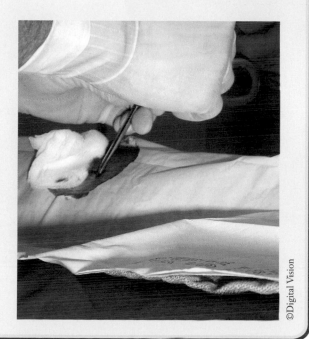

©Digital Vision

AEROBIC TRAINING AND BODY COMPOSITION

Body composition refers to the relative amounts of fat and lean weight. Although the **lean body weight** (body weight minus fat weight) is relatively unchanged with aerobic training, substantial loss of fat tissue is to be expected. One of the best-documented effects of training is the loss of unwanted fat, a transformation that reveals a trim, pleasing figure. Researchers use underwater weighing or skinfold calipers to measure percent body fat.

If you have 25 percent fat and weigh 120 pounds (54.4 kg), you have 30 pounds (13.6 kg) of fat and 90 pounds (40.8 kg) of lean body weight (LBW). If you jog 3 miles (4.8 km) a day, 5 days a week, you will burn about 1,650 calories per week (3 mi × 110 cal/mi × 5 days = 1,650 cal). In just 2 weeks, you'll burn 3,300 extra calories, almost a pound of fat (3,500 cal = 1 lb [.45 kg] of fat), or almost 2 pounds a month. In the process, you will lower your percent body fat and your body weight with only a slight increase in LBW. We'll say much more about body composition and fat loss in chapters 12 and 13.

AEROBIC TRAINING AND THE SKELETAL SYSTEM

Bones, ligaments, and tendons respond to the stress placed on them. Adaptations follow every change in function. For bones, increased weight-bearing activity leads to a denser, stronger structure designed to counteract the new level of stress. Inactivity leads to reabsorption of calcium and loss of bone density. Increasing age and inactivity create a dangerous combination, especially for females. Bone demineralization, or osteoporosis, begins early in adult life (30 to 40 years of age) and becomes more serious after menopause. Lack of activity hastens the weakening of bones. Weight-bearing activity causes bone tissue to become stronger and denser. But excessive training along with weight loss or menstrual irregularities (amenorrhea, or absence of menstruation) can cause early and possibly irreversible osteoporosis. Calcium intake may be helpful, but it won't do much good without the stress of moderate weight-bearing exercise.

Moderate activity also strengthens ligaments, tendons, and other connective tissue, such as the covering of muscle. By gradually increasing the workload, you can make tissues tough enough to withstand the normal demands of activity and resist damage during slips, trips, and falls.

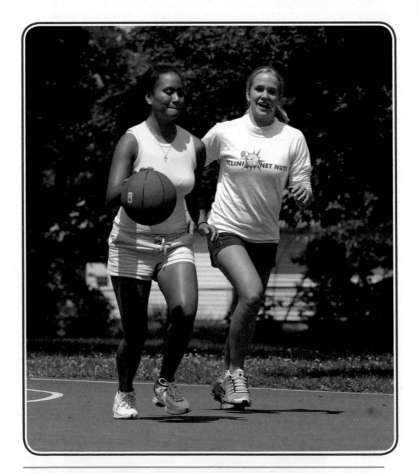

■ Regular, moderate activity can strengthen connective tissues, which can prevent injuries.

TRAINING SUPPLY AND SUPPORT

The respiratory, circulatory, nervous, endocrine, and other systems supply and support the activities of muscles. Aerobic training affects them in the following ways:

- Increases the efficiency of respiration and the endurance of respiratory muscles.
- Improves blood volume, distribution, and delivery to working muscles.
- Improves cardiovascular efficiency (increases stroke volume and cardiac output while decreasing resting and exercise heart rates).
- Fine-tunes nervous and hormonal control mechanisms.

Respiratory System

Aerobic training doesn't alter the size of the lungs, but it does improve the endurance and efficiency of breathing muscles, allowing greater use of inherited capacity (see figure 7.7). Training reduces the residual volume, the portion of lung capacity that goes unused. Residual volume increases with age and inactivity, and this decline of lung volume eventually compromises exercise capacity. The human respiratory system is overbuilt for its task, however, so people don't notice the gradual decline at first. Aerobic training slows the decline, ensuring adequate respiratory capacity throughout life.

Training also enhances the efficiency of respiration, so the trained person needs fewer breaths to move the same volume of air. Ventilation is the amount of air moving in or out of the lungs. It is the product of respiratory rate (or frequency) times the volume of air in each breath (tidal volume):

Ventilation (expired air in liters per minute) = frequency × tidal volume

Consider values for trained and untrained subjects jogging on a treadmill:

Untrained: 60 liters per minute = 30 breaths × 2 liters per breath

Trained: 60 liters per minute = 20 breaths × 3 liters per breath

The trained person moves more air with fewer breaths and is able to move more air at maximal ventilation (150 L/min or more, versus 120 or less for the untrained). Slower, deeper breaths are more efficient because they allow more of each breath to reach the portion of the lungs where oxygen and carbon dioxide are exchanged (alveolar sacs). Training also improves diffusion of oxygen from the lungs into the blood. Diffusion depends on good ventilation and adequate blood flow in the capillaries.

Cardiovascular System

Red blood cells and hemoglobin transport oxygen. We have long known that aerobic fitness is closely associated with total hemoglobin, and that blood volume and hemoglobin improve with training. We have also learned that the loss of blood volume that occurs with detraining is closely correlated with the reversal of important cardiovascular adjustments, leading to a higher resting heart rate and decreased stroke volume (Coyle, Hemmert, and Coggan 1986). Thus, the increase in blood volume that occurs with training is likely responsible, at least in part, for so-called cardiovascular changes. These changes may be secondary to training-induced increases in blood volume. Blood volume may increase 10 to 15 percent with training, raising the volume from 5 liters to 5.5 or even 5.75 liters.

Training-induced changes in blood volume are likely responsible, at least in part, for so-called cardiovascular changes.

A large portion of the enhanced cardiovascular function of endurance athletes is due to their high blood volume and its effect on cardiac function, increased hemoglobin and stroke volume, and decreased heart rate and blood viscosity (Gledhill, Warburton, and Jamnik 1999). Training-induced changes in blood volume have been reported to account for approximately 47 percent of the improvements in $\dot{V}O_2$max, and the results were similar for continuous or interval training (Warburton et al. 2004).

For years, we knew that endurance training led to a reduction in the heart rate at rest and at submaximal workloads and to an increase in the stroke volume, the amount of blood pumped with each beat of the heart. That is why we used the term *cardiovascular* to describe training effects. Training leads to an increase in the size of the left ventricle, but only during the filling stage, or **diastole** (increased left ventricular end diastolic volume [LVEDV]) (see figure 7.8). This change takes place with some thickening of the heart muscle and subtle alterations in its oxidative enzyme capacity. The efficient, trained heart pumps more blood each time it beats, at rest or during exercise. Therefore, it can beat at a slower rate. The heart is a pump that ejects much of the blood that enters its chambers. Put more blood into the chamber, and more comes out.

The volume of blood that the heart pumps with each beat depends on the blood volume and size of the left ventricle. A fibrous sac (pericardium) encloses the heart, limiting its size. When the sac was removed from dog hearts, the animals were able to train and increase their stroke volume and cardiac output (cardiac output equals heart rate multiplied by stroke volume) a whopping 20 percent (Stray-Gunderson 1986). You can't risk removal of your pericardium (an infection could lead to heart failure), but you can increase blood volume with training. This seems to lead to increases in stroke volume and cardiac output, as well as decreases in resting and exercise heart rates. Does the heart rate go down because the stroke volume goes up, or vice versa? You'll soon see.

Aerobic training appears to have subtle effects on the dimensions of heart muscle and on aerobic enzymes and mitochondria. The trained heart is better able to use fat as a source of energy, perhaps because training enlarges the diameter of coronary arteries and improves the oxygen supply to heart muscle. Another important contributor to stroke volume and cardiac output is the redistribution of blood from digestive and other organs to working muscles. Blood vessels in active muscles dilate, whereas those in nonworking muscles and organs constrict, directing blood where it is needed during exercise and helping to maintain high stroke volume. Training improves this ability to redistribute blood. Training also seems to enhance delivery of blood to skeletal muscle fibers by the capillaries. Trained muscles have a higher ratio of capillaries to fibers

Heart Muscle Fibers

Adult rats engaged in up to 13 weeks of high-intensity treadmill training and then were detrained. Training led to increases in heart muscle contractile capacity and $\dot{V}O_2$max, and the improvements were correlated to fiber length. When training stopped, training-induced improvements in $\dot{V}O_2$max decreased 50 percent in 2 weeks, and leveled off at 5 percent above sedentary controls after 4 weeks of detraining. Heart muscle fiber length declined along with $\dot{V}O_2$max, and remained 9 percent above sedentary levels after 4 weeks. Other measures of contractile capacity regressed completely within 2 to 4 weeks of detraining (Kemi et al. 2004). A close association exists between heart muscle dimensions, contractile capacity, arterial relaxation, and aerobic fitness. Of course, some portion of this association may be due to training-induced alterations in blood volume.

(Blomqvist and Saltin 1983). Because trained muscle fibers increase in diameter, the rise in capillaries may be necessary to maintain short diffusion distance from the capillary to the interior of the muscle fiber.

Nervous System

Training has several subtle but important effects on the nervous system. These include improved economy and efficiency of movement and improved efficiency of the cardiovascular system. The economical athlete uses less energy to perform at a given speed. Hours of practice lead to relaxed and efficient use of force to achieve results. This economy is especially evident in skilled tasks such as swimming and cross-country skiing, but it also occurs in running and cycling. Trained distance runners use 10 percent less energy than untrained runners when running at a given speed.

The nervous system, which controls heart rate and the constriction and relaxation of blood vessels, participates in another adjustment that may help solve the question of why heart rate and stroke volume change with training. In 1977, Saltin published a simple but elegant experiment in which subjects trained one leg on a bicycle ergometer, while the other leg served as an untrained control (see figure 8.3). Pre- and posttest measures of oxygen intake and oxidative enzyme activity demonstrated that changes occurred only in the trained leg. In other words, the training was specific. Furthermore, the heart rate response to exercise was significantly lower for the trained leg compared with the control, or untrained, leg.

Saltin reasoned that the improvements in the trained muscles were responsible for the lower heart rate response. Mitchell and associates (1977) demonstrated that small nerve endings located in muscle fibers are able to sense conditions in the muscle and modify the heart rate response to exercise through connections to the cardiac control center in the brain. Thus, it appears that the influence of training on the muscle may alter cardiovascular responses—that the reduced heart rate can be traced to improved metabolic condition in trained muscles. When the heart beats slower, it has more time to fill, allowing improved stroke volume.

This interpretation suggests that some of the well-documented effects of training are actually by-products of changes in the skeletal muscles. When we consider these changes with the increase in blood

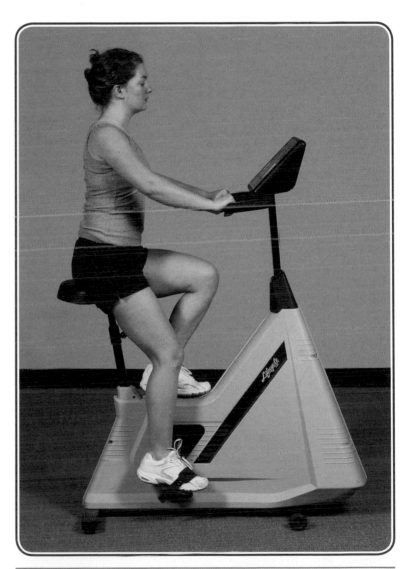

FIGURE 8.3 Subject trains one leg while the other leg serves as an untrained control.

volume and redistribution of blood, which combine to put more blood into the heart, we understand why training leads to a decrease in exercise heart rate and an increase in stroke volume. Therefore, it appears that some so-called cardiovascular effects of training are due to changes in the muscles being trained, that these changes are specific, and that training doesn't easily transfer from one leg (or one activity) to another. These conclusions also explain why we never use the term *cardio* to describe aerobic exercise.

Endocrine System

The endocrine system includes the many glands whose secretions, or hormones, are distributed by the circulation. The effects of training include the following:

- Adjustments in hormonal response
- Increased sensitivity to certain hormones
- Important metabolic adjustments

Many hormones are involved in the regulation of energy. Epinephrine, cortisol, thyroxine, glucagon, and growth hormone raise blood sugar, whereas insulin is the only hormone capable of lowering blood sugar. The pancreas secretes insulin when blood sugar levels rise, such as after a meal, helping tissues take up the sugar. The others are secreted when blood levels are low, as in vigorous exercise. Epinephrine and growth hormone also are involved in the mobilization of fat from adipose tissue, whereas insulin leads to fat deposition. Endurance training lowers the need for insulin because the muscle can take up sugar during exercise, even in the absence of insulin (as in diabetes). Training seems to increase receptor sensitivity to insulin, leading to more efficient use of hormones and energy.

Fat Metabolism

Years ago, animal and then human studies demonstrated improved fat utilization following training. Trained muscle is better suited to use fat as a source of energy, thereby conserving limited supplies of carbohydrate (glycogen) in muscle and the liver. A key finding was the enhancement of beta oxidation, an enzymatic process that systematically chops two carbon fragments from fat (free fatty acids), initiating the release of energy stored in fat to produce ATP. Along with this improvement in fat metabolism is a near doubling of stored fat (triglyceride) in trained muscle fibers. On top of all this, training leads to improvement in fat mobilization.

Fat Mobilization

Epinephrine is available from two sites, the adrenal gland and the nerve endings of the sympathetic nervous system. Like most other hormones, epinephrine acts on receptors located in the surface membrane of its target organ, in this case, adipose tissue. The hormone initiates a series of steps leading to the breakdown of triglyceride fat and the release of free fatty acids (FFA) into the circulation (see figure 8.4). The FFA then travel to working muscles or the heart, where they can be used to fuel contractions. During vigorous exercise, lactic acid produced in the muscles seems to inhibit the action of epinephrine, thereby reducing the FFA available for energy. Under these conditions, the muscle must use limited supplies of muscle glycogen for energy.

Training improves the oxidative ability of muscles, leading to less lactic acid production and greater fat mobilization and fat metabolism (Hollo-

We'll say it again: The ability to utilize fat may be one of the most important outcomes of the active life and fitness.

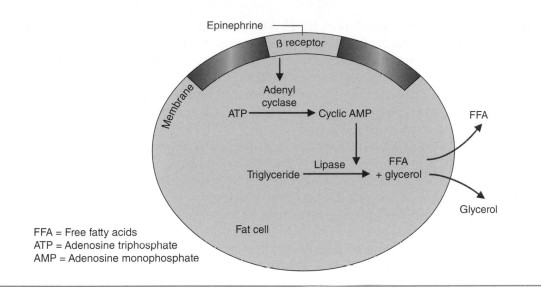

FIGURE 8.4 Mobilization of free fatty acids from adipose tissue. Lactic acid inhibits the influence of epinephrine on the fat cell and blocks the mobilization of fat.

Adapted from B.J. Sharkey, 1975, *Physiology and physical activity* (New York: Harper and Row).

szy et al. 1986). Trained people appear to be able to mobilize fat even when lactic acid is elevated (Vega deJesus and Siconolfi 1988). The result is improved access to a major source of energy, some 50 times more abundant than carbohydrate! The enhanced utilization of fat has significant health benefits beyond those related to fitness and performance. We'll say it again: The ability to utilize fat may be one of the most important outcomes of the active life and fitness.

SPECIFICITY OF TRAINING

An activity such as jogging recruits muscle fibers uniquely suited to the task. Slow jogging recruits slow fibers. The metabolic pathways and energy sources are also suited to the task. Daily jogging recruits the same fibers and pathways repeatedly, leading to the adaptive response known as the training effect.

Training leads to changes in aerobic enzyme systems in muscle fibers, so it is easy to see why those changes are specific. In the early stages of training, the inability of the muscles to use oxygen limits performance. Later on, as the fibers adapt and can use more oxygen, the burden shifts to the cardiovascular system, including the heart, blood, and blood vessels. Then the cardiovascular system becomes the factor that limits performance (Boileau, McKeown, and Riner 1984).

Training gains don't automatically transfer from one activity to another. Training effects can be classified as peripheral (in the muscle) and central (heart, blood, lungs, hormones). Central effects may transfer to other activities, but peripheral changes are unlikely to transfer. Central changes in blood volume and redistribution, however, may aid performance in another endurance activity. However, keep in mind that one-leg training studies show that some part of the heart rate (and stroke volume) change is due to conditions within the muscle fibers, conditions that are relayed

*The outcomes of training are directly related to the activity employed as a **training stimulus**.*

to the cardiac control center (Saltin 1977). These changes are specific and do not transfer from one activity to another.

Concentrating your training on the movements, muscle fibers, metabolic pathways, and supply and support systems that you intend to use in an activity or sport makes sense. This approach does not imply that athletes should ignore other exercises and muscle groups. Additional training is necessary to avoid injury and boredom, to achieve muscle balance, and to provide backup for prime movers when they become fatigued. In spite of the widespread affection for the term *cardiovascular fitness* (or *cardio*), the evidence suggests that the concept is overrated. Muscle is the target of training.

Finally, if exercise and training are specific, then testing must be specific if it is to reflect the adaptations that occur with training. This proposition means that you should not use a bicycle to test a runner, and vice versa. Training is so specific that the best test for hill runners is an uphill treadmill test. How do we test the effects of training on dancers? We don't. When studies compare runners and dancers on a treadmill test, runners exhibit higher $\dot{V}O_2$max scores. If that is true, why do runners poop out in aerobic dance, cycling, or swimming? The answer is that the effects of training are specific. At present, there is no widely accepted way to make an accurate assessment of the effects of aerobic, ballet, modern, or other dance forms.

AEROBIC FITNESS FIELD TESTS

One way to estimate your aerobic fitness is with a simple, inexpensive field test. If you are a walker, use the 1-mile (1.6 km) walking test to estimate your $\dot{V}O_2$max. If you are a runner, you can use the 1.5-mile (2.4 km) running test. Be sure to take the health-screening questionnaire (form 3.1, page 60) before engaging in either test.

Walking Test

The Rockport Walking Test uses the time for a 1-mile (1.6 km) walk and some personal information to estimate the $\dot{V}O_2$max. Walk the measured course as quickly as possible and then substitute the time (to the nearest hundredth of a minute), posttest heart rate, and other information in the following equation.

$$\dot{V}O_2\text{max} = 132.853 - (.0769 \times \text{weight in lb } [.03488 \times \text{weight in kg}])$$
$$- (.3877 \times \text{age in yr}) + (6.315 \times \text{sex } [0 \text{ for female}, 1 \text{ for male}])$$
$$- (3.2649 \times \text{time } [\text{min to the nearest 100th}]) - (.1565 \times \text{HR at end of test})$$

The result in milliliters per kilogram per minute is highly correlated to a laboratory measure of aerobic fitness (Kline et al. 1987).

Running Test

The 1.5-mile (2.4 km) running test requires a near-maximal effort. If you've been inactive, precede training with an adjustment to activity (walking), and then begin 6 to 8 weeks of training for the test. If you're over the age of 45, consider a medical examination, especially if you have two or more cardiovascular risk factors. Be sure to warm up and stretch before the test. The time for the 1.5-mile (2.4 km) run is used to predict aerobic fitness and is based on the oxygen cost of running (see figure 8.5).

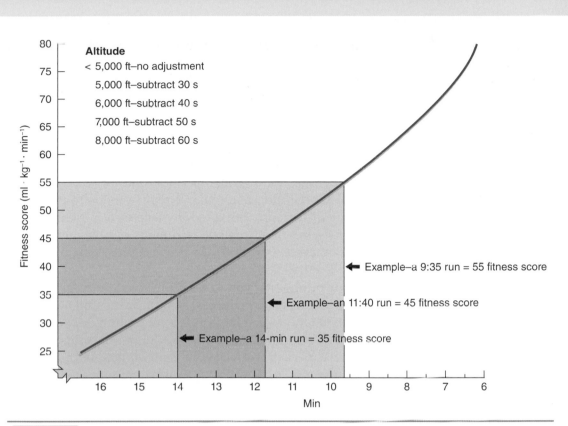

FIGURE 8.5 1.5-mile (2.4 km) aerobic fitness test.

Note: Subtract altitude adjustment from 1.5-mile (2.4 km) run time. Then use the graph to find your score.

Adapted from B.J. Sharkey, 1997, *Fitness and work capacity*, 2nd ed. (Missoula, MT: USDA Forest Service).

Sources: Balke 1963, Cooper 1968, Sharkey and Gaskill 2007, Daniels 1977, pers. comm.

SUMMARY

Aerobic fitness, defined as the ability to take in, transport, and use oxygen, is a measure of exercise intensity. The second lactate threshold, which defines the upper limit of sustainable aerobic exercise, is a measure of **exercise duration** and is an excellent predictor of endurance performance in events lasting from 30 minutes to several hours. The first lactate threshold defines the level of work or sport that you can sustain for prolonged periods. Heredity and training, as well as other factors such as age, sex, and body fat, influence all the dimensions of aerobic fitness and performance. Factors such as your current health, diet, hydration, level of rest, and **acclimatization** to heat and altitude also influence your ability to perform an endurance event. Few of us ever reach our potential for fitness and endurance, and no laboratory test exists to pinpoint this potential. World-class athletes train daily for years to be the best that they can be. Most of us must be content to do the best we can within the time constraints imposed by family, profession, community, and other responsibilities. The best time to start training is as you approach puberty. The second best time to start is today.

In this chapter, we've looked at the effects of aerobic training. We've shown that muscles undergo specific adaptations when an exercise recruits them over a period long enough to overload their oxidative pathways. As aerobic pathways improve, muscles use oxygen more efficiently and burn more fat. Maximal aerobic fitness (VO_2max) and lactate thresholds rise. The metabolic efficiency is relayed to the cardiac control center in the brain, which results in a slower heart rate, more filling time, and greater stroke volume. Increased blood volume and improved distribution provide ample blood for the heart to pump. Because so many adaptations take place in the muscle, training should be specific to its intended use.

Because training is so specific, you should select an appropriate activity for aerobic training. Fat metabolism and cardiovascular benefits are enhanced in regular, moderate activity that employs major muscle groups for extended periods, but not when different muscles are engaged in a series of short lifting bouts (i.e., circuit weight training). Fat metabolism and cardiovascular benefits are also enhanced in some intermittent aerobic activities, in which an ever-changing series of movements maintains aerobic metabolism. Subjecting bones to regular, moderate stress, as in weight-bearing and resistance exercises, maintains bone mineral content.

Choose an activity that you enjoy or one that you want to improve. Long, slow training improves the ability of SO fibers to use fat as an energy source. Faster and necessarily shorter training recruits fast-twitch (FOG) fibers. High-intensity training may also have more effect on the cardiovascular system. Your approach to training depends on your goals. Train more slowly for distance, faster for speed. You can combine both by going easy and then increasing pace near the end of the workout. German distance coach Ernst Van Aaken advocated a 20:1 slow-to-fast ratio for his elite athletes (1976). For example, on a 5-mile (8 km) run, you can pick up the pace for the last quarter mile (the last .4 km). This short distance provides some speed training at a time when you are well warmed. We like this approach because it limits the discomfort associated with elevated lactic acid. Training doesn't have to hurt to be good, as you'll see in the chapter 10, which provides a prescription and programs to get you started. Chapter 14 provides additional guidance to help you reach your potential.

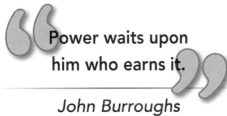

> "Power waits upon
> him who earns it. "
>
> *John Burroughs*

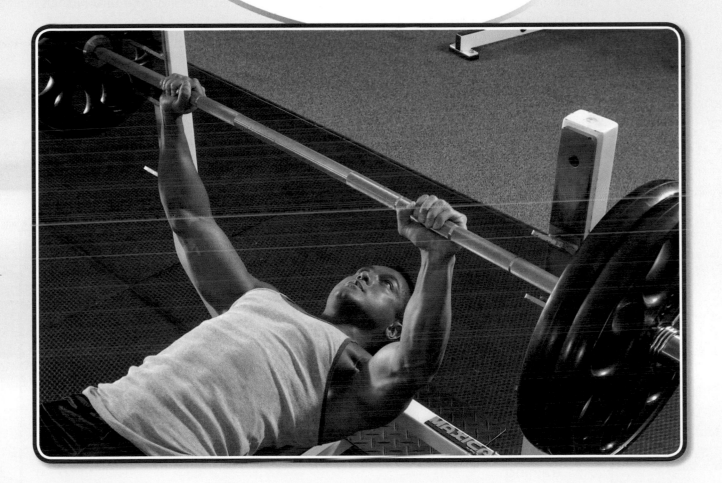

Many years ago, muscular fitness occupied an awkward position on the fringe of the fitness movement. We recognized its contributions to performance in sport and some forms of work, but we lacked conclusive evidence linking muscular fitness with health and the quality of life. That situation has changed, and we can now say with confidence that both aerobic fitness and muscular fitness contribute substantially to health. Muscular fitness training increases muscle mass, the furnace that burns fat. Exercises that improve muscular fitness help prevent osteoporosis. Attention to muscular fitness is essential if you are to avoid the lower back problems and repetitive motion injuries that plague millions of Americans. Continued participation ensures the capacity for independence and mobility in your postretirement years.

The essential components of muscular fitness are strength, **muscular endurance**, and flexibility. Other important components include power, speed, **agility**, and balance. With most physiological capabilities, you either use them or lose them, and that is certainly true for muscular fitness. Strength, endurance, flexibility, power, agility, and balance all decline with age. But the rate of decline is much slower for those who remain active. And numerous studies show that we have the capability to build strength even into our 90s (Fiatarone et al. 1994)!

But don't wait until you are 90 to experience the pleasures and rewards of muscular fitness. Begin now. You will soon notice that you can do tasks more easily. Your muscles will be firmer and your tummy will be flatter. You will feel better about yourself and life in general.

Young folks use muscular fitness to improve performance in a favorite sport or activity, or to look good in a bathing suit. Middle-aged people rely on abdominal tone and flexibility exercises to prevent or minimize lower back problems. Older folks employ strength and endurance activities to retain bone density and to remain active and independent, capable of performing important activities of daily living. In recent years, we have learned that

This chapter will help you do the following:

- Identify the components of muscular fitness
- Understand the factors that influence strength
- Differentiate between strength and muscular endurance
- Understand the importance of flexibility
- Determine how muscular fitness contributes to health, total fitness, and performance
- Understand how a bout of training leads to changes in muscles
- Identify the specific changes that result from strength or endurance training
- Evaluate the importance of flexibility exercises
- Understand how to minimize muscle soreness
- See how speed and power training improve performance
- See how core training contributes to health and performance

muscular fitness training (e.g., resistance or weight training) is a good way to avoid the crippling bone demineralization known as osteoporosis and maintain the muscle that you need to burn fat and to sustain mobility well into retirement years. So, if you intend to remain active after retirement, you'd better add muscular fitness training to your fitness program.

Chapter 7 describes the structure and function of muscle. This chapter begins by considering the primary components of muscular fitness—strength, muscular endurance, and flexibility—called so because they are the ones most related to health. We'll cover other components, such as speed, power, agility, balance, and coordination, later in the chapter.

MUSCULAR STRENGTH

Strength is important when your occupation demands it, in certain sports, and—surprisingly—for those over 60 years of age. During the early part of our lives, as we age, strength declines at a slow pace, especially if we use it. But sometime after 55 years of age, the rate of decline accelerates. Throughout our years, we need some strength to avoid acute or chronic injury, to meet emergencies, and to engage fully and independently in life. We need strength to change a flat tire, to shovel the walk, and to lift and carry infants, laundry, or groceries. Lack of muscular fitness leads to less activity, which hastens the loss of strength, and so on, creating a vicious cycle that ends in a nursing home. But you can reverse this cycle and remain strong and independent well into your eighth decade.

Strength is defined as the maximal force that can be exerted in a single voluntary contraction. Most of us possess more strength than we are able to demonstrate. In a fascinating experiment, Ikai and Steinhaus (1961) showed that significant increases in strength could be elicited with a gunshot, shouting, drugs, or hypnosis during a contraction. Untrained people inhibit the full expression of strength. **Inhibitions** reside in the brain and in inhibitory muscle receptors. One effect of strength training is to reduce inhibitions and allow a fuller expression of available strength.

> **M**ost of us possess more strength than we are able to demonstrate.

Strength, then, is not an absolute value. It is subject to change, and this makes the subject of strength training extremely interesting. When strength improves, how much of the improvement is because of reduced inhibitions and how much is from changes in muscle tissue? Can we find a way to increase strength without spending a lot of time with weights?

The force that you exert in a maximal voluntary contraction depends on a number of factors, such as inhibitions, muscle mass or cross-sectional area, the number of contracting fibers and their contractile state (length, fatigue), and the mechanical advantage of the bony lever system. Most of these are easy to explain. More fibers equal more girth and more force. The stretched muscle exerts more force (probably because of elastic recoil and favorable alignment of contractile proteins), while the rested muscle exerts more force than a fatigued one. Mechanical factors conspire to magnify force or speed. Several other factors (sex, age, fiber type, and training) deserve more attention.

Sex

Until early adolescence (age 12 to 14), boys are not much stronger than girls. Thereafter, the average male gains an advantage that persists throughout life. Is the difference due to the increase in the male hormone testosterone at puberty? Perhaps; the average male has 10 times the testosterone of the average female. Testosterone is an anabolic (growth-inducing) steroid that helps muscles become larger. College women have 50 to 60 percent of the arm and shoulder strength and 70 percent of the leg strength of their male counterparts. But a

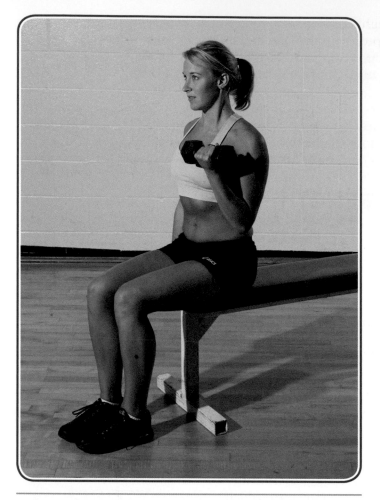

■ Strength training can greatly improve women's upper body strength.

relationship doesn't imply cause and effect. The relationship of strength and testosterone might also be related to a third factor. For example, the hormone may make men more aggressive and willing to train harder.

Consider another confounding possibility—body fat. Young women average twice the percentage of fat as men (25% versus 12.5%). When you look at strength per unit of lean body weight (body weight minus fat weight), women have slightly stronger legs, whereas their arm strength remains 30 percent below the values for men. Wilmore (1983) suggests that because women use their legs as men do (walking, climbing stairs, bicycling), their leg muscles are similar in strength. Because fewer women use their arms in heavy work or sport, their strength lags behind in this area. Thus, judging women the weaker sex may be a mistake. As more women engage in upper body strength training for sport or occupational purposes (law enforcement, firefighting, construction), their strength will certainly come closer to that of men. In fact, testing by the authors with cross-country skiers showed that elite female athletes had 97 percent of the upper body power of male athletes per unit of lean body mass, suggesting that when women train their upper bodies, they can develop upper body power that is comparable with men.

Muscle size and strength do go together for both sexes, however, and the average male is larger than the average female. Most studies indicate a force of 4 to 6 kilograms per square centimeter of muscle girth. To estimate muscle girth in the upper arm, we should measure **subcutaneous fat** and bone size as well, because they will be part of the total circumference. All other things being equal, the larger muscle is the stronger one, but not necessarily the most successful in work or sport.

Age

Strength reaches a peak in the early 20s and declines slowly until about age 60. Thereafter, the rate of decline usually accelerates, but it doesn't have to. When people use their strength, it hardly declines at all, even into the 60s. Champion weight lifters have achieved personal records in their 40s. Auto mechanics retain grip strength into their 60s. Training before puberty leads to improvements that are mostly due to changes in the nervous system (**neurogenic** factors include reduced inhibitions and learning how to exert force). Training after puberty combines nervous system changes with changes in muscle tissue (**myogenic changes**). Because testosterone levels decline in old age, many physiologists thought that older people would be able to achieve only neurogenic changes when they engaged in strength training. A study of very elderly people (72 to 98 years), however, has shown that

Training at any age maintains or improves strength, especially when diet is adequate.

resistance training leads to increased strength, muscle mass, and mobility (Fiatarone et al. 1994). Elderly people who perform strength training achieve increases in protein synthesis, strength, and muscle size, and improvements in activities of daily living (Frontera and Bigard 2002). Training at any age maintains or improves strength, especially when diet is adequate. We'll say more about both later on.

Muscle Fiber Types

Chapter 7 notes the presence of two fiber types, slow-twitch and fast-twitch. The larger, faster contracting fast-twitch fibers have greater potential for rapid development of tension. People with a higher percentage of fast-twitch fibers have greater potential for power development. Studies of human muscle tissue reveal that power lifters have twice the area of fast-twitch fibers that nonlifters do. The size can be attributed to heredity and to training. The effect of strength training on muscle fiber types has yet to be completely resolved. Current evidence indicates that both types grow larger with training, but growth of the fast fibers is more pronounced. Strength training improves the capabilities of both types, but doesn't seem to change one type into another.

Although resistance training may not change slow fibers into fast fibers, we are learning that, besides heredity and training, several other factors may influence muscle mass and strength. A study shows a positive correlation between birth weight and adult grip strength for 2,775 men and women, even when adjusted for adult body size and social class. The study suggests that birth weight has an important influence on the number of muscle fibers established at birth, and that even in middle age (53 years of age), compensating **hypertrophy** may be inadequate. As the inevitable loss of muscle fibers proceeds with aging, the deficit in fibers could threaten the quality of life (Kuh et al. 2002).

MUSCULAR ENDURANCE

An additional component of muscular fitness is muscular endurance. Muscular endurance means the ability to persist. We define and measure it as the **repetition** of submaximal contractions or submaximal holding time (static or isometric endurance). Muscular endurance is essential for success in many work and sport activities. When you have the strength to perform a repetitive task, additional improvement in performance depends on muscular endurance, the ability to persist. As mentioned earlier, stronger fast-twitch fibers fatigue more readily. Thus, endurance and strength are not highly related, except when a very heavy load is used in an endurance test.

Muscular endurance is essential for success in many work and sport activities.

We use the term *muscular endurance* to differentiate it from other uses of the concept of stamina, such as aerobic endurance. A person may develop considerable endurance in small muscles, such as a barber who develops the finger flexors, without achieving any noticeable effect on the heart or respiratory systems. Although barbers are likely to have great endurance in the muscles of their fingers, their aerobic fitness may be poor. Muscular endurance resides in metabolic adaptations and neuromuscular efficiency of the fibers used in the activity.

Let's spend a moment contrasting muscular endurance and strength, which are quite different in physiological terms. We achieve muscular endurance by repetitive contractions of muscle fibers. Repetitive contractions require a continuous supply of energy, and muscle fibers with aerobic (oxidative) capabilities (slow, oxidative fibers, or SO, and fast, oxidative-glycolytic fibers, or FOG) are suited to the job. Repetitive contractions enhance aerobic enzymes, mitochondria, and fuels needed for repetitive contractions.

Strength comes from lifting heavy loads a few times. As we have said, the effects of strength training are most noticeable in fast-twitch fibers. Training effects include increases in contractile proteins (actin and myosin) and tougher connective tissue. Increased strength comes from greater cross-sectional area, which means that more contractile protein is available to exert force. The type of training and the physiological effects of endurance and strength training are quite different. Keep that in mind as you plan your program. Endurance is important for practice, training, and performance. Repetition leads to skill, and repetition requires endurance, so endurance is one of the keys to success in sport or work.

FLEXIBILITY

Flexibility is the range of motion through which the limbs are able to move. Skin, connective tissue, and conditions within joints restrict range of motion, as does excessive body fat. Injury can occur when a limb is forced beyond its normal range. Improved flexibility reduces this potential. Range of motion increases when joints and muscles are warm.

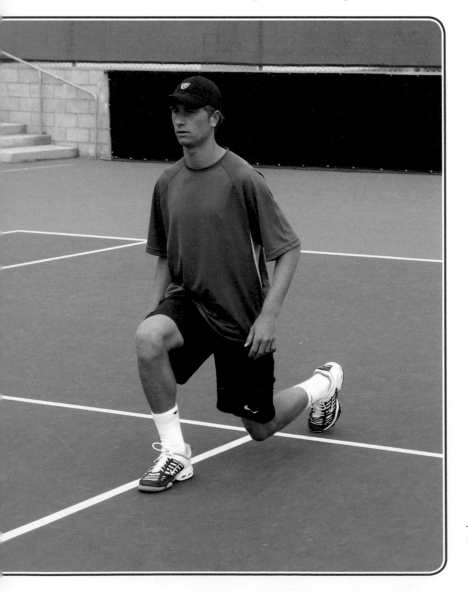

Stretching exercises are successful after a warm-up but before vigorous effort. Stretching after exercise, during the cool-down period, may reduce **delayed-onset muscle soreness (DOMS)** and improve flexibility for the next workout. Stretching before subsequent activity certainly reduces feelings of tightness and discomfort. Flexibility exercises are important when you are training for strength or endurance. They help you maintain the range of motion that might otherwise decrease. Most runners turn to stretching to make the pastime more enjoyable. Calf, hamstring, groin, and back muscles can become tight and sore, especially after an increase in intensity or duration of training. Stretching may enhance enjoyment and limit discomfort. We have found that the need for stretching increases with age.

Does stretching improve performance? Some studies found that stretching before competition could diminish performance. However, a review of over 100 studies (Kay and Blazevich 2012) concluded that short static stretches (held under 30 sec) had no adverse effect on

■ Stretching warm muscles before and after training and between training sessions may reduce muscle soreness.

performance. Notice that stretching did not improve performance. Improved range of motion is important in activities such as gymnastics, diving, and dancing, where range of motion is essential. It may help in wrestling or in golf. But, for the rest of us, elaborate stretching programs may be a waste of time.

Yoga has gained popularity as a way to achieve relaxation and meditative states. When stripped of its mystical elements, yoga emerges as a safe, enjoyable, and relaxing flexibility program. The benefits are typically limited to flexibility. Little evidence supports claims of improved aerobic fitness or significant gains in strength or muscular endurance.

Many fitness instructors believe that flexibility contributes in work and sport. Lack of flexibility may be a factor in the development of acute and chronic injuries, repetitive trauma, and lower back problems. Studies of military recruits show that static stretching did not influence total injury rates. But the incidence of muscle and tendon injuries and lower back pain were significantly lower in the stretching group (Amako et al. 2003). The value of stretching in injury prevention may be more problematic. When the sport demands high range of motion in a joint, stretching seems to be valuable. But when the activity consists of low intensity or contraction cycles (jogging, cycling, swimming), the need for a very compliant muscle–tendon unit is less. In these cases, stretching has no beneficial effect on injury prevention (Witvrouw et al. 2004). In addition, when 34 elite runners were examined for flexibility (sit-and-reach test) and running economy, the least flexible runners were the most economical (Jones 2002). Evidence is insufficient either to endorse or to disapprove of routine stretching before or after exercise to prevent injuries in competitive or recreational athletes (Thacker et al. 2004). Some of us may profit from regular stretching exercises. Older folks have a special need, because connective tissue becomes less elastic with age.

Lack of flexibility may be a factor in the development of acute and chronic injuries, repetitive trauma, and lower back problems.

SPEED

Speed may be the most exciting ingredient in sport. It requires rapid acceleration, which involves the contraction of fast-twitch muscle fibers. **Speed of movement** includes reaction time and movement time. Reaction time (the time from the stimulus, such as a starting gun, until the beginning of the movement) is a function of the nervous system. We can't change the speed of nerve-impulse transmission along a neuron. Thus, the only way to achieve significant improvement in reaction time is by increasing awareness of important stimuli and by repeating appropriate responses, which reduces processing time of the **central nervous system (CNS)**. In sports, coaches use special drills to improve reaction time.

Speed of movement = reaction time + movement time

Movement time, the interval from the beginning to the end of the movement, may improve (decrease) with appropriate strength and power training. The key to success lies in the principle of specificity: The movement must be specific to the sport. If you want to throw a baseball with greater velocity, train with light weights at a fast speed (e.g., throw a weighted ball). If you are a shot-putter, throw heavier weights as fast as possible. Specificity applies to the rate of movement and the resistance employed, which means that training should simulate the action as closely as possible.

How much can you improve? Remember what we've said about fast-twitch fibers: You'll need a high percentage to be fast. If you don't have more than 50 percent fast fibers, don't despair. You may never be as fast as those with a high percentage, but you can improve your movement time by following the principles presented in the next chapter. But don't conclude that continued improvements in strength will always lead to improvements in movement time. Strength is related to speed when movement is resisted (as in football and shot put), but less so when resistance is light (as in the tennis serve). And remember, speed—like strength—is task specific. The speed of arm movement is not necessarily related to leg speed. Some people may be quick with their hands but, because of lack of training or skill or because of excess weight, may be slow of foot. Improved skill and strength training reduce the time it takes to complete a movement.

POWER

Football coaches often talk about power. Power is a combination of strength (force) and velocity or speed. A lineman needs explosive power to move his opponent. But power is important in every sport that requires speed and acceleration. Even cycling and cross-country skiing require power. Power is defined as work divided by time, or the rate of doing work.

$$\text{Power} = \text{force} \times \text{distance} \div \text{time, or } F \times D \div T = \text{force} \times \text{velocity (velocity} = D \div T)$$

Power combines strength (force) and velocity or speed (distance divided by time). A person who is able to do more work than someone else in the same unit of time has more power. A person who moves 100 kilograms 1 meter in 1 second has done 100 kilogram-meters of work per second. If you move the same load 2 meters in 1 second or 1 meter in .5 second, you've exhibited twice as much power. Thus, power is related to strength and velocity (distance divided by time). If you improve them, you'll increase power.

Power is important in a number of sports, but nonathletic adults seldom need it. If you want to increase your power for cycling, skiing, basketball, or some other sport, remember the principle of specificity. Even runners can increase power by lifting weights, running uphill, and running against resistance. They can increase speed by using high-speed repetitions in power training or by running downhill. We'll provide a prescription for power training in chapter 11.

AGILITY AND SKILL

Agility is the ability to change position and direction rapidly, with precision and without loss of balance. It depends on strength, speed, balance, and coordination. Agility is undeniably important in the world of sport, but it is also useful in helping people avoid embarrassment or injury in recreational activities and in potentially dangerous work situations. Because agility is associated with specific skills, no one test predicts agility for all situations. You can improve agility with practice and experience. Excess weight hinders agility, for obvious reasons. Extreme strength isn't a prerequisite, nor is aerobic fitness. But because agility deteriorates with fatigue, aerobic and muscular endurance can help maintain agility for extended periods, such as a long tennis match.

Coordination implies a harmonious relationship, a smooth union or flow of movement in execution of a task. In striking the tennis serve, one develops force sequentially. As momentum from the body turn approaches its peak, the arm extends at the elbow, and maximum racket speed finally occurs with the snap of the wrist. If the forces are added in the wrong sequence, the movement appears uncoordinated.

Although a certain amount of coordination may be inherited (as with the natural athlete), skill is achieved with practice, practice, and more practice. Repetition of a skill leads to decreases in synaptic resistance in the nervous system, increasing the likelihood and accuracy of the practiced movement and eventually making the movement automatic. Correct practice is crucial. Repetition of the wrong movement will form a bad habit that is hard to break. Seek professional instruction as you endeavor to improve your skill.

Practice makes permanent: Perfect practice makes perfect.

Because every skill is specific, we must learn each individually. Ability in tennis doesn't ensure success in badminton, squash, or racquetball. Skill doesn't transfer between sports as readily as we once thought it did. Another feature of coordination or skill will become apparent as you train for fitness. Skilled performers work efficiently; they don't waste movement or energy. A skilled runner uses less energy at a given speed. A skilled worker often can outproduce a coworker who is stronger and more fit. We can learn skill, coordination, and technique. With proper skill, we make best use of leverage and large-muscle groups, thereby avoiding injury and fatigue of smaller muscles.

Because every skill is specific, we must learn each individually.

BALANCE

Balance can be static or dynamic. **Static balance,** as measured by a test such as the stork stand (standing on one foot with hands on hips and eyes closed), measures the ability to maintain balance while stationary. Balance is important in activities like diving, gymnastics, and mountain climbing. You can improve balance with specific training. It may decline with age or inactivity, or as the result of illness or even head trauma. **Dynamic balance** is the ability to maintain equilibrium while in motion. Balance depends on the ability to integrate visual input with information from the semicircular canals in the inner ear and from muscle–joint receptors. Although measuring and predicting its role is difficult, dynamic balance certainly contributes to sport performance.

Evidence indicates that people can improve their balance through participation in

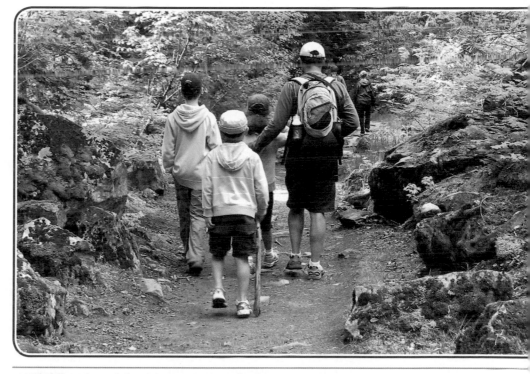

■ Childhood participation in sports and other movement experiences can improve balance.

sports and a variety of movement experiences, especially during childhood. Leg strength is a factor in dynamic balance, especially in the elderly (Spirduso 1995). Elderly practitioners of tai chi exhibited better joint proprioception and balance control than sedentary subjects did, but when they were compared with elderly golfers, the active groups were similar in dynamic standing balance control (Tsang and HuiChan 2004). Active older males subjected to a 6-week balance intervention program showed little improvement in static or dynamic balance. An active life appears sufficient to maintain balance, even in older adults (Lail et al. 2004).

Because balance is probably task specific, practice of the specific activity is likely the best way to improve balance and performance. Having football or basketball players engage in aerobic dance or ballet classes is likely to result in a profound cultural experience for both the players and the teacher, and the classes are sure to make the athletes better dancers. Whether the classes will improve the players' performance on the field or court has yet to be demonstrated. We can safely say that few, if any, top basketball professionals developed their moves around an arabesque, entrechat, or glissade. And none whom we've seen shoot fouls in the fifth position!

BENEFITS OF MUSCULAR FITNESS

How does training lead to changes in muscle fibers? How does a muscle fiber know the difference between strength and endurance training? Part of the answer to these questions is related to the training stimulus, the characteristic of training that leads to specific adaptations. Strength improves when you apply sufficient tension to the muscle fiber and its contractile proteins. The tension required seems to be above two-thirds of the maximal force of the muscle. If you do contractions that require little tension, you won't gain much strength. Contraction time, the total number of repetitions, also seems to influence the development of strength (Smith and Rutherford 1995). By doing more contractions you obtain better results, up to a point. The number of contractions probably depends on your level of training, nutrition, and genetic endowment. You will receive benefits from any form of strength training, as long as you exert enough tension for a sufficient number of repetitions (or time).

$$\text{Strength} = \text{tension} \times \text{time (number of sets and repetitions)}$$

STRENGTH TRAINING EFFECTS

In training, we often speak of the overload principle, which states the following:

- For improvements to take place, workloads have to impose a demand (overload) on the body system (above two-thirds of maximal force for strength).
- As adaptation to loading takes place, more load must be added.
- Improvements are related to the intensity (tension for strength), duration (repetitions), and frequency of training.

Overload training leads to adaptations in the muscles according to the type of training. Here again, the principle of specificity applies, as it did with aerobic training. The adaptation to strength training includes increased size because of increases in contractile proteins (actin and myosin) and tougher connective tissue. These and other adaptations allow the muscle to exert more force.

The specific adaptations to muscular endurance training include improved aerobic enzyme systems, larger and more numerous mitochondria (increased mitochondrial density), and more capillaries. All these changes promote oxygen delivery and utilization within the muscle fiber, thereby improving endurance (Jackson and Dickinson 1988). Fatiguing repetitions somehow stimulate the muscle fiber to become better adapted to use oxygen and aerobic enzymes for the production of energy (adenosine triphosphate, or ATP) to sustain contractions. If you perform many repetitions, you become better able to use fat as a source of energy.

We do not entirely understand how the strength or endurance training stimuli bring about the appropriate changes. But from what we know about how cells work, the training stimulus probably signals the nucleus to make messenger RNA (mRNA). This messenger is shaped by the DNA and sent into the muscle fiber to order the production of specific proteins (contractile protein for strength training, aerobic enzyme protein for endurance training). Structures in the muscle fiber called ribosomes receive the message and begin to produce the protein needed to adapt to the training stimulus. Another RNA (transfer RNA, or tRNA) gathers up the amino acids needed to construct the desired protein, transports them to the ribosome, and places them in the growing chain of amino acids that become a specific protein. Because DNA forms RNA, the training stimulus must somehow influence the nuclei (one muscle fiber has many). We don't know whether tension, metabolic activity, hormones, or a combination of factors signal the nuclei; therefore, we are unable to trick the muscle into getting stronger or building endurance without training. So, you'll have to pursue the prescriptions in chapter 11 to improve your muscular strength or endurance.

Table 9.1 reviews the effects of each type of training. The table shows that high-resistance training leads to the development of strength and that low-resistance repetitions lead to muscular endurance. It also suggests that questions remain regarding the effects of training

Table 9.1 Strength–Endurance Continuum

	Strength	Short-term (anaerobic) endurance	Intermediate endurance	Long-term endurance
Outcome	Maximum force	Brief (2–3 min) persistence with heavy load	Persistence with intermediate load	Persistence with lighter load
Prescription	4–8RM (slow) 3 sets rest >3 min	15–25RM 3 sets rest 1–3 min	30–50RM 2 sets rest <1 min	Over 100RM 1 set —
Improves	Contractile protein ATP and CP Connective tissue	Some strength and anaerobic metabolism (glycolysis)	Some endurance and anaerobic metabolism Slight improvement in strength (for untrained)	Aerobic enzymes Mitochondria Oxygen and fat utilization
Doesn't improve	Oxygen intake Endurance	Oxygen intake	—	Strength

RM = maximum repetitions

ATP = adenosine triphosphate

CP = creatine phosphate

that falls between strength (high resistance and low repetitions) and endurance (low resistance and high repetitions). Use the table to help identify your training goals. Later in the chapter, we will explain how to add power to your muscular fitness training program.

Strength contributes to performance in work and sport, and strength training puts stress on bones, which leads to stronger bones and lower risk of osteoporosis. You can also use strength training to tone muscles, to improve your appearance, and, within hereditary limits, to enhance your shape. In addition, strength training will certainly help you lead an active and vigorous life, well beyond retirement years. How does this simple mode of exercise produce such remarkable results?

Strength training, also called resistance training or weight training, involves high resistance and low repetitions and leads to the following adaptations:

- Increased contractile protein (actin and myosin)
- Tougher connective tissue
- Reduced inhibitions
- Contractile efficiency
- Possible increase in number of muscle fibers
- Increase in muscle mass and cross-sectional area (hypertrophy)

• *Contractile protein.* Years ago, Gordon (1967) compared the effects of strength and endurance training on muscle proteins. Researchers throughout the world have since corroborated the results. Strength training adds to the portion of the muscle that generates tension, the contractile proteins. Endurance training, on the other hand, enhances the energy supply system, the aerobic enzymes (all enzymes are constructed of proteins). But the most surprising outcome of Gordon's study was the observation that strength training brought about a decline in endurance enzymes, and that endurance training led to a decline in contractile protein. Thus, if you train only for strength or endurance, you could lose a bit of the other. This aspect of specificity shouldn't surprise us too much—the size and strength of your thigh muscles increase during weight training, but decline somewhat when you return to distance running.

Strength training adds to the portion of the muscle that generates tension, the contractile proteins.

• *Connective tissue.* Connective tissue and tendons grow in size and toughness when you place them under tension. This increased toughness in tendons may help quiet the inhibitory influence of the muscle receptor known as the tendon organ, a receptor sensitive to stretching. The increase in thickness of connective tissue contributes some to the growth, or hypertrophy, of the muscle.

• *Nervous system.* Some of the effects of strength training occur in the nervous system. With experience, we seem to have fewer inhibitions, both in the central nervous system and from muscle receptors. Prac-

New Fibers?

We once believed that the number of muscle fibers was set at birth and was not subject to change. Van Linge (1962) transplanted the tendon of a small rat muscle into a position where it would have to assume a tremendous workload. He studied the rat muscle after he had subjected it to a period of heavy training and found that the transplanted muscle had doubled its weight and tripled its strength. Furthermore, the heavy workload stimulated the development of new muscle fibers. Research indicates a role for satellite cells in muscle hypertrophy. They seem to aid regeneration of injured cells and may contribute to the formation of new fibers (Barton-Davis, Shoturma, and Sweeney 1999).

tice (repetition) allows us to be more efficient, more skilled in the application of force. Thus, practice alone accounts for some of the improvement in the early stages of training. This notion may explain why involuntary contractions brought on by an electrical stimulator do not equal the results obtained with voluntary contractions. Involuntary contractions may elicit changes in the muscle, but they don't teach the nervous system how to contract (Massey et al. 1965).

• *Muscle fibers.* The ability to look at samples of human muscle before and after training has led to some fascinating questions. Can strength training lead to the formation of additional muscle fibers?

Studies on human muscle suggest that we may be able to increase the number of muscle fibers when overloaded fibers split to form new fibers. This finding, however, is still the

Flexibility Effects

To understand the effect of training on range of motion, we must first consider the limits of flexibility. The tough connective tissue that covers muscles is a major restriction to range of motion, as are the joint capsule and tendons. Thus, training must concentrate on altering these limits. Flexibility decreases with age and inactivity. Some injuries may be more likely as flexibility decreases, and lower back problems are associated with poor flexibility (back, hamstrings) and weak abdominal muscles. On the other hand, enhanced flexibility may improve performance in some sports, especially those with obvious flexibility components (gymnastics, diving, wrestling).

Increased muscle and joint temperatures increase flexibility, as do specific stretching exercises. Stretching gradually leads to minor distensions in connective tissue, and the summation of these small changes can dramatically improve range of motion.

Years ago, flexibility exercises conjured up images of vigorous bobbing and jerking movements, but times have changed. Today, we engage in static stretching or dynamic stretching, such as sport-related swinging of the golf club. The reason for the change is the stretch reflex. A rapid stretch invokes a stretch reflex, and the reflex calls forth a vigorous contraction of the muscle. Because a vigorous contraction is the opposite of what we are seeking, we must avoid explosive stretching and learn the gentle art of static stretching. See chapter 11 for stretching instructions.

subject of scientific debate. And we would never suggest that you will form new fibers as the result of ordinary strength training. But athletes who spend hours each day lifting weights or who use hormones (anabolic steroids, growth hormone) to promote extra growth may be able to increase the number of muscle fibers. Note, however, that anabolic steroids have been found to lower HDL cholesterol and increase the risk of heart disease.

ENDURANCE TRAINING EFFECTS

Endurance training, which involves low resistance and high repetitions, leads to the following adaptations:

- Increased aerobic enzymes
- Increased mitochondrial density
- Increased capillaries
- More efficient contractions
- Possible changes in fiber type (e.g., fast-twitch to slow-twitch)

We've already mentioned the effects of endurance training on aerobic enzymes, particularly those involved in fat metabolism, on mitochondria, and on capillaries. Aerobic pathways that are more efficient are able to provide more energy from fat, thereby conserving muscle glycogen as well as blood glucose, which is the preferred fuel of the brain and nervous system. As a result, muscles that once fatigued in minutes become able to endure for hours. Some of the effects of endurance training take place in the nervous system. Skilled, more efficient movement conserves energy, thereby contributing to endurance. But most documented effects of muscular endurance training seem to focus on muscle fibers.

Evidence suggests that the aerobic enzyme improvements noted in endurance training may be an early stage in the eventual transformation of fast-twitch to slow-twitch muscle fibers. Pette (1984) has reported metabolic (enzyme) and then structural changes in muscle following prolonged endurance training (electrical stimulation). Studies of rat and rabbit muscle show that fast fibers first take on improved oxidative capabilities and eventually assume the contractile properties of slow-twitch fibers. We do not yet know if these fiber-type changes occur in humans.

We do know that successful distance runners have as high as 80 percent slow-twitch fibers. Is that high percentage due to fiber-type transformation or to heredity? At present, it appears that endurance training can improve the aerobic or oxidative capabilities of all fibers, and that fast-twitch fibers become more able to use oxygen. These studies demonstrate that muscle is extremely adaptable and that it can adjust to the demands imposed on it.

METHODS OF TRAINING

What is the best method to train for strength or endurance: static, dynamic, or isokinetic? The answer depends on what you are training to accomplish, the goal of your training. If you just want to get stronger, almost any method will work. If you want to gain strength to improve performance in work or sport, your training should be specific to your goal. We conducted a study in which college women trained with weights (isotonic), isokinetic devices, or calisthenics. The isotonic group did best on lifting tests, and the calisthenics group scored best on calisthenics tests. The isokinetic training group, which gained strength on the isokinetic devices, came in third on the other two tests. This study showed the importance of training in the manner in which you will eventually use the strength (Sharkey et al. 1978).

- Static (isometric) training. Based on an early study conducted in Germany (Hettinger and Müller 1953), static training was popular until studies finally compared isometrics with traditional weightlifting and found that static contractions came in a distant second. Isometric contractions don't provide a sense of accomplishment through lifting something. They elevate blood pressure, and they are seldom specific to the training goal. Isometrics do have some uses: in rehabilitation (when that is all that the patient can do), for work at the sticking point of a lift, and for activities that require **static strength** or endurance (e.g., archery or rock climbing). More recently, isometric contractions have been used in conjunction with weightlifting to produce better results.

- Dynamic (isotonic) training. Isotonic contractions (weightlifting) gained popularity when DeLorme and Watkins (1951) outlined a formula for success. Simply stated, the formula called for high-resistance, low-repetition exercise. People still use variations of that formula to develop **dynamic strength**. Free weights and weight machines are readily available in most health clubs. And lifting free weights remains the method of choice for most serious athletes and bodybuilders.

- Isokinetic training. Isokinetic exercises combine the best features of isometric (near maximal force) and isotonic (full range of motion) training. With the appropriate device, the exerciser can overload the muscles with a near maximal contraction throughout the range of motion and control the speed of contraction. The problem, if one exists, seems to be the lack of specific devices for many sports skills (see figure 9.1) and the cost of sport-specific equipment. But as more devices are developed for specific sports, isokinetic training may become even more popular.

No single method is best for strength or endurance training. Free weights are inexpensive and versatile, but they require more supervision for safety. Weight machines are convenient and require less supervision. Isokinetic devices are effective, but are costly and limited in their application. But unlike weightlifting, isokinetic training doesn't cause muscle soreness. Thus, people can do it in conjunction with other activities without adversely affecting performance.

A note of caution before we go on: Be sure that the training program you adopt is appropriate to your level of fitness and ability. What is best for beginners doesn't work for athletes, and vice versa. In psychology, many theories are based on research conducted on college freshmen and rats. In exercise physiology, numerous studies have been conducted on "gym rats," college students enrolled in activity classes. Studies that compare various

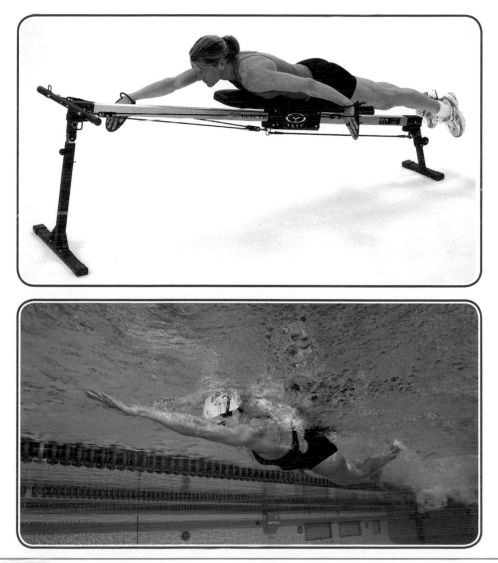

FIGURE 9.1 The swim bench provides a sport-specific way to train swimming strokes.

Top photo courtesy of www.vasatrainer.com.

forms of strength training on gym rats all seem to yield similar results: With beginners who follow the prescription, anything works. But that finding doesn't predict how the method will work on athletes or others with high levels of strength, and it doesn't prove that the increased strength will improve performance. We know how to improve strength. Now we need to find out how much strength a person needs to improve performance and how best to train to get results (chapter 11).

MUSCLE SORENESS

The muscle soreness that becomes evident 24 hours after you overdo training (delayed-onset muscle soreness, or DOMS) may be due to slight tears in connective tissue, to uncontrolled contractions or spasms of individual muscle fibers, to muscle fiber damage, or to the lingering effects of metabolic by-products. We are reasonably certain that soreness is not due to leftover lactic acid, which is eliminated within an hour of cessation of effort. We do know that certain types of exercise (but not isokinetic) lead to soreness that often persists for days and can make subsequent activity less enjoyable. Komi and Buskirk (1972) compared two types of strength training: **concentric contraction** (as in ordinary flexion) and eccentric (in which the muscle is under high tension as it lowers an overload). Subjects in the eccentric group, the group that lowered the weight, complained of muscle soreness, whereas the other group did not (see figure 9.2). So if you begin a weightlifting program and plan to lower the weights, be prepared for some soreness.

You may be surprised to know that the eccentric group in the Komi and Buskirk study gained a bit more strength, a common finding in eccentric training studies, probably because you can let down more weight than you can lift (hence, the muscle is under more tension). But before you get excited about eccentric training, remember what we keep saying about specificity: Unless your sport or job calls for letting down heavy loads, the training may not help performance as much as regular weight training will, and you are certain to get muscle soreness with **eccentric contractions**.

You can diminish soreness by beginning with light weights and progressing gradually. Avoid maximal lifting, all-out running, or ballistic movements such as hard throwing or serving at the start of the season. Be patient. Experience shows that we are seldom patient enough; therefore, we need a way to reduce soreness. Stretching has been shown to reduce muscle discomfort (deVries and Housh 1994), so stretch after a warm-up and after exercise and whenever you feel tight or sore. If your legs are stiff and sore during a long flight, go to the rear of the plane and stretch. If other passengers see you trying to push down the wall of the galley, don't be embarrassed. Fitness enthusiasts will understand that you are experiencing the pleasure and relief of a good static stretch.

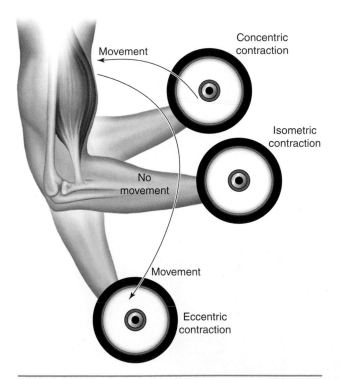

FIGURE 9.2 Eccentric contraction happens when a muscle lengthens during contraction, such as lowering a dumbbell, or downhill running or hiking. It is more likely to cause muscular microdamage, leading to delayed onset muscle soreness, than is concentric (shortening) or isometric (holding length constant) muscle contraction.

Muscle soreness is correlated with submicroscopic muscle damage, accumulation of fluid (edema), and diminished strength that may persist up to 2 weeks. The damage may occur in older or otherwise susceptible muscle fibers. Recovery is faster and soreness diminishes after successive bouts of exercise. Leakage of the muscle enzyme creatine kinase (CK) suggests membrane damage. Because soreness peaks 1 or 2 days after the effort and the enzyme levels peak 2 or 3 days later, the cause of muscle soreness is still unclear (Newham 1988). Fortunately, DOMS occurs only during the start-up phase, and the symptoms disappear within a few weeks, reappearing only after a long layoff or the vigorous start of a new activity. Indeed, exercise-induced muscle soreness seems to inoculate the body from subsequent discomfort for up to 6 months following the initial soreness (Nosaka et al. 2001).

> **M**uscle soreness is correlated with submicroscopic muscle damage, accumulation of fluid (edema), and diminished strength that may persist for up to 2 weeks.

FORCE–VELOCITY RELATIONSHIP

Years ago, while attempting to make some sense of the confusing and sometimes contradictory research on strength and speed, we noticed that strength and speed seemed to be related when heavy loads were used in the test of speed. When little resistance was used, strength and speed were not related. In an effort to generalize the findings to other areas of work and sport, we turned to a well-known physiological principle: the force–velocity relationship.

It has long been known that velocity of shortening in a contraction is greatest with no load or resistance. As the resistance increases, the velocity of shortening decreases (see figure 9.3). We thought that the force–velocity relationship could help simplify basic principles about how and why muscles should be trained for force, speed, or power. From reading the available literature, we concluded that strength training would improve heavily loaded movements, but would have little effect on the velocity of unloaded movements, and vice versa. Imagine our delight when we happened on studies that confirmed the hypothesis!

Ikai (1970) demonstrated that training for strength alone led to increased strength and velocity with heavy loads. He also found that training for speed alone improved velocity with light loads, but did nothing for strength or velocity with heavy loads. Most interesting of all was the finding that training with intermediate loads (30%–60% of maximal strength) at the highest speed possible led to improvements in force, speed, and power. Years later, this finding was corroborated when Kanehisa and Miyashita (1983) confirmed the specificity of velocity in training. They trained three groups at either slow-, medium-, or high-speed contractions. The slow-speed group improved in leg-extension strength at slow speeds, and the fast group improved in the force that they could exert at fast speeds. But only the intermediate-speed group was able to improve at all speeds. Power training (15–25 repetitions at 30%–60% of maximal strength, as fast as possible) may be the way to train when you desire speed or power (see table 9.2). Does that throw out the concept of specificity?

If you are preparing for the shot put, a sport in which both force and speed are important, you should train for strength, since you will need a considerable amount of it. If high speed is your primary

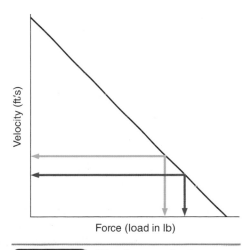

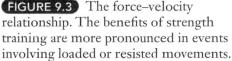

FIGURE 9.3 The force–velocity relationship. The benefits of strength training are more pronounced in events involving loaded or resisted movements.

Table 9.2 Training for Power

	Power with heavy load	Power with moderate load
Prescription	8–12RM FAP* 60% of max	15–25RM FAP 30% of max
Sets	3 sets	2–3 sets
Rest	3 min	1–2 min
Improves	Some strength Neural recruitment ATP and CP Connective tissue	Some muscular endurance Neural recruitment Strength
Doesn't improve	Oxygen intake	Oxygen intake

*FAP = fast as possible. Training is sport or activity specific, and may require specialized equipment to allow explosive movement.

goal, as in pitching a fastball, train for speed. Power training could help performance in both. The power prescription is ideal for sports like cross-country skiing, a power and endurance sport that requires hundreds of little explosions to power the skier uphill. The principle of specificity does not imply that you should avoid other types of training, only that training must eventually mimic the movements of the sport to obtain the best results.

A final note concerning the use of isotonic and especially isokinetic training for speed, strength, and power development is in order. Both techniques adapt to the advice that we've just provided. By reducing resistance below 30 percent of maximal, you can increase the velocity of contractions. By increasing resistance above 60 percent, you'll focus on force development.

When power (force times velocity) is required, contract as fast as possible with weights in the range of 30 to 60 percent of maximal. Although isokinetic contractions seem ideally suited for strength or power development, it is possible that you can develop both strength and power with weight-training equipment or even with calisthenics and **plyometrics** that follow prescriptions provided in chapter 11.

PRELOAD AND ELASTIC RECOIL

Before we leave the subject of power, we want to acquaint you with one of the secrets of athletic performance. It took us years to realize that a well-known fact of muscle physiology—that a muscle exerts more force when it is stretched just before contraction—describes how muscles are meant to work. The stretch, or preload, does several things: It aligns contractile elements (crossbridges) in muscle for maximal force, takes slack out of the system, and stores elastic energy in the muscle–tendon complex. Studies of the force and efficiency of contraction indicate that this stretch-shortening cycle is the way that muscle works most efficiently (Komi 1992).

Here's how it works in a vertical jump. First, you sink at the knees to stretch the thigh muscles. Then, you immediately contract the stretched muscles and quickly convert the preload into elastic recoil as you jump. To see how effective the combination of preload and elastic recoil is, compare that jump with one in which you eliminate the preload. Sink to the starting position, stop for a full second, and then jump. Without preload and elastic recoil, the results are inferior. The preload and elastic recoil combination works whenever you are able to preload just before contraction. It happens in running at the ankle and thigh, in cross-country skiing, in tennis during the serve, and, of course, in weightlifting, where it has been called cheating! Often, the preload and elastic recoil combination happens automatically. If it doesn't, see whether you can use it to provide more power, or the same power with less effort. Done properly, it contributes to power and economy of movement.

> **S**tudies of the force and efficiency of contraction indicate that this stretch-shortening cycle is the way that muscle works most efficiently.

CORE TRAINING

An important development in muscular fitness training is a focus on the core, the central portion of the body. Core exercises recruit one or more large-muscle areas (abdominal, back, chest, shoulders, hips), involve two or more primary joints (multi-joint), and are a high priority for health and performance (Baechle, Earle, and Wathen 2000). A moderate amount of core training seems essential for lower back health. More is necessary for those in physically demanding occupations, such as construction, firefighting, law enforcement, and the military (Sharkey and Davis 2008). The relationship of core fitness to performance in sport is less well established. Logic tells us that we must develop the **core muscles** as we train the muscles of the arms and legs.

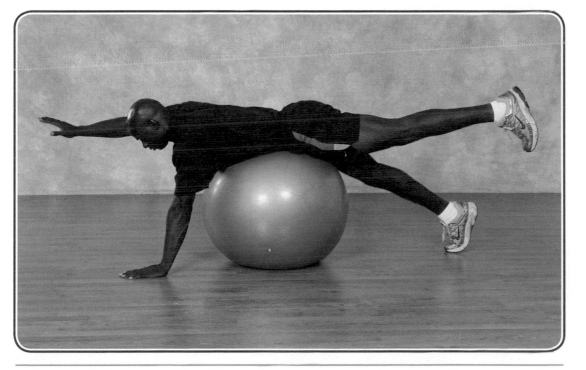

■ Strong and balanced muscles of the trunk permit better transfer of power from one part of the body to another or to an external object, such as a golf ball. Here, a participant exercises on a stability ball.

Willardson (2007) reviewed research evaluating the use of core training by athletes. His summary suggests varying the core exercises to fit the training period. During the recovery and off-season periods, small-load exercises with isometric Swiss balls and long tension times are recommended. During preseason and in-season periods, sport-specific free-weight exercises performed while standing on a stable surface are recommended for increases in core strength and power. He further recommends balance-board and stability-disc exercises, performed in conjunction with plyometric exercises, to improve propriocep-tive and reactive capabilities, which may reduce the likelihood of lower extremity injuries.

MUSCULAR FITNESS FIELD TESTS

Maintaining adequate strength throughout life is important to our ability to live indepen-dently and enjoy life to the fullest. We can measure and develop strength in several ways, each of which is highly specific to how we use strength and should dictate the mode of training and testing.

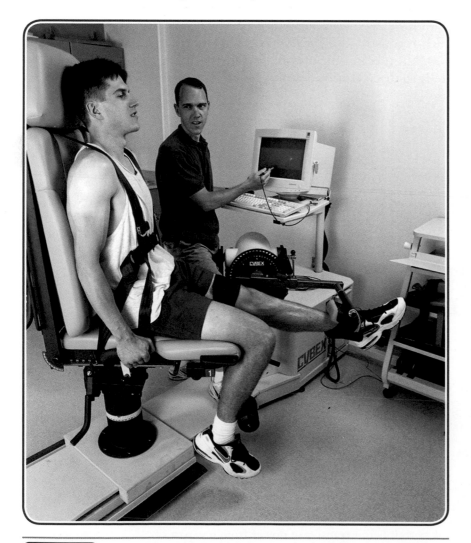

FIGURE 9.4 Isokinetic strength testing is important for sports medicine and rehabilitation.

Using muscular power during movement is called dynamic strength. Dynamic strength, also called **isotonic strength**, is defined as the maximal weight that a person can lift one time. This amount is actually a measure of strength at the hardest part of the lift, usu-ally the beginning. Because the mechanical advantage of your mus-cle-lever system changes, a lift such as a forearm curl becomes easier after you overcome the initial resis-tance and angle of pull. Dynamic strength measurements are related to performance in sport and work. Weightlifting with machines or free weights is the common form of isotonic training. (*Iso* means same, and *tonic* means tone.)

Another measure of strength is static strength. A person demon-strates static strength by exerting maximal force against an immov-able object. Also called **isometric strength**, it is specific to the angle at which it was trained. Static strength doesn't necessarily reflect dynamic strength or strength throughout the range of motion. You train by exerting near maxi-mum force against an immovable object. (*Metric* means length, so *isometric* means same length—the muscle doesn't change length appreciably during the contraction.)

A popular measure of strength in clinical and rehabilitation settings is **isokinetic strength**, which is measured with expensive electronic or hydraulic apparatus. The equipment allows the exertion of maximal force throughout the range of motion, as well as the control of the speed of contraction. Although such devices have become popular testing aids, it is not yet clear to what extent strength throughout the range of motion is related to performance. (*Kinetic* means motion or speed, so *isokinetic* means same speed.) A number of sophisticated devices are available for isokinetic measurement of muscle force and power. Sports medicine specialists test knee extension and flexion strength, power, and endurance, and use isokinetic devices to rehabilitate athletes following knee surgery. **Variable (accommodating) resistance** devices are used to strengthen muscles and to prevent injuries (see figure 9.4).

Athletes may use free weights, isokinetic machines, and even isometric contractions to improve performance. Keep in mind that strength is specific to the method of training, to the speed of contractions, and to the angle used in training. Therefore, to obtain an accurate assessment of the effects of training, the method of testing should be specific to the mode of training. In other words, a static strength test will not accurately measure changes from dynamic strength training or vice versa.

You may wonder how you stack up in terms of muscular fitness (see table 9.3). If you want to assess your muscular fitness, be sure to warm up and do some stretching before you attempt a vigorous test. Or you may prefer to engage in some training before you do

Table 9.3 Muscular Fitness Tests

			MEN			WOMEN		
			Low	Medium	High	Low	Medium	High
Upper body	Strength	Chin-up*	<6	6–10	>10	<20	20–30	>30
	Endurance	Push-up	<20	20–40	>40	<10	10–20	>20
Trunk	Endurance	Sit-up	<30	30–50	>50	<25	25–40	>40
Leg	Strength	Leg press**	<220%	220–320%	>320%	<220%	220–300%	>300%
	Flexibility	Sit and reach	No	Yes	Beyond	No	Yes	Beyond
	Power	Vertical jump***	<17 in. (43 cm)	17–23 in. (43-58 cm)	>23 in. (58 cm)	<10 in. (25 cm)	10–15 in. (25-38 cm)	>15 in. (38 cm)
	Speed	40 m sprint	>7.5 sec.	7.5–6.0 sec.	<6.0 sec.	>9.0 sec.	9.0–7.5 sec.	<7.5 sec.

*Women do modified chin up.

**Percent of body weight.

***Low vertical jump is associated with a low percentage of fast-twitch fibers.

these or other tests. In the chapters that follow, we'll describe the effects of training and provide training prescriptions to help you improve your scores.

SUMMARY

We've introduced the components of muscular fitness and discussed their contributions to health and performance. We hope that you have decided to integrate muscular fitness into your activity program. You won't be sorry that you did. With improved muscular fitness, you will be better able to do yard work, to hike with a pack, to cycle or run uphill, to paddle a canoe, to cross-country and downhill ski, and more. The effects become more pronounced with every passing year. See what muscular fitness can do for you!

Research has shown that tension multiplied by time is the stimulus for strength development. How the tension is produced doesn't seem to matter. Legend tells of Milo from Crete, who began daily lifts of a young calf. As time passed and the animal grew, so did Milo's strength. More recently, study subjects have lifted weights, pulled rubber bands, squeezed bags of water, and suffered electrical stimulation to build strength. All these methods worked. We are beginning to understand how the stimulus leads to stronger, tougher, more efficient muscles. More important is our growing understanding of the distinction between strength and endurance in terms of training and cellular outcomes. We may soon be able to say how much strength or endurance is required to perform optimally in a sport or job.

By now, you know enough to design and carry out a muscular fitness program that will improve your appearance, health, and everyday performance. If you want to improve performance in work or sport, you'll find more help in chapter 14.

Improving Fitness

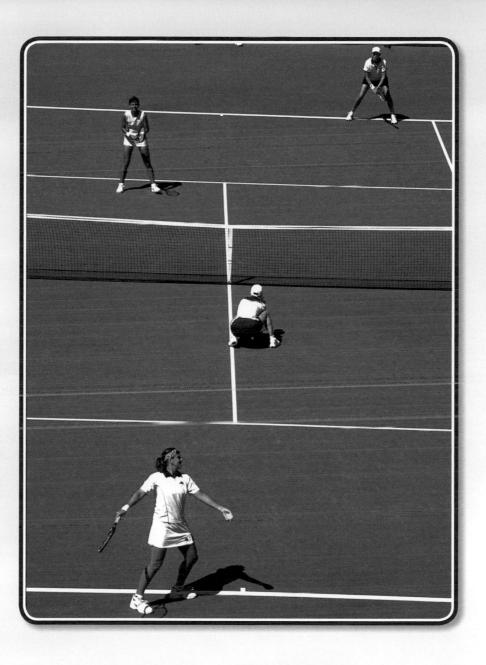

There are many ways to improve fitness: you can take the gentle approach and do it gradually, get somewhat faster results with a systematic approach, or you can rush the process, push it to the limit risking muscle soreness, overtraining, injury, or illness. This section describes the gentle and systematic approaches to improved fitness. It also illustrates the risks of overtraining and of increasing training intensity or load too rapidly.

Most individuals can improve aerobic fitness by gradually increasing the distance and pace of daily activities. Use this approach to train for hikes, bike rides, or fun runs. Senior citizens need to train for independent living, to play with the grandkids, or for travel. Improved muscular fitness is essential for seniors. Athletes and fitness enthusiasts utilize a systematic approach to training. In this section, we will outline the elements of these approaches and later provide more details in part V. Everyone should avoid overtraining and increasing intensity, duration, or training load too rapidly. Overtraining occurs when excess aerobic training causes a decline in immune response, opening the door to upper respiratory illness. Excessive muscular fitness training can cause severe muscular soreness, injury, and the risk of exertional rhabdomyolysis, a breakdown of muscle tissue that can cause kidney failure. Exercises must be prescribed and undertaken sensibly in order to realize the benefits and avoid potentially harmful side effects.

Aerobic Fitness Training

Steps for Success

"A journey of a thousand miles must begin with a single step."

Lao-Tzu

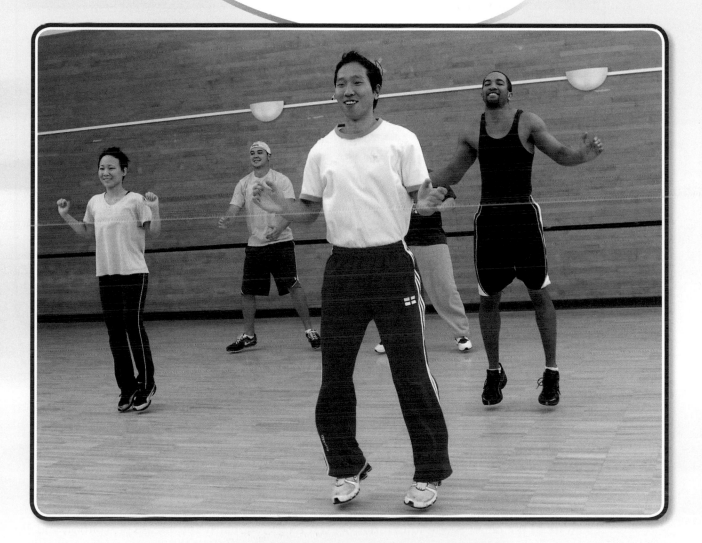

Many years ago, before we knew how to prescribe exercise, we chose from a number of unproven training systems that were based on the ideas and experience of well-known physicians, coaches, or educators. Then researchers began to identify the factors associated with improvements in fitness. Exercise prescriptions today are based on the results of thousands of studies. The dose of exercise that safely promotes the training effect is usually represented by the intensity, duration, and frequency of exercise. Research and clinical experience are adding to a carefully developed methodology for safe and effective prescription of exercise.

You earn aerobic fitness minute by minute, day by day, as you engage in appropriate training exercises. As with any treatment or drug, the exercises must be prescribed and taken with care if you are to realize the benefits and avoid potentially harmful side effects.

This chapter will help you do the following:

- Develop a personalized aerobic fitness prescription based on your level of fitness and training goals
- Use your heart rate or perceived exertion to determine exercise intensity
- Determine exercise duration using calories, minutes, or miles (kilometers)
- Decide on the appropriate frequency of exercise
- Understand how to achieve, maintain, and regain aerobic fitness
- Understand how to make training safe and enjoyable
- Apply your aerobic fitness prescription with walk–jog–run programs, cycling or swimming, or advanced training
- Select alternative ways to remain active and fit
- Deal with common exercise problems

FITNESS PRESCRIPTION

Throughout history, people have sought the health benefits believed to be associated with exercise, with prescriptions dating back to centuries-old Chinese and Roman documents. In the late 1800s, Dr. Dudley Sargent, physician and director of the Harvard college gymnasium, tested students and prescribed exercises to rectify weaknesses. Prescriptions improved only slightly until the 1950s, when researchers began to establish the link between lack of activity and heart disease. Since then, we have agreed on a definition of aerobic fitness, identified the factors that contribute to its improvement, and have become more aware of the benefits and limitations of exercise as a modality for disease prevention and rehabilitation. We now know how hard (intensity), how long (duration), and how often (frequency) one must exercise to achieve an aerobic training effect.

Figure 10.1 illustrates how to carry out the prescription on a given day. Begin every session with a warm-up to minimize soreness and risk of injury. Start with a gradual increase in exercise activity and then stretch. Pay attention to stretching the lower back, hamstrings, calf muscles, and any sore muscles. Muscle soreness shows up 24 hours after the start of a program, but diminishes soon thereaf-

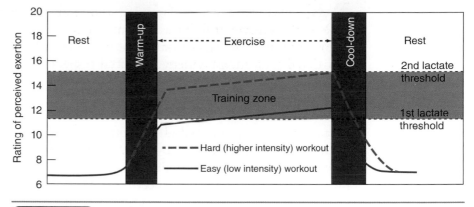

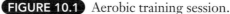

FIGURE 10.1 Aerobic training session.

ter. It won't return unless you lay off for months, increase intensity, or do a new activity. Follow the prescription during the aerobic portion of the session, and then be sure to cool down before you hit the shower. Easy jogging, walking, and stretching help lower body temperature, reduce metabolic by-products such as lactic acid, and dissipate the hormone norepinephrine, which could cause irregular heart rhythms.

To vary the program, take different routes, work at the upper edge of the training zone for short periods (i.e., hard and short) and the lower edge for longer periods (easy and long), or use another activity for variety (cross-training). As training progresses, the same pace will feel easier and more enjoyable. As fitness improves, the prescription needs to change, calling for more intensity, duration, or frequency. You'll find yourself going faster at the same level of perceived exertion. By then, you will have an idea of what you want to achieve from fitness, and you can decide what works and feels best to you.

Intensity

Intensity, the most important factor in the development of maximal oxygen intake ($\dot{V}O_2max$), reflects the energy requirements of the exercise, the rate of oxygen consumption, and the calories of energy expended per minute. Although the training heart rate is typically used to define intensity, other measures can be used (see table 10.1).

Table 10.1 Measures of Exercise Intensity

Intensity	Heart rate* (bpm)	RPE**	Cal/min***	METs****
Light	90–120	8–10	5	4.0
Moderate	120–150	11–14	10	8.1
Heavy	150–200	15–18	15	12.2

For any specific activity and intensity, the number of calories burned per minute depends on body weight; therefore, a heavier person burns more during a given exercise.

*Approximate range for a 20-year-old person. Subtract 1% for every 2 years after age 20.

**RPE = Rating of perceived exertion (6–20 scale).

***1 L of oxygen is equivalent to 5 cal/min.

****The MET, or metabolic equivalent, is a multiple of the resting metabolic rate. The resting rate is 1.2 cal/min (1 MET), so 12 cal/min = 10 METs for a 150-pound (68 kg) person. Each MET equals 3.5 ml oxygen per kilogram of body weight each minute, so the MET is adjusted for body weight.

A comprehensive review of training studies showed that maximal gains in aerobic fitness ($\dot{V}O_2$max) were achieved with high intensity (90% of $\dot{V}O_2$max or 95% of maximal heart rate), a duration of 35 to 45 minutes, and a frequency of four times per week (Wenger and Bell 1986). Less intensity produced respectable increases in $\dot{V}O_2$max with less risk of injury. But keep in mind that all these conclusions were based on changes in $\dot{V}O_2$max, acknowledged as a measure of intensity (Sharkey 1991). Although $\dot{V}O_2$max is important, better measures of endurance are available, such as the first and second lactate thresholds. Sustained training just above LT1 is effective at improving long-term endurance. Shorter (3 to 4 min) intervals just above LT2 contribute to improvements in the second lactate threshold, the one related to performance in races lasting from 15 minutes to 2 hours or more. But fitness and performance aren't the only goals. People can achieve health benefits, weight control, and improved appearance with moderate levels of intensity, duration, and frequency. Use the prescription in table 10.2 as a starting point, but don't be a slave to training. Adapt the program to meet your personal style and goals.

Athletes occasionally train at higher intensity or longer duration, and sometimes do two or even three workouts a day. Chapter 14 provides advice on advanced endurance training and insights into cross-training and other ways to make fitness enjoyable. Table 10.3 shows how some popular training activities fit the prescription.

Table 10.2　Aerobic Fitness Prescription

Activity category	RPE	Duration (calories)*	Frequency (days/wk)	Walking or running distance (to meet caloric needs)
Inactive	11–13	100–200	3–4	1–2 mi (1.6–3.2 km)
Moderately active	12–14	200–400	5–6	2–4 mi (3.2–6.4 km)
Very active	13–16	>400	≥6	>4 mi (6.4 km)

*Add or subtract 10% for each 15 lb over or under 150 lb (or 7 kg above or below 70 kg).

Table 10.3　Sample Aerobic Activities

Fitness category (ml · kg^{-1} · min^{-1})	Running Distance (mi [km])	Running Time (min)	Jogging Distance (mi [km])	Jogging Time (min)	Cycling Distance (mi [km])	Cycling Time (min)	Walking Distance (mi [km])	Walking Time (min)
Inactive	0.8–1.7 (1.3–2.7)	7–14	0.8–1.7 (1.3–2.7)	10–20	1.9–3.9 (3.1–6.3)	12–24	1.0–2.1 (1.6–3.4)	18–36
Moderately active	1.7–3.4 (2.7–5.5)	14–27	1.7–3.4 (2.7–5.5)	20–40	3.9–7.8 (6.3–12.6)	24–47	2.1–4.2 (3.4–6.8)	36–72
Very active	≥3.4 (≥5.5)	≥27	≥3.4 (≥5.5)	≥40	≥7.8 (≥12.6)	≥47	≥4.2 (≥6.8)	≥72

Adapted from B.J. Sharkey, 1997, *Fitness and work capacity*, 2nd ed. (Missoula, MT: USDA Forest Service).

Minimum Training Intensity

Early studies agreed that training had to exceed a certain minimum metabolic level or threshold if significant changes in aerobic fitness were to occur (see figure 10.2). In an early study, we trained young men at heart rates of 120, 150, and 180 beats per minute. The higher-intensity groups improved $\dot{V}O_2$max similarly, but the low-intensity subjects did not (Sharkey and Holleman 1967). Then we learned that training intensity depended on the person's level of fitness. Low-fit subjects made progress at lower intensities, whereas high-fit subjects had a higher training threshold (Sharkey 1970). The minimal training threshold, first called the aerobic threshold, is now known as the first lactate threshold (LT1). Training at the LT1 will feel like an intensity that you could easily sustain for a long time.

Maximum Training Intensity

Studies also defined an upper limit to training intensity. They showed that training above that level didn't yield additional improvements in $\dot{V}O_2$max. In recent years, we recognized that this upper limit of the training zone coincides with the second lactate threshold (LT2), once called the anaerobic threshold. When the activity exceeds the ability of the muscle to produce energy aerobically and blood lactate accumulates rapidly, the ability to sustain the exercise decreases, and limited aerobic training benefits occur. Stated another way, anaerobic exercise does not contribute substantially to the development of aerobic fitness.

Thus, the optimal **aerobic training zone** ranges from the first lactate threshold on the low end to the second lactate threshold, the point of diminishing returns. Training at the low end of the zone leads to changes in slow-oxidative muscle fibers, improvements in fat metabolism, and changes in LT1. Training at the high end of the zone recruits and benefits fast, oxidative-glycolytic muscle fibers and leads to central circulatory (cardiovascular) benefits. In addition, the high-intensity interval training that athletes use has been shown to raise LT2. This improvement in LT2 can take place without an increase in $\dot{V}O_2$max, especially among those who have already undergone extensive training.

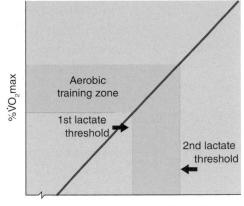

FIGURE 10.2 Aerobic fitness improves when you exercise within the aerobic training zone. This zone applies to aerobic fitness training. Endurance athletes generally do interval training just above the second lactate threshold and easy training near the first lactate threshold.

Training Heart Rate

Early training studies focused on the metabolic demands of training (liters of oxygen consumed or kilocalories of energy expenditure). Because heart rate is correlated to metabolism, it was used as a simple, inexpensive way to translate training information to the lay public. Unfortunately, over the years, the public and some fitness professionals have lost sight of this point. Today many mistakenly consider the training heart rate, not the sustained metabolism of a large muscle mass (e.g., legs), to be the goal of training. They believe that raising the heart rate, no matter how it is done, will improve fitness. For example, the elevation of the heart rate during weight training has led some to believe that circuit weight training can improve aerobic fitness. They ignore the fact that weight training engages each muscle group for only 20 to 30 seconds, far too short a time to prompt changes in the oxidative pathways of muscles. The training heart rate is a convenient external indicator of exercise intensity and oxygen consumption, but it isn't an end in itself. We'll show an alternative to using heart rate later in this chapter.

Aerobic Training Zone

The aerobic **training zone** is defined as the training intensity between the first and second lactate thresholds. Both thresholds are related to your level of activity and fitness. Inactive people have a low LT1. If normal daily activity seldom exceeds a slow walk, a brisk walk will exceed the threshold and elicit a training effect. Regular participation in high-intensity activity raises LT2, so highly active people have an elevated threshold and a higher training zone.

In the past, the training zone was based on a percentage of estimated maximal heart rate. Because maximal heart rate declines with age, we used both fitness level and age-adjusted maximal heart rate to determine the training zone.

Fitness (milliliters per kilogram per minute)	Training zone (percent maximal heart rate)
Low (under 35)	60 to 75 percent
Medium (35 to 45)	70 to 85 percent
High (over 45)	75 to 90 percent

If your maximal heart rate (HRmax) hasn't been measured, we estimate it with the following formula:

$$HRmax = 220 - age$$

Since maximal heart rate varies considerably (see table 3.3, page 61), we use estimated heart rate with caution. If the training zone feels too high, we urge people to back off to a more comfortable level. Your maximal heart rate estimate could be lower than expected, so if the zone feels too easy, we move it up a bit. Because of this variability and uncertainty, and because of new research findings, we decided not to emphasize use of heart rate to identify training intensity. Instead, we use the rating of perceived exertion (RPE) to define training intensity. Perceived exertion is determined with a simple rating scale that provides an estimate of exercise intensity (see table 10.4).

First developed by Swedish psychologist Gunner Borg (1973), perceived exertion has been validated and used in numerous studies (Robertson 2004). You can use the perceived exertion scale to establish exercise intensity at the start of exercise and maintain it throughout the workout (Kang et al. 2003), focusing on how you feel rather than on your heart rate. We provide two practical versions, along with related information that you can use to define levels of exertion. To estimate a common scale, simply remove the last zero from each heart rate in table 10.4.

The talk test is another way to determine whether you are within your zone. You should be able to carry on a conversation while you train, at least until you approach your second lactate threshold. Exercise doesn't have to hurt to be good.

Both thresholds are related to your level of activity and fitness. The first lactate threshold is related to activities that you regularly carry out. Sedentary people have LT1s similar to the oxygen cost of activities of daily living (walking, climbing stairs). People who are more active have higher thresholds. The greater the intensity of your long-duration activities, the higher the oxygen cost of your first lactate threshold. In other words, the first lactate threshold for an active person will be higher than that for a sedentary person. The second lactate threshold is related to the highest intensity aerobic activity that you perform regularly for at least several minutes. Regular participation in high-intensity activity raises LT2, so highly active people have elevated thresholds and higher training zones.

Table 10.4 Perceived Exertion: Evaluating Your Intensity Based on Breathing and Duration

Estimated heart rate	Breathing scale	Duration
60		
70	Can sing full songs	Could continue all day
80		Could continue 4–8 hours
90	Can sing partial verses	Could continue 3–4 hours
100		Could continue 2–3 hours
110	Can talk in full sentences	Could continue 1–2 hours
120		Could continue 45–60 minutes
130	Can talk in short sentences	Could continue 30–45 minutes
140		Could continue 20–30 minutes
150	Breathing hard, thinking clearly	Could continue 15–20 minutes
160		Could continue 10–15 minutes
170	Breathing very hard	Could continue 5–10 minutes
180		Could continue 2–5 minutes
190		Could continue 1–2 minutes
200		Could continue <1 minute

You can use perceived exertion to define your training zone. The data from a large multicenter research project indicate that the RPE can be used to estimate the lactate thresholds (Gaskill et al. 2001). The thresholds form the limits of the aerobic training zone.

First lactate threshold

- Talk in short to full sentences
- Could continue for 45 minutes to 2 hours

Second lactate threshold

- Breathing hard, but still thinking clearly
- Could continue for 10-30 minutes.

Use table 10.2 to determine your thresholds and aerobic training zone. To determine your first lactate threshold (LT1), complete a warm-up and then find a comfortable intensity (in any aerobic activity) that you can easily maintain for 1 to 2 hours. Hold that pace for 10 minutes and then see whether it fits the talk test. The activity should feel somewhat easy, and you should be able to talk in full sentences and keep going for at least an hour. If you want to know your heart rate at LT1, stop, immediately count the rate for 15 seconds, and then multiply by 4 for the rate per minute. This intensity defines your LT1, the bottom of your aerobic training zone. Generally, your aerobic training zone ranges from the LT1 heart rate to about 25 beats per minute higher.

To determine your second lactate threshold (LT2), increase your intensity until your heart rate is 25 beats above LT1. After about 5 minutes, check table 10.2. If the exertion feels hard, if you can maintain it for another 10 to 30 minutes, if you are on the verge of breakaway ventilation, and if you can't talk but can still think clearly, then you are near your second lactate threshold. If necessary, adjust the pace until the effort seems hard and meets all of the above criteria. Take your heart rate, note your pace (e.g., miles or kilometers per hour), and how you feel (breathing and so forth). You can carry on a conversation at the lower end of the zone (LT1), but you will be able to say only short phrases at LT2. We'll say more about the training zone later in this chapter.

In time, you won't need to check your heart rate because you'll know how it feels to be in the training zone (perceived exertion). We begin with a prescription, but as you learn more about exercise and your body, improve your fitness, and decide on your goals, you will outgrow the need for heart rates and training zones. The RPE is a simple way to judge exercise intensity on a numerical scale that correlates to heart rate, lactate thresholds, and other physiological variables. The RPE is a valid tool for the prescription of exercise (Steed, Gaesser, and Weltman 1994).

Heart Rates

We have elected to minimize use of heart rates in this edition of the book. For many, they are a needless distraction from the pleasures of exercise. If you enjoy the discipline of heart rate measurements, however, continue to use them. You can use a percentage of your maximal heart rate (e.g., HRmax = 220 − age) or the **heart rate reserve** formula (reserve = HRmax − resting HR) to identify your training heart rate. The heart rate reserve formula calculates a heart rate equal to the percentage of $\dot{V}O_2$max. For a heart rate equivalent to 70 percent of $\dot{V}O_2$max for a 50-year-old (220 − 50 = 170):

$$HR = [70\% \times (HRmax - resting\ HR)] + resting\ HR$$
$$= [70\% \times (170 - 70)] + 70$$
$$= 140\ bpm$$

By contrast, 70 percent of the maximal heart rate (170) equals 119 beats per minute, which is approximately equal to 55 percent of $\dot{V}O_2$max. The heart rate reserve is sometimes used to adjust for measured differences in the resting and maximal heart rates, and to avoid errors in the estimation of the training heart rate.

Duration

Exercise duration and intensity go hand in hand; an increase in one requires a decrease in the other. Duration can be prescribed in terms of time, distance, or calories. We mention all three to show how they relate, but we prefer to use the calorie because it is so educational. Food labels tell you how many calories you gain when you eat and drink (a double burger equals 550 cal; beer equals 150 cal). You should also know how much exercise it takes to balance your energy intake. Jogging 1 mile (1.6 km) burns 100 calories, so you'd have to jog almost 7 miles (11.2 km) to burn the calories consumed with the burger and beer. Doing the math makes you think!

An early training study showed that low-fit people can improve their fitness with as little as 100 calories of exercise per session (10 min at 10 cal/min) (Bouchard et al. 1966). Low-fit subjects need less intensity and duration than fit subjects do to elicit a training effect. But in time, as fitness improves, they should extend duration to 200 calories or more. Fitness pioneer Dr. Tom Cureton found that people needed higher expenditures to bring about significant improvement in cholesterol levels (Cureton 1969). Additional studies have shown that longer workouts (more than 35 minutes) produce greater fitness benefits (Wenger and Bell 1986), perhaps because the proportion of fat metabolized continues to rise for the first 30 minutes of exercise.

A study of 17,000 Harvard graduates provides another way to assess the importance of exercise duration. Paffenbarger, Hyde, and Wing (1986) found significant reduction in the risk of heart disease for graduates who averaged more than 2,000 calories of exercise per week. That translates into about 300 calories daily (400 cal/day in 5 days of exercise per week). Longer duration training leads to improved fat metabolism, which may be the major health benefit of exercise. Increase your training duration to gain significant fitness, weight control, and fat metabolism benefits, and to lower blood lipids. But we have no conclusive evidence to recommend workouts that exceed 60 minutes (or 600 cal) for health benefits, other than weight loss. Endurance athletes participate in longer workouts to improve stamina and performance, not for enhanced health benefits. In fact, an epidemiological study suggests that mortality rates, which decline with increasing exercise, begin to rise when energy expenditure exceeds 3,500 calories per week (Lee, Hsieh, and Paffenbarger 1995). Table 10.5 lists some guidelines for exercise duration.

Overload is the key to improvements in training. As fitness improves, we need to increase intensity and duration if we hope to continue improvements in $\dot{V}O_2$max and the lactate thresholds. Now let's see how to adjust training frequency as training progresses.

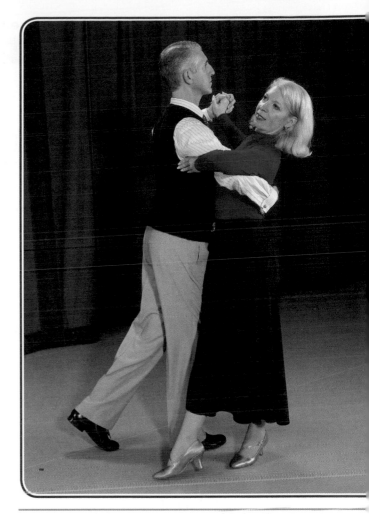

■ Low-fit people can improve their fitness levels with as little as 10 minutes of exercise per day.

Frequency

For low-fit people, three sessions a week on alternating days are sufficient to improve aerobic fitness (Jackson, Sharkey, and Johnston 1968). But as training progresses in intensity and duration, it must also increase in frequency if improvements are to continue (Pollock 1973). An extensive review of training studies found that changes in fitness are directly related to frequency of training when it is considered

Calorie

The calorie (technically a kilocalorie) is a unit of energy defined as the amount of heat required to raise the temperature of 1 kilogram of water 1 degree Celsius. We store calories when we eat and burn them when we exercise. Body weight influences caloric expenditure during exercise. A 180-pound (81.6 kg) person burns more calories running at a certain pace than one who weighs 150 pounds (68 kg). The first burns 136 calories per mile (85 calories per km), whereas the second burns 113 calories per mile (70 calories per km). In this book, caloric expenditures are based on a weight of 150 pounds; add or subtract 10 percent for each 15 pounds (6.8 kg) over or under 150 pounds. For example, add 20 percent to 113 calories to determine the cost for the 180-pound person (113 times .20 equals 22.6, plus 113 equals 135.6 calories).

Table 10.5 Duration per Training Session

Activity level	Walking distance	Calories*
Inactive	1–2 mi (1.6–3.2 km)	100–200
Moderately active	2–4 mi (3.2–6.4 km)	200–400
Very active	>4 mi (6.4 km)	>400

*Add or subtract 10% for every 15 lb above or below 150 lb (or 7 kg above or below 70 kg).

> **O**vertraining can lead to poor performance, overuse injuries, or illness through suppression of the immune system.

independent of the effects of intensity, duration, program length, and initial level of fitness (Wenger and Bell 1986). Six days per week is more than twice as effective as 3 days per week. So for fitness or weight control, consider more frequent exercise. Athletes engage in long sessions, or they train two or more times a day, two or three times a week. But they also observe the hard–easy principle, following hard or long sessions with easy or short ones. Failure to allow adequate time for recovery from training nullifies its effects; overtraining can lead to poor performance, overuse injuries, or illness through suppression of the immune system.

The body needs time to respond to the training stimulus, and some people find that they need more than 24 hours. As one of us reached his 60th year, he found that he needed more time to recover from extremely long or strenuous activity. Experiment with schedules to find one that suits you. Work out daily if you prefer, or try an alternate-day plan and increase duration. Whatever you do, be sure to schedule at least one day of relative rest or diversion each week. A colleague and former training partner once wrote, "We should approach running not as if we are trying to smash our way through some enormous wall, but as a gentle pastime by which we can coax a slow continuous stream of adaptations out of the body" (Frederick 1973, 20).

Activity level	Frequency (days per week)
Inactive	3–4 days
Moderately active	5–6
Very active	≥6*

*Athletes sometimes do two sessions per day, but always follow a hard day with an easy day.

Progression

"Make haste slowly" is a philosophy that works well for coaxing the gentle stream of improvements from your body. Training **progression** refers to how we gradually increase the overall training load. Although studies show the need to overload the body as fitness improves, few provide guidance on how to proceed. Gradual progress allows time for rest, recovery, and adjustments to training. Consider these guidelines. Meet the health goal by doing 30 minutes of moderate activity most days of the week. A brisk walk helps you meet this goal. If you have been sedentary, you may have to become active before you begin to train. Begin at the bottom of your training zone (somewhat easy) and find a comfortable duration. Remember, training does not need to be hard. Then, train 3 or 4 days per week, adjusting intensity and duration as you go. When you are ready, increase duration above what you have been doing, while staying at the same intensity. Work up to two longer sessions and one shorter session each week. Then you can increase frequency by adding an extra day with a short workout at a comfortable pace.

When you are feeling good, raise the intensity a bit, but try to avoid increasing the load too quickly. To increase intensity, replace a longer workout with one that is slightly harder (RPE of 11 to 13). Reduce the duration by increasing pace for 5 to 10 minutes and then slowing down to recover; repeat a few moderate intervals. Add intensity sessions gradually and pay attention to how your body responds. Then, repeat the cycle. Build on your progress and slowly increase duration, frequency, and intensity until you feel that you are where you would like to be.

After increasing duration, frequency, and intensity over several weeks, you should schedule an easier week for recovery, a process called **periodization**. You should also be willing to adjust your daily training plan. If you are tired, reduce the load by going shorter, easier, or maybe not at all. By progressing gradually and scheduling rest, you will achieve your goals. We all progress at different rates, so be patient and enjoy the journey.

Mode

Health benefits occur regardless of the exercise you select. Dr. Michael Pollock and associates compared the fitness and weight-control benefits of walking, running, and cycling. Sedentary middle-aged men trained for 20 weeks, all using the same intensity, duration, and frequency of exercise. Tests administered at the conclusion of the study indicated that all three groups improved similarly in fitness, body weight, and body fat (Pollock et al. 1975). No one mode of exercise is superior to others when the prescription is the same. The best exercise is the one that you enjoy and will continue to do regularly. As discussed earlier, however, improvements in fitness are specific to the manner of training. So if you want to improve your running, you should train by running. Swimming and cycling do surprisingly little to improve running, and vice versa, because many of the important changes take place only in the muscles used in training.

Periodization of Training

As your training proceeds, you'll want to use the progression technique that athletes use. Periodization describes the process of planning systematic variations and rest in the training program. Variation occurs at daily and weekly levels. This process ensures progression along with periods of relative rest and recovery. For example, you can increase training volume for several weeks and then back off for a week to recover. Repeat the pattern as training volume (intensity, duration, frequency) gradually increases. Periodization is used in aerobic and muscular fitness training. We'll show you how to use the technique in chapter 14.

Cross-Training

Will running enhance cycling or swim performance, or vice versa? Unfortunately, cross-training doesn't work that way; training must be specific to improve performance (Sharkey and Greatzer 1993). But there are several good reasons to use variety in training. One is to train for a multisport event like the triathlon. Another is to add variety and interest to your training. But the most important reason is to reduce impact and overuse in activities like running.

We've found that cross-training relieves the likelihood of nagging overuse injuries. And the variety eliminates the boredom of unrelenting training. We run and mountain bike in summer, with hiking, paddling, swimming, and even golf for diversion. Winter includes cross-country and downhill skiing as well as snowshoeing. Winter diversions include backcountry ski trips. We do one or two weightlifting sessions most weeks to maintain muscular fitness and try to improve or maintain performance. Fall and spring serve as transition periods, enhanced by new activities, new weather, and new locales. Try more than one mode of exercise to train some muscles while resting others. You'll like it!

Achievement

The key to the achievement of fitness goals is to make haste slowly. If you rush the process, the result may be painful, injurious, or worse. You need time to coax that slow, continuous stream of adaptations from the body. You'll experience improved energy and vigor within weeks. Improved self-concept and body image will follow, and performance will show change within a month. But don't view these exciting changes as a license for imprudent behavior. Athletes train for years to achieve dramatic results. Don't expect to undo years of inactivity or remove fat that accumulated over a decade in a few short weeks!

What progress can you expect when you follow your prescription? Although the ultimate achievement will depend on your genetic endowment (Bouchard et al. 1988), with time and effort, you can achieve your potential. Two factors, age and initial level of fitness, influence the rate of improvement (Sharkey 1970). Training during or just after puberty, a period of intense growth and development, leads to the greatest adaptations in the ability to take in, transport, and use oxygen ($\dot{V}O_2$max). Adolescent training may prompt a 30 to 35 percent improvement in aerobic fitness. Young adults are able to improve 20 to 25 percent. Trainability may decline slowly thereafter, but even a 70-year-old can expect a 10 percent improvement in fitness ($\dot{V}O_2$max). Greater improvements are possible at any age when significant weight loss is involved (Sharkey 1984).

> **Y**ou need time to coax that slow, continuous stream of adaptations from the body.

Because active people are closer to their genetic potential, they will not improve as much as their less-active and less-fit contemporaries. Complete inactivity, such as prolonged bed rest, provides a clean canvas for the demonstration of dramatic changes, perhaps as much as 100 percent improvement above bed-rest levels. Sedentary folks may improve more than 30 percent, whereas already trained athletes may have to accept 5 percent improvement or less, depending on age, proximity to genetic potential, and level of training.

The rate of improvement is dramatic at first, 3 percent per week for the first month, 2 percent per week for the second, and slowing to 1 percent or less thereafter. But although the improvement in aerobic fitness begins to level off after several months, the capacity to perform submaximal work continues to grow (see figure 10.3). Both the capacity for

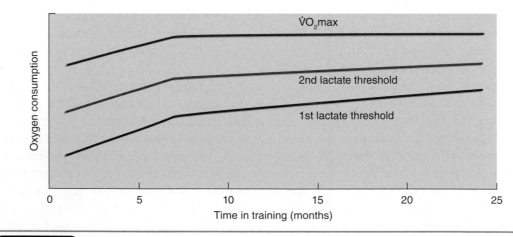

FIGURE 10.3 Training, aerobic fitness, and submaximal work capacity. With prolonged training, $\dot{V}O_2$max (aerobic fitness) begins to level off, but the capacity to perform submaximal work at the first and second lactate thresholds continues to improve.

prolonged work (first lactate threshold) and the upper limit of aerobic endurance (second lactate threshold) continue to increase after $\dot{V}O_2$max has reached a plateau. These submaximal capacities, not $\dot{V}O_2$max, define our capacity for work or sport.

A normally active middle-aged adult male with a fitness score of 40 milliliters per kilogram per minute may improve to 50. If he had started as an adolescent, with a fitness score of 55, and achieved a 30 percent improvement, he may have scored over 70 and been an outstanding athlete. If you started late, don't despair. You can still achieve dramatic improvements in endurance and energy. Most important are the improvements in submaximal capacities, changes that allow a once-sedentary person to climb a mountain or run a marathon. Besides improving your fitness, you are able to sustain a higher percentage of your maximal capacity and continue once-fatiguing activities indefinitely, without fatigue or discomfort. And the benefits extend beyond your regular mode of exercise to all your daily tasks. Fitness expands your horizons.

Maintenance

If you attain a level of fitness and performance that meets your needs, you may want to switch to a maintenance program. You'll be able to maintain your fitness with three sessions per week, allowing time to apply your newfound fitness in new pursuits. Maintenance has been studied several ways. One is to train to a level of fitness and then use various frequencies of training to see how much is required to remain at that level. Another is to cease training to see how quickly fitness

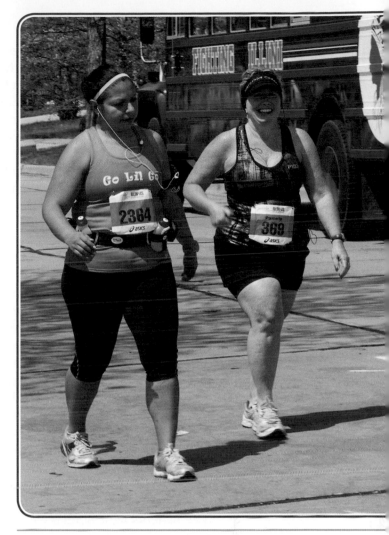

■ Even if you started late, you can dramatically increase your endurance and energy through training.

is lost. With some activity, fitness doesn't decline too rapidly, but with complete bed rest, it may drop as much as 10 percent a week (Greenleaf et al. 1976). You can maintain fitness with two or three sessions weekly, but the effort must be of the same intensity and duration as that used to achieve the improvements (Brynteson and Sinning 1973). Exercise of lower intensity but longer duration also seems to work, but it won't keep you tuned for a race. One workout of very long duration each week may help maintain fitness for a while; a combination of activities plus two or three training sessions is certain to do the job.

Researchers have used a more complex approach to study maintenance. By observing the effect of a single dose of training on specific aerobic enzymes, the researcher can plot the influence of training and determine its **half-life**, that is, the time it takes to lose one-half of the benefit. These studies suggest that the half-life of training ranges from 4.5 to 9.4 days (Watson, Srivastava, and Booth 1983). The half-life is used because it is difficult to tell when a biological effect, such as an increase in enzyme activity, returns to pretraining levels. So researchers measure the increase and the time that it takes to return to half that value. If half of the training effect is lost in 4.5 days, you'll want to train more frequently to maintain or improve fitness.

Regaining Fitness

Does a previously fit person regain fitness more quickly than one who has not been fit? Although the limited work in this area says probably not, our experience argues for a tentative maybe. The answer may depend on such factors as genetic potential, level of fitness, and extent of previous training. An extensive period of previous training may lead to changes that are retained longer than are alterations in aerobic enzymes and blood volume. Repetition of training will certainly lead to skill and economy of motion that makes subsequent activity seem easier.

But instead of worrying about how little it takes to achieve, maintain, or regain fitness, find activities that you enjoy and make them part of your life. Then you'll view activity as an essential and enjoyable part of every day. You'll be hooked on activity and fitness, and the rest will take care of itself.

TRAINING TIPS

People tell us that they would like to become more fit, but that they just don't have the time. We tell them how others make time for regular exercise, including the last seven U.S. presidents and many other busy people. The time has come for you to make time for regular fitness training. This chapter provides training tips, training programs, and other information that you'll need to make training safe, enjoyable, and effective. The programs in this chapter have proven cost-effective, providing maximum benefit for the time invested.

We'll begin with walking and running as modes of exercise because, for the time and cost, they provide excellent training stimulus. Intensity and duration are easy to control, and you can do the activities at any time, in almost any weather, with little investment in equipment. The equipment is light and easily transported on vacation or business trips. You can participate alone or in a group and can continue throughout life. A study of 72,488 female nurses found that brisk walking was inversely associated with the risk of heart disease; the relative risk declined as the amount of walking increased (Manson et al. 1999). The benefits were similar to those achieved with other forms of vigorous exercise, such as running. For these reasons and more, walking and running are fine ways to achieve and maintain aerobic fitness and its benefits.

What to Wear

Nothing is more important to your enjoyment than comfortable shoes, so don't economize when you buy footwear. Go to a reputable sporting goods dealer and seek advice from a knowledgeable salesperson. Avoid sale shoes at discount outlets unless you know something about the product. Buy a training shoe, not one built for competition. A firm, thick sole, good arch support, and a well-padded heel are essential. The sole should be firm but not terribly difficult to flex. A firm heel counter is also important. If blisters are a problem, try tube socks, a thin sock under a heavier one, or a balm on potential hot spots (try bag balm from a livestock outlet).

Walking and jogging don't require fancy clothing. Nylon or cotton shorts and a T-shirt are adequate in summer. For winter, a jogging suit serves until temperatures fall below 20 degrees Fahrenheit (minus 7 °C). Some runners prefer tights. Just remember that layers of lighter clothing are preferable to a single heavy garment. Add gloves and a knit cap in cold weather. A cap is important in cold conditions because you lose a large amount of heat from your head. When the wind blows, a thin windbreaker helps reduce heat loss. In extremely cold weather, you can wear tights and wind pants. Many runners continue in subzero (Fahrenheit) temperatures (minus 18 °C), which is safe if you are properly clothed, warmed up, and sensitive to the signs of **windchill** and **frostbite** (see chapter 15). For longer winter outings, we prefer polypropylene underwear to wick perspiration away from the skin, thereby avoiding rapid cooling. Add a pile vest and a windbreaker, and you are ready to go.

> **A** cap is important in cold conditions because you lose a large amount of heat from your head.

Technique

An upright posture conserves energy. Run or walk with your back comfortably straight, your head up, and your shoulders relaxed. When jogging, bend your arms, hold your hands in a comfortable position, and keep arm swing to a minimum. Pumping action will increase with more speed. Swing your legs freely from the hip with no attempt to overstride. Studies show that the stride that feels best is usually the most efficient as well.

Modern running shoes allow a heel-to-toe foot strike. Land lightly on the heel (or foot) and roll forward to push off the ball of the foot. For faster running, employ a slight forward lean, more knee lift, a quick and forceful push-off, and more arm action. New "five-fingered" shoes are reported to mimic barefoot running. They claim to imitate the biomechanics of being barefoot. At the time of this writing, there have been no independent research studies to confirm the claims or the value of barefoot running for the general population.

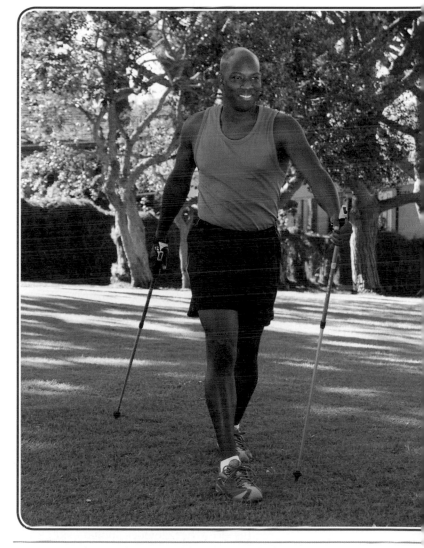

Time of Day

Exercise whenever it suits your fancy. Some people prefer to work out before breakfast, and others work out at midday or after work. A few night owls brave the dark in their quest for fitness; the run and shower help them sleep. Avoid vigorous exercise (except walking, cycling, or cross-country skiing) for an hour after a meal, when the digestive system requires an adequate blood supply. Some like to run during the lunch hour. If you have a problem at work in the morning, you'll often come back from the run with a solution. Unless you need time alone, consider training with a partner. If you find one with similar abilities, interests, and goals, you aren't likely to miss your workout.

■ Exercise during the time of day that works best for you.

Where to Walk or Run

Avoid hard surfaces for the early weeks of training. Walk or run in the park, on playing fields, on a golf course, or on a running track. Then you'll be ready to try the back roads or trails in your area. Varying your routes will help you maintain interest. When the weather prohibits outdoor exercise, try a mall, YMCA, or school gym, or choose an exercise supplement that you can do at home, such as running in place or skipping rope. We'll suggest other aerobic alternatives later in this chapter.

Pedometers

An inexpensive pedometer is an effective way to assess physical activity (Tudor-Locke et al. 2004). Use step goals (e.g., 10,000 steps per day) to motivate increased physical activity. Measure your stride length and set the pedometer. Then begin with a typical day and see how many steps you record. Add additional steps by parking farther from work, taking the stairs instead of the elevator, and taking a walk during your break. You will soon find ways to get 10,000 steps.

AEROBIC FITNESS OPTIONS

When you are unable to engage in your regular activity because of weather or injury, consider an alternative. These examples can also serve as a form of cross-training to reduce the impact of running. Many types of exercise devices are on the market; most end up gathering dust in the basement. Before you buy, use the device for several days and don't buy features that you don't need, such as fancy electronics (for good advice, go to www.acsm.org, the website for the American College of Sports Medicine). Finally, use a fan to make the indoor experience more enjoyable.

- *Bicycle.* A good stationary bicycle should be comfortable, and should offer good adjustment and controls and sufficient resistance to provide a training stimulus, now and in the future. Of course, the bike should also fit your significant other if he or she plans to use it. Some stationary bikes combine cycling with arm exercise, a good idea for someone with a condition like multiple sclerosis. The best allow leg, arm, or combined arm and leg exercise and include a flywheel for resistance and a fan for cooling. A low-cost alternative is a stand for your outdoor bike.

- *Treadmill.* Treadmills range from less expensive nonmotorized devices to sturdy motor-driven machines and devices that combine some arm exercise. Be sure that you like the feel of the machine, and that it is well built and guaranteed, and capable of sufficient elevation and speed to provide a training stimulus, now and in the future. Also, be aware that some machines may require a new electrical circuit in your home.

- *Cross-country ski device.* Ski simulators are widely advertised. Be sure that you try before you buy. Then buy a reputable brand known for durability. Consult the want ads in your local paper for a secondhand device.

- *Rowing machine.* Better-quality models use a flywheel instead of adjustable shock absorbers to control resistance. Rowing machines combine upper and lower body work (as do other devices such as ski simulators). The combined exercises allow you to burn more calories per minute than you do with leg-only exercise, without raising the perception of exertion.

- *Stair climber.* Popular in health clubs, these are now available for home purchase. Look for a sturdy, brand-name model with a good warranty.
- *Elliptical device.* An effective device for reducing impact forces during aerobic exercise, elliptical trainers are becoming popular at health clubs. Again, look for a brand-name device with a good warranty.
- *Rope skipping.* A skipping rope is inexpensive and easy to transport. It can be done anywhere, and it accommodates a wide range of intensity and skill. When you stand on the center of the rope, the ends should reach your armpits. Use a length of number 10 sash cord or buy a jumping rope and go for it. Just be careful to avoid overexertion while you are learning the skills.
- *Racewalking.* This Olympic event is an interesting alternative to running. The distinctive heel-to-toe gait is a complex skill that takes time to learn properly. For instructions and training programs, consult a good book, such as *USA Track & Field Coaching Manual* (2000) from Human Kinetics (www.hkusa.com).
- *Other alternatives.* Other aerobic alternatives include slide boards, aerobic dance, step aerobics, some martial arts, swing or Western dance, and the best low-impact activity, swimming. Runners can swim or they can run in the deep end of the pool while they wait for injuries to heal. In other words, you have no excuse for stopping exercise because of weather or injury.

You have no excuse for stopping exercise because of weather or injury.

EXERCISE RISKS

Previously inactive adults often encounter problems when they begin to exercise. You can avoid such problems if you make haste slowly. It took you years to get out of shape, and you won't be able to reverse the trend overnight. Plan for gradual progress; at the start, too little may be better than too much. After several weeks, when your body has begun to adjust to the demands of vigorous effort, you'll be ready to increase your exercise intensity or duration. Another way to avoid exercise problems is to warm up before each session. Careful attention to warming up and stretching eliminates many of the nagging complications that plague less patient people. Don't forget to cool down after each workout.

Prevention is the best way to deal with exercise problems. When a problem arises, treat the cause, not just the symptom. If your knee hurts, put ice on it, but don't stop there. Find out why it hurts (e.g., old shoes) and correct the problem.

Common Injuries

You can deal with many of the injuries that threaten to diminish your enjoyment of training. People who engage in regular exercise may experience the following problems, but by taking a few precautions, you can prevent minor injuries before they arise.

- *Blisters.* Blisters are minor burns caused by friction. You can prevent them by using properly fitted shoes, appropriate socks (double-layer or tube socks), and a lubricant (e.g., bag balm) on potential hot spots. At the first hint of a potential blister, cover the area with duct tape, that's right, duct tape. We've found that a tape job can last for several days of backcountry hiking or skiing. Treat advanced cases with a sterilized hollow needle. Release the fluid, treat with an antiseptic, circle the area with a foam rubber donut, and go back to work. Keep a blister prevention kit in your locker or gym bag and always carry the kit on hiking trips.

• *Muscle soreness.* Delayed-onset muscle soreness (DOMS) develops about 24 hours after you perform a new or more vigorous exercise. DOMS occurs in the muscles involved and may be due to microscopic tears in the muscle or connective tissue, to swelling, or to localized contractions of muscle fibers (Armstrong 1984). You can minimize the soreness by phasing into a sport gradually. Mild stretching and warming up make subsequent activity less painful. Massage seems to reduce the discomfort. The good news is that DOMS is a temporary inconvenience that inoculates you from further discomfort for several months—at least until you start a new sport.

• *Muscle cramps.* A cramp is a powerful involuntary contraction that results when the muscle refuses to relax. Normally, the nervous system tells muscles when to contract and when to relax, but when the normal control fails, the result can be painful. Immediate relief comes when you stretch and massage the cramped muscle. But that process does not remove the underlying cause of the involuntary contraction. Salt and calcium are involved in the chemistry of contraction and relaxation. Hot temperatures and **dehydration** seem to predispose muscles to cramps. Attend to fluid and electrolyte replacement during activity in hot weather.

• *Bone bruises.* Hikers and joggers sometimes get painful bruises on the soles of their feet. You can avoid such bruises with careful foot placement and quality footwear. Cushioned inner soles and gel- or air-sole shoes can aid in reducing the repetitive shocks that lead to bruises. A bad bruise can last for weeks. Ice may lessen discomfort, and padding may allow some activity. When bruises occur, examine your shoes. It may be time to replace them or try a cushioned heel cup or inner sole.

• *Ankle problems.* Treatment for a sprained ankle involves RICES (see the subsequent list). Ice the ankle immediately, preferably in a bucket of ice water. Ice several times a day, and in between, rest and elevate the ankle. Use a wrap to stabilize and maintain compression. When possible, use high-top shoes to prevent ankle problems. Tape or lace-on supports may allow some activity after the swelling subsides.

> **R**est
>
> **I**ce
>
> **C**ompression
>
> **E**levation
>
> **S**tabilization

• *Calf or Achilles tendon injuries.* Do not ignore a pulling sensation in the calf or Achilles tendon. Treat minor pulls with rest, ice, and gel heel cups. Return to activity cautiously; a serious pull can take weeks to heal. Prevent calf or Achilles problems with adequate stretching, good footwear, and a gradual warm-up.

• *Shin splints.* Pain on the front portion of the shinbones is known as **shin splints**. It can be caused by inflammation of the tibialis anterior muscle, its membrane, or the bone it attaches to, or a spasm of the inflamed muscle. Rest, compression wraps, deep massage (toward the heart), ultrasound, and anti-inflammatory drugs (e.g., ibuprofen) provide some relief. Prevention involves gradual adjustment to training, avoidance of hard running surfaces, occasional reversal of direction when running on a curved track, use of the heel-to-toe foot strike, resistance exercises, and stretching.

• *Knee problems.* Research suggests that running doesn't harm a healthy knee; indeed, it can improve cartilage health (Urquhart et al. 2011). Unfortunately, many of us run on less-than-healthy knees, knees already afflicted with osteoarthritis. Heavy physical loading (occupation or sport) increases the risk of knee osteoarthritis, and cumulative physical stress has a deleterious effect on the joint (Manninen et al. 2002). A high-school football injury left one of us with an arthritic knee. The knee is ACL deficient, and the cartilage was removed 40 years ago. Surprisingly, Brian continued to run with the help of weight training to stabilize thigh and hamstring muscles, cycling to add strength and endurance without trauma, and a nonsteroidal anti-inflammatory drug (NSAID), such as ibuprofen, to quiet inflammation and discomfort in the degenerative joint. Overuse (e.g., a long hike or run) called for a bit more of the NSAID until things cooled down. Recently, he had a total knee replacement.

If you experience runner's knee or some other problem, correct the cause while you treat the symptom. Try new shoes or arch supports. Alternate between two pairs of shoes if you run a lot, one with padding for sore feet and the other with a flexible sole for sore legs. If these ideas don't help, consult an athletic trainer or a podiatrist who specializes in sports medicine. Specialists may recommend orthotics to alleviate a foot problem. These plastic inserts can correct pronation and reduce some knee pain.

• *Stitch.* The side pain called a **stitch**, usually blamed on food or fluid in the digestive system, may be due to tugging of ligaments that attach the gut to the diaphragm. A treadmill study induced the stitch by giving the subjects a drink and then used several techniques to reduce their discomfort. Bending forward while tightening the abdominal muscles, exhaling through pursed lips, or tightening a belt around the waist were dramatically effective treatments. The authors suggested that the results were consistent with a ligamentous origin for the stitch (Plunkett and Hopkins 1995).

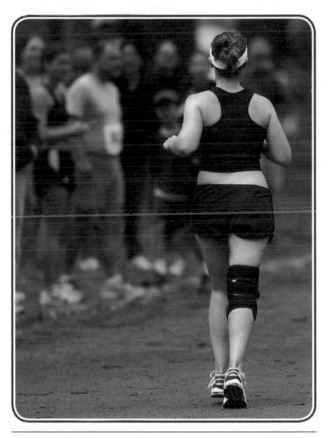

■ Prevent pain from interrupting your training by correcting the causes and treating the symptoms of knee problems.

Overuse Syndromes

If you go too far or too fast too soon, if you forget to stretch or warm up, if you have muscle imbalances, if one leg is shorter than the other, or if you have weak feet, you are bound

NSAIDs

Careful use of the nonsteroidal anti-inflammatory drugs (NSAIDs) aspirin and ibuprofen helps minimize many nagging problems and some big ones. With a doctor's advice, one of us started taking aspirin more than 40 years ago to quiet that painful knee. Then we learned that one small pill a day reduces blood clotting and the risk of heart attack. Aspirin also reduces the little strokes (transient ischemic attacks) that become more prevalent with age. Ibuprofen, which is good for muscle and joint pain, has been associated with lower risk of Alzheimer's disease. Both drugs cause stomach irritation, and some people are allergic to aspirin. When taken in small doses with food to minimize stomach irritation, aspirin or ibuprofen offers amazing relief for the price.

Aspirin reduces pain and inflammation by inhibiting the production of cell hormones called prostaglandins. Exercise causes prostaglandin production, which can cause soreness. A single NSAID before exercise can reduce the need for larger doses afterward. Judicious use of NSAIDs keeps many aging athletes active long after others have given up. Because ibuprofen interferes with some heart-health benefits of aspirin, you should not take them at the same time.

to have overuse problems now and then. Use ice for all acute strains and sprains. Keep an ice pop in the freezer (tape a tongue depressor upright in a disposable cup filled with water and put it in the freezer) and use it several times a day to reduce inflammation and hasten recovery. Rub the problem area with ice or Arnica salve. You'll be amazed by your rapid return to activity.

Exercise Hazards

Sedentary behavior is bad for your health (Owen et al. 2010). Regular, moderate physical activity is an established aid to health, fitness, weight control, and longevity. All of us understand the term *regular*, but the concept of *moderate* requires definition. Moderate exercise for an athlete may be hazardous for the sedentary adult. We can define moderate exercise as a level likely to bring about improved fitness without exposing the person to the hazards of strenuous effort.

Sudden Vigorous Exercise

Failure to warm up before vigorous exercise can result in electrocardiogram abnormalities, regardless of the fitness or age of the subject. Researchers found abnormalities in 31 of 44 apparently healthy firefighters tested on a vigorous treadmill test. The findings indicated inadequate blood flow in the coronary arteries and lack of oxygen to the heart. A warm-up consisting of a 5-minute jog prevented the problem (Barnard et al. 1972). Athletes aren't the only ones who need to warm up. Anyone performing vigorous work or exercise can benefit. Calisthenic warm-ups are common among factory workers in Europe and Japan, but less common in the United States. Although most workers can and should warm up, it is hard for law enforcement officers to do before chasing a suspect. For this reason, police officers should do all they can to keep fit and healthy.

Stressful Exercise

Stress is something that a person perceives as a threat. The body reacts to the threat by secreting a group of hormones that assist the mobilization of energy and prepare the body for combat or retreat (fight or flight). The body does not differentiate between physical and mental threats; it reacts similarly to each. An important exam may be stressful to a medical student, and a canoe trip could be stressful to a nonswimmer. Stress accelerates clotting time of the blood, which is good for a soldier in battle or a boxer in the ring, but bad for an adult with atherosclerosis, for whom a clot could block the flow of blood to the heart. Although exercise is not inherently stressful, studies indicate that unfamiliar, exhausting, and competitive exercise can be stressful for some people.

- *Unfamiliar exercise.* A person's first skiing or mountain-climbing experience may be stressful, but the stress diminishes as skill and confidence grow. We found faster clotting time on a subject's first treadmill test, but normal clotting after weeks of experience, when the test was no longer perceived as a threat (Whiddon, Sharkey, and Steadman 1969). Early experiences in unfamiliar or threatening exercise situations, such as whitewater kayaking, should be preceded with less-threatening introductions, such as a session in a pool.

- *Exhausting exercise.* In experiments on dogs, a Japanese researcher found that exhaustion could be stressful (Suzuki 1967). A bike-riding attendant took the animals for runs of various intensities and durations. Only exhausting runs increased the secretion of stress hormones. The researcher concluded that nonexhausting exercise need not be stressful. Of course, the dogs' fears of being left behind may have caused at least some of the stress associated with exhaustion.

- *Competitive exercise.* Years ago, researchers at Harvard University studied stress responses to various types of competition in rowers. Crew members did not perceive the strenuous effort of practice as a threat, but they did demonstrate increased hormone levels after either a time trial or a competitive race. The nonexercising coxswain also exhibited a stress response after the competitive event. The researchers concluded that exercise by itself was not stressful, but that the excitement of competition did elicit the response, with or without exertion (Hill, Goetz, and Fox 1956).

For many, the excitement of sport keeps them active.

The hormones of the stress response are required for the full mobilization of resources and the maximal performance of the athlete. We would never suggest that healthy men or women avoid the excitement of unfamiliar, exhausting, or competitive activity. Previously inactive people, however, should prepare for participation with gradual adaptation to the stress involved. In time, the unfamiliar becomes familiar, training reduces exhaustion, and the athlete within learns to cope with the physical and psychological requirements of competition.

Indeed, adults regularly engage in stressful activities. For many, the excitement of sport keeps them active. Those who thrive on challenge, excitement, or exhaustion do so after long periods of preparation. Aging athletes continue to practice and train so that they can remain competitive. If you want to become involved in competitive tennis, distance running, or mountain biking, give yourself time to adjust to the demands. Improve your fitness and skill as you prepare for your first exposure. Set reasonable goals and never take the results too seriously.

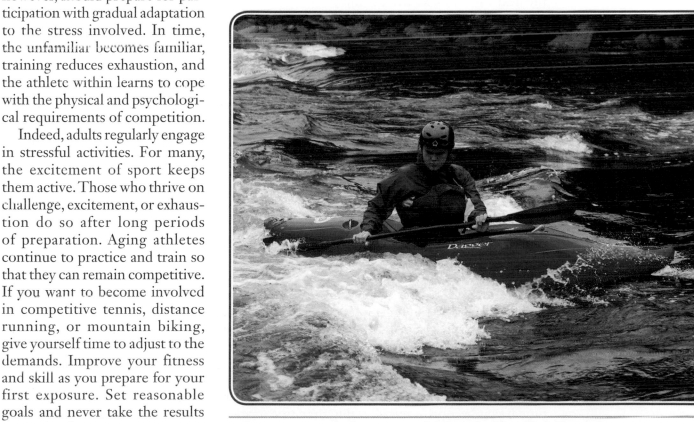

■ Learn new types of exercise gradually to avoid potential hazards.

SAMPLE AEROBIC FITNESS PROGRAMS

Your fitness prescription gives you freedom to tailor a program to meet your specific needs. You have a wide choice of exercise, many options in the length of time that you choose to exercise, and several alternatives for the intensity of the activity. Some people prefer a detailed, step-by-step approach. For this reason, we've included some walk–jog–run programs. All forms for this section may be found at the end of the chapter.

We'll describe programs for three levels of ability: a starter program for those making the transition to activity, an intermediate program, and one for those in higher fitness categories. The President's Council on Physical Fitness and Sport (1975) prepared the starter program, which appeared in the booklet *An Introduction to Physical Fitness.*

Starter Walk–Jog Programs

This program is suitable for beginner and intermediate exercisers. Use the walk or walk–jog test to determine your current level of fitness and where you should begin. Follow the instructions, and you will soon be moving to the next level.

Walk Test

The object of this test is to determine how many minutes (up to 10) you can walk at a brisk pace, on a level surface, without undue difficulty or discomfort. If you can't walk for 5 minutes, begin with the red walking program. If you can walk more than 5 minutes, but less than 10, begin with the third week of the red walking program. If you can walk for the full 10 minutes but are somewhat tired as a result, start with the white walk–jog program. If you can breeze through the full 10 minutes, you're ready for bigger things. Wait until the next day and take the 10-minute walk–jog test that follows.

Walk–Jog Test

In this test, you alternately walk 50 steps (left foot strikes the ground 25 times) and jog 50 steps for a total of 10 minutes. Walk at the rate of 120 steps per minute (left foot strikes the ground at 1 sec intervals). Jog at the rate of 144 steps per minute (left foot strikes the ground 18 times every 15 seconds). If you can't complete the 10-minute test, begin with the third week of the white program. If you can complete the 10-minute test, but are tired and winded as a result, start with the last week of the white program before moving to the blue program. If you can perform the 10-minute walk–jog test without difficulty, start with the blue program.

Red Walking Program

Start with this program, doing each activity every other day at first (see form 10.1). The first week, you'll walk at a brisk pace (RPE = 10–11) for 5 minutes, or for a shorter time if you become uncomfortably tired. Walk slowly for 3 minutes. Then walk briskly again for 5 minutes or until you become uncomfortably tired. The second week of the program is the same, but you increase your pace as soon as you can walk 5 minutes without soreness or fatigue. During the third week of the program, you'll increase your brisk walking to 8 minutes. Increase your pace in the fourth week. When you've completed the fourth week of the red program, begin at the first week of the white program.

White Walk–Jog Program

In this program, you'll begin by walking at a brisk pace for 10 minutes, or for a shorter time if you become uncomfortably tired (see form 10.2). After a slow walk or rest, you'll resume the brisk pace. The second week will increase the amount of time spent walking at a brisk pace. The third week takes you to 30 minutes of walking, most days of the week, the minimum level of activity suggested for health by the Centers for Disease Control and American College of Sports Medicine. The fourth week will incorporate jogging short distances, and the fifth week increases the jogging. Do each activity at least four times a week. When you've completed the fifth week of the white program, begin the first week of the blue program.

Blue Jogging Program

In this program, you'll increase the amount of time spent jogging each week (see form 10.3). Do each activity five times a week, as indicated. Although 30 minutes is the minimum time needed for health benefits, the Institute of Medicine has recommended 1 hour of daily activity to achieve greater health benefits and to maintain body weight, so you'll want to work toward the intermediate program.

Intermediate Jog–Run Program

If you've followed the red, white, and blue programs or are already reasonably active, you're ready for the intermediate program (see form 10.4). You're able to jog 1 mile (1.6 km) slowly without undue fatigue, rest 2 minutes, and do it again. Your sessions consume about 250 calories.

You're ready to increase both the intensity and the duration of your runs. You'll be using the rating of perceived exertion to determine intensity. You'll begin by jogging 1 mile (1.6 km) in 12 minutes, and when you finish this program, you may be able to complete 3 miles (4.8 km) or more at a pace approaching 8 to 10 minutes per mile (5–6 min/km). Each week's program includes three phases—the basic workout, longer runs (overdistance), and shorter runs (underdistance). If the program for a particular week seems too easy, move ahead; if it seems too hard, move back 1 or 2 weeks. On most of the days, you'll jog in intervals and walk to recover. For example, on Tuesday of the first week, begin by jogging .25 to .5 mile (.4 to .8 km) slowly. Then try to jog .5 mile (.8 km) in 5 minutes, 30 seconds, walk to recover, and repeat. Next, jog .25 mile (.4 km) in 2 minutes, 45 seconds, and then walk to recover. Repeat three more times. Finally, jog .25 to .5 mile (.4 to .8 km) as you did in the beginning of the workout. On Thursday, jog 1 mile (1.6 km) in 12 minutes, walk to recover, and repeat. Remember to warm up and cool down as part of every exercise session.

Advanced Running Program

This section is for the well-trained person. We'll provide some suggestions for advanced training, but keep in mind that there is no single way to train. If you enjoy underdistance training, use it. If you find that you prefer overdistance, use that approach. By simply picking up the pace as you approach the end of a long run, you'll receive the optimal training stimulus. Moreover, because the speed work is limited to a short span near the end of the run, discomfort is brief.

Consider the following suggestions to help make your training session safe and productive.

- Always warm up before you run.
- Stretch after warming up.
- Periodically train at RPE of 15 to 16.

- Vary the location, intensity, and distance of your runs (long or short, fast or slow, hilly or flat).
- Set distance goals:

Phase 1	20 miles (32.2 km) per week
Phase 2	25 miles (40.2 km) per week (ready for 3 to 5 mi, or 4.8 to 8 km, road races)
Phase 3	30 miles (48.3 km) per week
Phase 4	35 miles (56.3 km) per week (ready for 5 to 7 mi, or 8 to 11.3 km, road races)
Phase 5	40 miles (64.4 km) per week
Phase 6	45 miles (72.4 km) per week (ready for 7 to 10 mi, or 11.3 to 16.1km, road races)
Phase 7	More than 50 miles (80 km) per week (ready for longer races such as the half marathon—13.1 mi, or 21.1 km)

- Don't be a slave to your goals, and don't increase weekly distance unless you enjoy it.
- Run 6 days per week if you like. Otherwise, try an alternate-day schedule with longer runs.
- Try one long run (not more than one-third of weekly distance) on Saturday or Sunday.
- Try two shorter runs if the long ones seem difficult. Try 5 plus 5 instead of 10.
- Every third or fourth week, do an easier week as a way to recover physically and mentally.
- Keep records if you like. You'll be surprised! Record date, distance, and comments. Note morning pulse and body weight. At least once per year, check your performance over a measured distance to observe progress. Use a local road race or the 1.5-mile (2.4 km) run test (see chapter 8). Check your fitness several times per year.
- Don't train with a stopwatch. Wear a wristwatch so that you'll know how long you've run.
- Increase speed as you approach the finish of a run.
- Always cool down after a run.

Cycling Program

This program uses a training menu to guide your progress (see form 10.5). The weekly training menu includes the following:

Monday	Easy distance—Ride at a comfortable pace (RPE = 13).
Tuesday	Pace—Cycle at a brisk pace (RPE = 15).
Wednesday	Hills—Include hills to build stamina (RPE = 14).
Thursday	Intervals—Push harder for brief intervals (RPE = 15). Increase to RPE = 16 after 4 weeks.
Friday	Overdistance—Go easy to develop endurance (RPE = 11).
Saturday	Variety—Try a different activity (e.g., tennis or hiking) or ride a trail.
Sunday	Rest—or try a light activity (e.g., gardening or walking).

After 8 weeks, design your own program using elements from this plan or others that you enjoy. Plan a long trip with friends and do your training rides together.

Note: When using a stationary bicycle, use a fan for ventilation or place the bicycle in a cool room to enhance the experience and allow a full workout (VanSchuylenbergh, VandenEynde, and Hespel 2004).

Swimming Program

This program assumes a certain amount of skill in swimming (see form 10.6). If the program seems too difficult for your level of ability, scale it down and take lessons to improve your skill and efficiency.

The weekly training menu includes the following:

Monday	Easy distance—Go easy at a comfortable pace (RPE = 12).
Tuesday	Pace—Swim at a firm pace (RPE = 15).
Wednesday	Arms or legs—Swim with arms or legs only (RPE = 13).
Thursday	Intervals—Swim harder for brief intervals (RPE = 15). Increase to RPE = 16 after 4 weeks.
Friday	Overdistance—Relax on a longer swim (RPE = 11).
Saturday	Variety—Try a different activity or water games (e.g., water polo).
Sunday	Rest—Try a light activity (e.g., gardening or walking).

When you have completed 8 weeks, design your own program using the types of training that you most enjoy. You could even decide to engage in cross-training or train for the triathlon (see chapter 14).

SUMMARY

This chapter summarizes the findings of hundreds of studies that have contributed to our knowledge of the factors associated with the development of aerobic fitness. Manipulation of intensity, duration, and frequency of exercise brings about improvements in fitness. Until recently, virtually all studies relied on the same measure of improvement, $\dot{V}O_2max$, which is a measure of exercise intensity. So it is not surprising that most studies favor intensity as the most important factor in the training prescription. If your goal is to raise $\dot{V}O_2max$, emphasize intensity, at least some of the time.

But if your goal is health, or the capacity to endure for extended periods, you should give equal attention to another important dimension of fitness—duration, as measured by time or distance. Long-duration exercise raises LT1 and ensures the utilization of fat as a source of energy, a development that has distinct health benefits. If your goal is performance, you should include some training at or near your second lactate threshold. Remember, training must be specific to its intended purpose if you are to achieve optimal results.

Intensity is important, but excessive emphasis on intensity can take the joy out of regular activity. Athletes don't train hard every day, and you shouldn't either. That is why we encourage you to move beyond the objective approach of heart rates and training zones to the subjective, in which you use perceived exertion and listen to your body. Adopt the active life gradually and enjoy the experience, the adaptations, and the amazing results.

The second part of this chapter presents training tips, training programs, aerobic alternatives, and advice on how to handle some common training problems. You are welcome to adopt one of the programs or to use your aerobic prescription and fashion your own approach. We're often amazed by the ingenious and personal approaches that some folks devise, such as the retired zoology professor who regularly climbed the mountain behind our campus, both for exercise and to observe the flora and fauna. Years ago, before it was in vogue, he used ski poles to exercise his arms while lowering the load on his legs. The poles become even more important on the return trip, relieving stress on his knees during the steep descent. His creative adaptation extended his range and saved his knees for many years of enjoyable outdoor exercise.

Another way to avoid common problems is to include attention to muscular fitness training, as presented in the next chapter.

Form 10.1   Red Walking Program

Week	Sunday	Monday	Tuesday	Wednesday	Thursday	Friday	Saturday
1	Brisk walk 5 min Slow walk/ rest 3 min Brisk walk 5 min	Off	Brisk walk 5 min Slow walk/ rest 3 min Brisk walk 5 min	Off	Brisk walk 5 min Slow walk/ rest 3 min Brisk walk 5 min	Off	Brisk walk 5 min Slow walk/ rest 3 min Brisk walk 5 min
2	Off	Brisk walk 5 min Slow walk/ rest 3 min Brisk walk 5 min	Off	Brisk walk 5 min Slow walk/ rest 3 min Brisk walk 5 min	Off	Brisk walk 5 min Slow walk/ rest 3 min Brisk walk 5 min	Off
3	Brisk walk 8 min Slow walk/ rest 3 min Brisk walk 8 min	Off	Brisk walk 8 min Slow walk/ rest 3 min Brisk walk 8 min	Off	Brisk walk 8 min Slow walk/ rest 3 min Brisk walk 8 min	Off	Brisk walk 8 min Slow walk/ rest 3 min Brisk walk 8 min
4	Off	Brisk walk 8 min Slow walk/ rest 3 min Brisk walk 8 min	Off	Brisk walk 8 min Slow walk/ rest 3 min Brisk walk 8 min	Off	Brisk walk 8 min Slow walk/ rest 3 min Brisk walk 8 min	Off

From B.J. Sharkey and S.E. Gaskill, 2013, *Fitness and health, seventh edition* (Champaign, IL: Human Kinetics).

Form 10.2   White Walk–Jog Program

Week	Sunday	Monday	Tuesday	Wednesday	Thursday	Friday	Saturday
1	Brisk walk 10 min Slow walk/ rest 3 min Brisk walk 10 min	Brisk walk 10 min Slow walk/ rest 3 min Brisk walk 10 min	Off	Brisk walk 10 min Slow walk/ rest 3 min Brisk walk 10 min	Off	Brisk walk 10 min Slow walk/ rest 3 min Brisk walk 10 min	Off
2	Brisk walk 15 min Slow walk/ rest 3 min Brisk walk 10 min	Off	Brisk walk 15 min Slow walk/ rest 3 min Brisk walk 10 min	Off	Brisk walk 15 min Slow walk/ rest 3 min Brisk walk 15 min	Off	Brisk walk 15 min Slow walk/ rest 3 min Brisk walk 15 min
3	Brisk walk 10 min Rest 3 min Brisk walk 15 min	Moderate walk 30 min	Brisk walk 10 min Rest 3 min Brisk walk 15 min	Moderate walk 30 min	Brisk walk 10 min Rest 3 min Brisk walk 15 min	Moderate walk 30 min	Off
4	Jog 10 s (25 yd) Walk 1 min (100 yd) 12×	Off	Jog 10 s (25 yd) Walk 1 min (100 yd) 12×	Off	Jog 10 s (25 yd) Walk 1 min (100 yd) 12×	Off	Jog 10 s (25 yd) Walk 1 min (100 yd) 12×
5	Off	Jog 20 s (50 yd) Walk 1 min (100 yd) 12×	Off	Jog 20 s (50 yd) Walk 1 min (100 yd) 12×	Off	Jog 20 s (50 yd) Walk 1 min (100 yd) 12×	Jog 20 s (50 yd) Walk 1 min (100 yd) 12×

Walk briskly at an RPE of 10 to 11. Jog at an RPE of 13 to 15. Meters = yards (1 yd= ~1 m).

From B.J. Sharkey and S.E. Gaskill, 2013, *Fitness and health, seventh edition* (Champaign, IL: Human Kinetics).

Form 10.3   Blue Jogging Program

Week	Sunday	Monday	Tuesday	Wednesday	Thursday	Friday	Saturday
1	Jog 40 s (100 yd) Walk 1 min (100 yd) 9×	Jog 40 s (100 yd) Walk 1 min (100 yd) 9×	Off	Jog 40 s (100 yd) Walk 1 min (100 yd) 9×	Jog 40 s (100 yd) Walk 1 min (100 yd) 9×	Off	Jog 40 s (100 yd) Walk 1 min (100 yd) 9×
2	Jog 1 min (150 yd) Walk 1 min (100 yd) 8×	Jog 1 min (150 yd) Walk 1 min (100 yd) 8×	Jog 1 min (150 yd) Walk 1 min (100 yd) 8×	Off	Jog 1 min (150 yd) Walk 1 min (100 yd) 8×	Jog 1 min (150 yd) Walk 1 min (100 yd) 8×	Off
3	Jog 2 min (300 yd) Walk 1 min (100 yd) 6×	Jog 2 min (300 yd) Walk 1 min (100 yd) 6×	Off	Jog 2 min (300 yd) Walk 1 min (100 yd) 6×	Jog 2 min (300 yd) Walk 1 min (100 yd) 6×	Off	Jog 2 min (300 yd) Walk 1 min (100 yd) 6×
4	Jog 4 min (600 yd) Walk 1 min (100 yd) 4×	Off	Jog 4 min (600 yd) Walk 1 min (100 yd) 4×	Jog 4 min (600 yd) Walk 1 min (100 yd) 4×	Off	Jog 4 min (600 yd) Walk 1 min (100 yd) 4×	Jog 4 min (600 yd) Walk 1 min (100 yd) 4×
5	Jog 6 min (900 yd) Walk 1 min (100 yd) 3×	Jog 6 min (900 yd) Walk 1 min (100 yd) 3×	Off	Jog 6 min (900 yd) Walk 1 min (100 yd) 3×	Jog 6 min (900 yd) Walk 1 min (100 yd) 3×	Off	Jog 6 min (900 yd) Walk 1 min (100 yd) 3×
6	Jog 8 min (1,200 yd) Walk 2 min (200 yd) 2×	Off	Jog 8 min (1,200 yd) Walk 2 min (200 yd) 2×	Jog 8 min (1,200 yd) Walk 2 min (200 yd) 2×	Off	Jog 8 min (1,200 yd) Walk 2 min (200 yd) 2×	Jog 8 min (1,200 yd) Walk 2 min (200 yd) 2×
7	Jog 10 min (1,500 yd) Walk 2 min (200 yd) 2×	Jog 10 min (1,500 yd) Walk 2 min (200 yd) 2×	Off	Jog 10 min (1,500 yd) Walk 2 min (200 yd) 2×	Jog 10 min (1,500 yd) Walk 2 min (200 yd) 2×	Off	Jog 10 min (1,500 yd) Walk 2 min (200 yd) 2×
8	Jog 12 min (1,760 yd) Walk 2 min (200 yd) 2×	Off	Jog 12 min (1,760 yd) Walk 2 min (200 yd) 2×	Jog 12 min (1,760 yd) Walk 2 min (200 yd) 2×	Off	Jog 12 min (1,760 yd) Walk 2 min (200 yd) 2×	Jog 12 min (1,760 yd) Walk 2 min (200 yd) 2×

Walk briskly at an RPE of 11 to 12. Jog at an RPE of 13 to 15. Meters = yards (1 yd= ~1 m).

From B.J. Sharkey and S.E. Gaskill, 2013, *Fitness and health, seventh edition* (Champaign, IL: Human Kinetics).

Form 10.4 Intermediate Jog–Run Program

Week	Monday	Tuesday	Wednesday	Thursday	Friday	Saturday and Sunday
1	1 mi jog (13–14). Walk 3–4 min 2×.	1/2 mi slow jog (13). 2× 1/2 mi (14). 4× 1/4 mi (15). 1/2 mi slow jog (13).	2 mi slow jog (13).	1 mi jog (13–14). Walk 3–4 min 2×.	1/2 mi slow jog (13). 2× 1/2 mi (14). 4× 1/4 mi (15). 1/2 mi slow jog (13).	2 mi slow jog (13).
2	1 mi jog (13–14). Walk 3–4 min 2×. Your mile time should be about 10–15 s faster than week 1.	1/2 mi slow jog (13). 1/2 mi (14). 2× 1/4 mi (16). 2× 1/4 mi (15). 4× 220 yd (15-16). 1/2 mi slow jog (13).	Brisk walk 30–60 min (12).	1 mi jog (13–14). Walk 3–4 min 2×. Your mile time should be about 10–15 s faster than week 1.	1/2 mi slow jog (13). 1/2 mi (14). 2× 1/4 mi (16). 2× 1/4 mi (15). 4× 220 yd (15–16). 1/2 mi slow jog (13).	2 1/4 mi slow jog (13) or brisk walk 30–60 min (12).
3	1 mi jog (13–14). Walk 3–4 min 2×. Your mile time should be about 5–10 s faster than week 2.	1/2 mi slow jog (13). 1/2 mi (15). 4× 1/4 mi (14). 4× 220 yd (16). 4× 100 yd (16). 1/2 mi slow jog (13).	2 1/2 mi slow jog (13) or brisk walk 30–60 min (12).	1 mi jog (13–14). Walk 3–4 min 2×. Your mile time should be about 5–10 s faster than week 2.	1/2 mi slow jog (13). 1/2 mi (15). 4× 1/4 mi (14). 4× 220 yd (16). 4× 100 yd (16). 1/2 mi slow jog (13).	2 1/2 mi slow jog (13) or brisk walk 30–60 min (12).
4	1 mi jog (13–15). Walk 3–4 min 2×. Your mile time should be about 5–10 s faster than week 3.	1/2 mi slow jog (13). 2× 1/2 mi (14). 4× 1/4 mi (16). 4× 220 yd (15). 1/2 mi slow jog (13).	2 3/4 mi slow jog (13) or brisk walk 45–70 min (12).	1 mi jog (13–15). Walk 3–4 min 2×. Your mile time should be about 5–10 s faster than week 3.	1/2 mi slow jog (13). 2× 1/2 mi (14). 4× 1/4 mi (16). 4× 220 yd (15). 1/2 mi slow jog (13).	2 3/4 mi slow jog (13) or brisk walk 45–70 min (12).
5 Easier week	1 mi jog (13–14). Walk 3–5 min 2×. Your mile time should be about the same as the previous week.	Off	3 mi slow jog (13).	1 mi jog (13–14). Walk 3–5 min 2×. Your mile time should be about the same as the previous week.	1/2 mi slow jog (13). 1/2 mi (15). 4× 1/4 mi (16). 4× 220 yd (15). 4× 100 yd (14). 1/2 mi slow jog (13).	Brisk walk 45–70 min (11–12).
6 Harder week	1 1/2 mi jog (13–15). Maintain same pace as weeks 4 and 5.	1/2 mi slow jog (13). 2× 1/2 mi (15). 4× 1/4 mi (16). 4× 220 yd (15). 4× 100 yd (16). 1/2 mi slow jog (13).	3 mi slow jog (13), increasing the pace the last 5–8 min (15).	1 1/2 mi jog (13–15). Walk 5–6 min 2×. Maintain same pace as weeks 4 and 5.	1/2 mi slow jog (13). 2× 1/2 mi (15). 4× 1/4 mi (16). 4× 220 yd (15). 4× 100 yd (16). 1/2 mi slow jog (13).	4 mi slow jog (13).

(continued)

Week	Monday	Tuesday	Wednesday	Thursday	Friday	Saturday and Sunday
7 Medium week	1 mi jog (14–15). Walk 3–5 min 2×. Your mile time should be about 5–10 s faster than the previous 3 weeks.	1/2 mi slow jog (13). 2× 1/2 mi (15). 3× 1/4 mi (16). 3× 220 yd (15). 1/2 mi slow jog (13).	3 mi slow jog (13).	1 mi jog (14–15). Walk 3–5 min 2×. Your mile time should be about 5-10 s faster than the previous 3 weeks.	1/2 mi slow jog (13). 2× 1/2 mi (15). 3× 1/4 mi (16). 3× 220 yd (15). 1/2 mi slow jog (13).	3 1/2 mi slow jog (13).
8 Hard week	1 mi jog (15). Walk 3–5 min. 1 mi jog (14) 2×. The first mile of each set should be slightly faster than week 7.	1/2 mi slow jog (13). 2× 1/2 mi (15). 4× 1/4 mi (16). 4× 220 yd (16). 4× 100 yd (15). 1/2 mi slow jog (13).	3 1/2 mi slow jog (13) .	1 mi jog (15). Walk 3–5 min. 1 mi jog (14) 2×. The first mile of each set should be slightly faster than week 7.	Off	5 mi slow jog (13).
9 Easy week	1 mi jog (14). Walk 3–5 min 2×. Your mile time should be about the same as week 7.	1/2 mi slow jog (13). 2× 1/2 mi (15). 3× 1/4 mi (15). 4× 220 yd (16). 4× 50 yd (16). 1/2 mi slow jog (13).	3 mi slow jog (13).	1 mi jog (14). Walk 3–5 min 2×. Your mile time should be about the same as week 7.	1/2 mi slow jog (13). 2× 1/2 mi (15). 3× 1/4 mi (15). 4× 220 yd (16). 4× 50 yd (16). 1/2 mi slow jog (13)	4 mi slow jog (13).
10 Harder week	1 1/2 mi jog (13–15). Walk 4–6 min 2×. Maintain same pace as week 9.	1/2 mi slow jog (13). 2× 1/2 mi (16). 3× 1/4 mi (14). 4× 220 yd (17). 1/2 mi slow jog (13).	4 mi slow jog (13), increasing the pace the last 8–10 min (15).	1 1/2 mi jog (13–15). Walk 4–6 min 2×. Maintain same pace as week 9.	1/2 mi slow jog (13). 2× 1/2 mi (16). 3× 1/4 mi (14). 4× 220 yd (17). 1/2 mi slow jog (13).	6 mi slow jog (13).
11 Medium week	1 mi jog (14–15). Walk 3–5 min 3×. Your mile time should be about 10 s faster than week 10.	1/2 mi slow jog (13). 4× 1/2 mi (15). 4× 1/4 mi (16). 2× 220 yd (17). 1/2 mi slow jog (13).	4 mi slow jog (13).	Off	1/2 mi slow jog (13). 4× 1/2 mi (15). 4× 1/4 mi (16). 2× 220 yd (17). 1/2 mi slow jog (13).	5 mi slow jog (13).
12 Hard week	1 1/2 mi jog (13–15). Walk 4–6 min 2×. Maintain same pace as week 11.	1/2 mi slow jog (13). 5× 1/2 mi (16). 4× 1/4 mi (15). 4× 220 yd (16). 2× 100 yd (17). 1/2 mi slow jog (13).	4 mi easy jog (13), increasing the pace the last 8–10 min (15).	1 1/2 mi jog (13–15). Walk 4–6 min 2×. Maintain same pace as week 11.	1/2 mi slow jog (13). 5× 1/2 mi (16). 4× 1/4 mi (15). 4× 220 yd (16). 2× 100 yd (17). 1/2 mi slow jog (13).	6 mi slow jog (13–14).

Values in parentheses are RPE units (see table 10.4). Meters = yards (1 yd= ~1 m). Kilometers = miles × 1.61.

From B.J. Sharkey and S.E. Gaskill, 2013, *Fitness and health, seventh edition* (Champaign, IL: Human Kinetics).

Form 10.5   Weekly Cycling Program

Day	Week							
	1	2	3	4	5	6	7	8
Monday	30 min	40	50	40	50	60	70	60
Tuesday	2 × 10 min	2 × 15	2 × 20	3 × 10	3 × 15	3 × 20	4 × 10	4 × 15
Wednesday	15 min	20	25	20	2 × 15	2 × 20	2 × 25	3 × 20
Thursday	3 × 3 min	3 × 4	3 × 5	3 × 6	4 × 3	4 × 4	4 × 5	5 × 5
Friday	60 min	70	80	75	90	100	110	120

Always wear a helmet; ride easy to warm up.

Pace: Ride 10 min, relax and recover, ride another set. Hills: Include some standing, but try to keep RPE = 14. Intervals: Ride one, cycle easy to recover, and ride the next. Overdistance: Ride easy; stop for rest and fluids every 30 min.

From B.J. Sharkey and S.E. Gaskill, 2013, *Fitness and health, seventh edition* (Champaign, IL: Human Kinetics).

Form 10.6   Weekly Swimming Program

Day	Week							
	1	2	3	4	5	6	7	8
Monday	15 min	20 min	25 min	20 min	25 min	30 min	35 min	30 min
Tuesday	2 × 5 min	2 × 6 min	2 × 7 min	2 × 8 min	3 × 6 min	3 × 7 min	3 × 8 min	4 × 5 min
Wednesday	5 min/each	6 min/each	7 min/each	8 min/each	9 min/each	10 min/each	11 min/each	12 min/each
Thursday	3 × 3 min	3 × 4 min	3 × 5 min	3 × 4 min	4 × 3 min	4 × 4 min	4 × 5 min	5 × 4 min
Friday	25 min	30 min	35 min	40 min	35 min	40 min	45 min	50 min

Use good goggles. Warm up well on Tuesday, Wednesday, and Thursday, and swim easy laps after these workouts. Pace: Swim slowly or walk in the water to recover between sets. Arms and legs: Use a kickboard or flotation device for support. Intervals: Swim slowly or walk to recover between sets.

From B.J. Sharkey and S.E. Gaskill, 2013, *Fitness and health, seventh edition* (Champaign, IL: Human Kinetics).

Muscular Fitness Training

Lifetime Mobility

> " The two kinds of people on earth . . . are the people who lift and the people who lean. "
>
> *Ella Wheeler Wilcox*

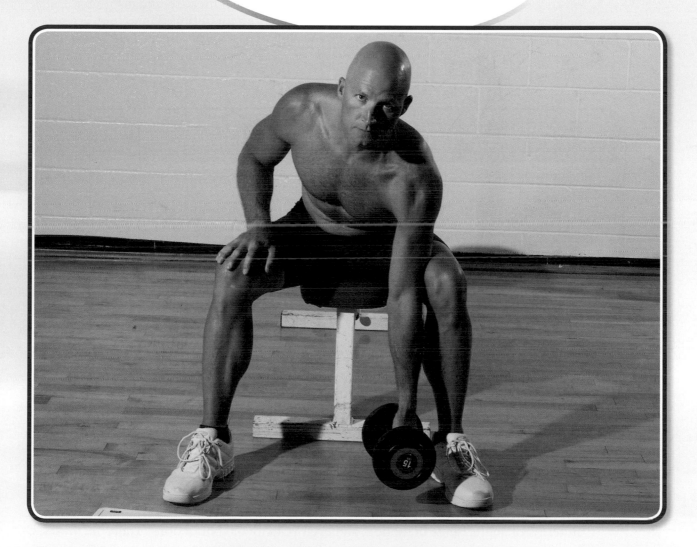

By now, you have some idea of the benefits and applications of muscular fitness. First are the health benefits. All of us need flexibility and abdominal exercises to prevent lower back problems. We all need core training to reduce the risk of injury and improve performance. Try to maintain a regular schedule. If you don't, you are likely to become one of many people (millions in the United States alone) whose days are diminished by preventable back pain and other problems. Those at risk for osteoporosis should plan a prevention program that consists of moderate weightlifting along with weight-bearing aerobic activity. Middle-aged people must understand how muscular fitness contributes to muscle mass, mobility, and the quality of life, especially after retirement. They should begin long before they retire and continue the rest of their days.

Of course, people seek to improve muscular fitness for many other reasons. Some become involved to correct posture or perceived deficiencies of figure or physique (e.g., to look good at the beach). Body shaping and bodybuilding motivate others. To decide on a program, you may want to evaluate your current level of muscular fitness. If you are dissatisfied, if you have room for improvement, or if you want to enhance performance in work or sport, use the prescriptions, select your mode of exercise, and get going. You'll be happy to learn that muscular fitness doesn't require a lot of time. Unless you are seeking high levels of strength or endurance, you should be able to achieve health and other benefits with 2 or 3 weekly sessions of 30 minutes each. You can maintain muscular fitness with 1 or 2 sessions per week.

*T*his chapter will help you do the following:

- Develop training prescriptions for muscular strength, endurance, and power
- Take precautions and follow guidelines to make training safe and effective
- Improve and maintain core fitness
- Adopt a program to maintain lower back health

MUSCULAR STRENGTH FITNESS PRESCRIPTION

Research has identified safe, proven prescriptions for each component of muscular fitness. You may fulfill the prescription with calisthenics, free weights, or weight machines. You'll get results with hydraulic devices, accommodating or variable-resistance equipment, or old-fashioned free weights. The key to improving strength is to place the muscle under tension for a sufficient amount of time (repetitions and sets). Your level of muscular fitness and how you intend to use the strength will dictate how you should train. If you are untrained, use 60 percent of maximal strength (one **repetition maximum,** or **RM**). Increase to 80 percent RM as you become trained (Rhea et al. 2003). Training is specific in terms of angle, range of motion, and even velocity of contractions. Train the muscles and movements that you want to improve. In designing your program, consider the factors described in the following sections.

Warm-Up

Warming up is as important for you as it is for your car. During winter months, you can't just jump into the old pickup and expect instant performance. You start the engine and wait a few seconds while the oil pressure rises. Then you drive slowly to avoid overloading the engine until it heats up. In the case of the human body, muscle is the engine, and increased muscle temperature improves enzyme activity and energy utilization. By slowly increasing heart rate, respiration, and muscle temperature, you avoid wasteful and uncomfortable anaerobic metabolism early in the workout. And by slowly warming and stretching the muscles, you reduce the risk of discomfort or injury. Begin with a brisk walk, increasing to an easy jog. Use any aerobic exercise or do light lifting exercises to warm up, and then do your stretching routine prior to lifting.

A 5-minute warm-up before exercise and a cool-down afterward will enhance your enjoyment of the experience and increase the likelihood that you will be able to participate the following day without discomfort. Remember that muscular fitness is only part of total fitness. No program is complete without a well-planned aerobic fitness regimen.

If you engage in calisthenics, weight training, or isokinetics, keep the following points in mind:

- Ease into the program with lighter weights and fewer sets. Begin with 15 to 25RM and gradually increase the load to 10RM resistance.

- Avoid holding your breath during a lift. Doing so can cause a marked increase in blood pressure and the work of the heart. Holding your breath also restricts the return of blood to the heart and the flow of blood in the coronary arteries that serve the heart muscle (just when your heart needs more oxygen, it gets less—a dangerous situation, especially for older, untrained people). Severe breath holding and straining can increase intra-abdominal pressure and cause a hernia.

- Exhale during the lift and inhale as you lower the weight.

- Always work with a companion or spotter when using free weights.

- Alternate muscle groups during a session; alternate arm and leg exercises. Allow 2 to 3 minutes of recovery time between sets of the same exercise.

- You should keep records of your progress. Test for maximum strength every few weeks (see form 11.1 for a log to keep track of progress). Also record body weight and fat, and important dimensions (chest, waist, biceps, and so on). Vary the program; each fourth week should be somewhat easier to allow recovery.

Experienced lifters use a process called periodization that usually includes several cycles of training. Athletes may train strength in the off-season, endurance in the preseason, and power in the early competitive season. Because progress begins to level off after 2 months, you may want to change the program every 8 weeks, or when you reach a plateau or get bored. In chapter 14, we will show you how to use periodization in muscular fitness training to improve performance in sport.

Date	Chin-ups	Sit-ups	Push-ups				Other					

Date	Body weight	Waist	Chest		Other measurements			

FORM 11.1 Muscular Fitness Log

From B.J. Sharkey and S.E. Gaskill, 2013, *Fitness and health, seventh edition* (Champaign, IL: Human Kinetics).

Repetitions

We've known how to prescribe strength training since the early 1950s, when DeLorme and Watkins (1951) published their analysis of progressive resistance exercise. This report and more recent studies have confirmed the need for lifters to use a resistance that they cannot lift more than 12 times (~10RM). When more repetitions are possible, the load must be increased, hence the term *progressive resistance*. A comprehensive review of the literature leads to the conclusion that there is no optimal number of repetitions. Anything between 2 and 12RM yields success, as long as each set is in fact the maximal number of repetitions possible (Fleck and Kraemer 1997). Of course, working at the higher number of repetitions is safer, so 8 to 12 repetitions are usually prescribed for all but the most serious lifters.

Move the weight at a slow to moderate rate, always maintaining control. Breathe out as you lift and inhale as you lower the weight. Although some have recommended very slow lifts (10 sec/rep), studies have not confirmed the value of this approach.

Sets

Although a study with adult recreational lifters suggests that a single set provides an adequate training stimulus (Hass et al. 2000), other studies show that 3 sets of up to 10RM yield as much as 50 percent more training stimulus (Kramer et al. 1997). A review of 140 training studies showed that 4 sets per muscle group elicited maximal strength gains in trained and untrained people (Rhea et al. 2003). However, a prudent approach for the newcomer is to begin with 1 set of each exercise, progress to 2, and then perform 3 sets as strength develops. Proceed to 4 sets if you have specific training goals, such as an improvement in leg strength for alpine skiing.

Allowing time to recover after each set of repetitions is important. For strength training, 2 to 3 minutes is recommended. For muscular endurance, 1 minute is recommended. Inadequate rest will diminish strength gains.

Frequency

One of the early studies to compare different training frequencies (Barham 1960) found that 3- or 5-day-per-week formats were superior to 2 days per week, but that the 3- and 5-day programs were not significantly different from each other. In their 1997 review, Fleck and Kraemer concluded that the majority of research indicates that three training sessions per muscle group per week is the minimum frequency that causes maximum gains in strength. Apparently, untrained people need 48 hours to recover from a training bout and to adapt to the training stimulus. One analysis indicated that untrained people can achieve maximal gains by training each muscle group 3 days a week, whereas trained people do best with 2 days per week (Rhea et al. 2003). Of course, trained athletes participate in a more demanding program (see chapter 14).

The basic prescription for strength is as follows:

- Three sets of 8 to 12RM (with slow movement and adequate recovery time)
- Workout performed three times per week (every other day).

RM = repetition maximum: The number of repetitions that you can maximally do with a given weight. A weight that you can lift only one time is a 1RM weight, while a weight that you can lift eight times would be an 8RM resistance.

Heavier weights of 1 to 7RM may result in faster strength gains, but may also increase the likelihood of injury.

In practice, many lifters prefer to vary the program by changing the number of repetitions per set. Some begin at 10RM, then go to 8, and end at 6. For safety, we recommend that you begin with more reps and less weight and avoid high weights (low RM) (see table 11.1). Just remember to increase the resistance when you are able to do more than 10 reps in all 3 sets. **Progressive resistance training** suggests that you always try to increase the load. In general, this is true. We recommend that you add resistance as necessary (to stay below 10RM) for 2 to 3 weeks. Then do a week with lighter weights and reduce the frequency to two sessions per week. This easier week promotes muscle recovery and long-term gains.

Achievement

Although strength doesn't increase rapidly, you can expect the following:

- Your rate of increase will range from 1 to 3 percent per week, with previously untrained people increasing at a faster rate. With hard training, some people may temporarily achieve a rate of 4 to 5 percent improvement per week.
- The rate of improvement will decrease or level off as you approach your potential maximal strength. Take 1 or 2 easy weeks and then resume strength training (at less than 10RM) to reach a higher plateau.
- The rate of improvement may decrease if you combine strength training with strenuous aerobic training.
- Improvement will take place only in the muscle groups that you train.
- Your gains will be smaller if you fail to maintain adequate protein and energy in your diet. Increase protein intake if you are on a weight-loss diet.
- A previously sedentary person on an adequate diet can expect to increase strength 50 percent or more in 6 months. Hard training could lead to similar gains in less time.

Maintenance

You can maintain strength with lower volume and frequency of training, as long as intensity (resistance) remains high. One session per week will maintain strength for 6 weeks

Table 11.1   Prescriptions for Components of Muscular Fitness

Component	% 1RM	Reps	Sets	Recovery	Speed of movement
Strength	70–90%	6–12**	3–4	2–3 min	Slow
Endurance—short term	<60%	15–25	3	1–2 min	Moderate
Endurance—intermediate	<50%	20–30	2–3	1 min	Moderate
Endurance—long term	<40%	>30	1–3	<1 min	Sport specific
Power	30–60%	15–25	3	2–3 min	Fast as possible
Hypertrophy*	50–75%	10–20	3–6	1 min	Moderate

*Sought by bodybuilders, hypertrophy is an increase in muscle mass and cross-sectional area.

**Trained athletes may use 1–5RM with longer rest.

or more. Two sessions will ensure maintenance for a prolonged period, depending on the level of strength that you achieved before beginning the maintenance program.

With normal activity, you will retain most of your newly gained strength for up to 6 weeks after cessation of training, and you will retain half the strength that you gained for up to 1 year. When you resume training, you'll return to previous levels with less effort, perhaps because of the learning that took place in earlier training. Studies on older people show that strength declines very slowly in muscle groups that they use regularly. Thus, an investment in strength could pay dividends later in life. Of course, we recommend that you set aside at least 8 weeks each year (and as many as 12) to maintain or improve strength, and to continue a maintenance program (1 or 2 times per week) thereafter. Find a season that suits your schedule and follow a program. As the years pass, you'll be glad that you did.

Dietary Needs

Diet can exert positive effects on the development of muscular fitness. Carbohydrate and protein intake significantly alters circulating metabolites and the hormonal environment, including insulin, testosterone, growth

> **S**tudies on older people show that strength declines very slowly in muscle groups that they use regularly.

Strength and Aerobic Training

A 1980 study concluded that combining strength training with aerobic training diminished strength, but not the aerobic outcomes (Hickson 1980). Strength training is most effective in fast-twitch muscle fibers, whereas endurance training is likely to influence slow and fast fibers. Endurance training interferes with maximal strength development by causing fast, glycolytic fibers to convert to FOG fibers and attenuated hypertrophy (Putman et al. 2004). Yet other work indicates that concurrent strength and aerobic endurance training does not impair adaptations in strength or muscle hypertrophy (McCarthy, Pozniak, and Agre 2002). And in studies of older subjects, concurrent strength and aerobic training were each as effective as either strength or endurance training alone. The authors suggested that combining strength and aerobic training for older subjects may be more effective in optimizing functional fitness than are programs that involve only one component of fitness (Wood et al. 2001). Glowacki and colleagues (2004) suggested that concurrent strength and endurance training in untrained subjects did not interfere with strength development, but might hinder development of aerobic capacity. A 2010 review of concurrent strength and resistance training in endurance athletes concluded that high-volume, heavy-resistance strength training protocols combined with endurance training can enhance long-term (>30 min) and short-term (<15 min) endurance capacity both in well-trained people and highly trained top-level endurance athletes (Aagaard and Andersen 2010). They reported increases in the proportion of fast-twitch muscle fibers, gains in maximal muscle strength, improved rate of force development and possible enhancements in neuromuscular function. Both research and empirical data suggest that you incorporate reasonable amounts of both strength and endurance training into your program.

How Much Strength?

Strength may be related to performance in your work or sport. Don't assume, however, as many have, that if some is good, more is better. In most activities, performance improves with strength, but only to a point. Thereafter, you may be wasting your time or diminishing performance with excessive attention to strength. The trick is to know how much is enough. When strength is optimal for the sport, move on to other important phases of training. Just be sure to maintain the necessary strength with 1 or 2 sessions each week.

How much strength is sufficient? The answer differs according to the sport. For an endurance sport such as swimming or cross-country skiing, strength is adequate when the force needed in a single contraction (e.g., the arm pull in swimming) is below 40 percent of your maximal for that movement. If you exert 20 pounds of force in the average arm pull, you need approximately 50 pounds of force (2.5 × 20 lb) in a single maximal pull. More strength will not contribute to performance; if the arm pulls through too quickly, you'll go slower, not faster. So, if strength is adequate, move on to endurance training. For daylong work, strength is adequate when the force that you need is at or below 20 percent of your maximal. If a loaded shovel weighs 10 pounds, you'll need 50 pounds of force (5 × 10). We'll say more about strength and performance in chapter 14.

hormone, and cortisol, thereby influencing muscle protein response to training (Volek 2003). Postexercise intake of carbohydrate and protein is associated with muscle growth. Furthermore, the need for protein increases in strength training. Although sedentary people need .8 gram of protein per kilogram of body weight per day, serious weightlifters can use 1.4 to 1.8 grams per kilogram, as well as sufficient energy to avoid breakdown of muscle mass (Lemon 1995). You should take energy or protein snacks after a training session. Consume sufficient protein and carbohydrate calories and avoid rapid weight loss during muscular fitness training. We'll say more about diet and nutrition in chapters 12 and 13.

MUSCULAR ENDURANCE FITNESS PRESCRIPTION

We've pointed out how strength and endurance are different and why endurance may be more important than a high level of strength, presuming that you have adequate strength. The main difference between training for strength and training for endurance is the level of tension in the muscle and, consequently, the resistance used and number of repetitions possible. Lighter weights (less than 66% of maximum strength) don't provide much stimulus for strength development, but if you do enough repetitions, you will develop muscular endurance.

Years ago it was believed that training with fewer than 10RM developed strength, whereas training with more than 10RM developed endurance. We wondered if the body really made such fine distinctions. Studies have added to our knowledge of strength and endurance and the territory that lies between. Studies in our lab (Washburn et al. 1982) and others (Anderson and Kearney 1982) show that 15 to 25RM will still develop some strength (1% per week versus 2%–3% with 6 to 10RM for strength training), along with short-term or anaerobic endurance. Table 11.1 summarizes muscular fitness prescriptions for strength, endurance, and power. As the number of repetitions increases, less strength and more endurance develops.

The number of repetitions that you need depends on several factors. What are you training for? Are you training for short-term (anaerobic) endurance or long-term endurance? Your training should be specific to the way in which you will use it. Emphasize speed when necessary. Do many repetitions when you need long-term endurance with less resistance. When the activity involves moderate resistance, lift heavier weights and do fewer repetitions. For short (less than 2 min) and intense activities, train with 15 to 25RM to get short-term or anaerobic endurance. If your goals are vague and time is short, use fewer repetitions to avoid boredom. Follow the appropriate endurance prescription and observe the precautions mentioned for strength training. Because the loads are lighter, muscle endurance training is safer than strength training, and it is probably more suited to the everyday activities of the average adult.

Circuit Weight Training

Circuit weight training (CWT) involves a series of resistance exercises designed to promote strength and muscular endurance. The CWT circuit, with short rest intervals between sets, is intended to raise energy expenditure and heart rate and, according to some fitness practitioners, to improve aerobic fitness. Although this popular technique will improve strength and muscular endurance, its effect on aerobic fitness is slight (3%–5%). A set of 10 repetitions of an exercise such as a forearm curl is not sufficient to overload the oxidative system of the muscle. So its effect on aerobic fitness is far less than the 20 to 25 percent improvement derived from sustained large-muscle activity such as cycling or running. Aerobic fitness improvements are greater when you jog between sets.

CWT is an effective way to achieve muscular fitness goals, but whether the rest interval between sets is short (20 sec) or long (60 sec), the effect on energy expenditure or aerobic fitness is modest at best (Haltom et al. 1999). Do CWT if you like, but if you want the most from muscular and aerobic fitness training, focus on each one individually.

Achievement

Muscle endurance is trainable. Although going from two to four chin-ups is difficult (that takes strength), improving from 20 to 40 push-ups is easy (that takes endurance). When you have sufficient strength for the task, gains in endurance come with relative ease. Subjects in the Washburn study improved 10 percent per week in short-term endurance when they trained with 15 to 25RM. On an upper body endurance test, short-term (anaerobic) endurance training was more effective than strength training was, improving short-term endurance 70 percent versus 50

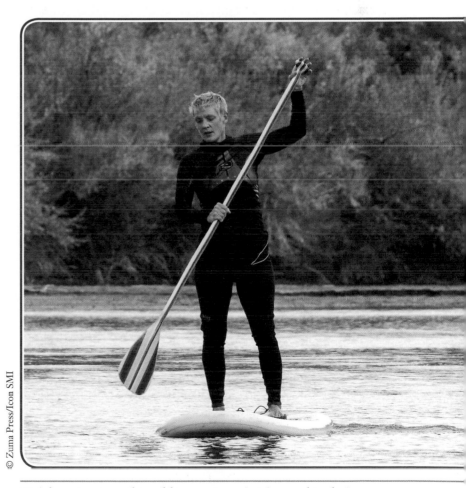

© Zuma Press/Icon SMI

■ Adequate strength enables you to maintain good technique during practice.

> *Improvement in endurance enhances most adult activities.*

percent for strength training. When strength is adequate, improvement in endurance enhances most adult activities. Tennis and skiing require hours of practice, and good practice requires endurance. The fatigued tennis student usually practices a sloppy version of the skill, and a fatigued skier carries a higher risk of injury.

How do you know if your strength is adequate for an activity? If you can perform an activity 10 times the way you would in the sport, you probably have adequate or functional strength. If you have enough strength to hit 10 tennis shots, or ski a series of turns down the slope, you may want to work on muscular endurance. If you struggle with the activity, you may need to develop additional strength and then concentrate on endurance.

Of course, your genetic endowment and your devotion to training will dictate your ultimate progress. If you have a high percentage of slow-twitch muscle fibers, your potential for muscular endurance is excellent. If you do not, don't despair. Training will improve the endurance capabilities of slow and fast fiber types. Although you may not be a world-class endurance athlete, you will come closer to your potential.

Dietary Needs

The best endurance performances occur when muscle fibers are well supplied with glycogen. And glycogen levels are highest when you follow a high-carbohydrate diet. Scandinavian studies have shown that a full day of alpine skiing can deplete muscle glycogen stores. If you dine on steak and salad after skiing, your muscles will not be ready to perform the following day. By doing all that you can to replace muscle glycogen, you will be able to ski all day and still have energy for après-ski. More important, you will be less likely to fatigue, fall, and be injured. Take energy snacks throughout the day and begin energy replacement immediately after activity, with several hundred calories of a carbohydrate–protein mix (ratio of 4 g of carbohydrate for 1 g of protein) (Ivy et al. 2002). Then continue with the high-carbohydrate **performance diet** indicated in chapter 12.

SAMPLE MUSCULAR FITNESS PRESCRIPTIONS

Many ways exist to improve your muscular fitness. This section covers a number of the common methods. We start with calisthenics, which you can do anywhere with limited equipment, and then move on to resistance training. Because of the need for individualized programs, we do not offer step-by-step programs. Rather, we refer you to table 11.1 for general guidelines on muscular fitness training. For performance programs, we encourage you to read about periodization in resistance training in chapter 14.

Calisthenics

Calisthenics include a wide range of exercises, such as push-ups, chin-ups, and sit-ups. The strength-training prescription calls for high resistance and low repetitions, so you may have to add additional resistance when you are able to do more than 10 repetitions (more than 10 repetitions will build short-term endurance, but not much strength). You can overload the push-up in several ways. For example, have someone place a hand on your back to increase the resistance or put your feet on a chair to place more weight on the arms. You could also do variations, such as fingertip push-ups or power push-ups (push up and clap hands). Just remember that as the number of repetitions exceeds 10, you are shifting toward endurance training. You can use calisthenics to train for both.

Knee Push-Up

A good chest and triceps exercise for beginners is the knee push-up. With hands outside your shoulders and knees bent, push up, keeping your back straight. Do as many as possible.

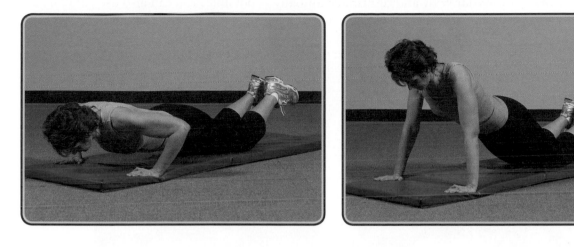

Push-Up

The push-up is an intermediate exercise. With hands outside your shoulders, push up, keeping your back straight. Return until your chest almost touches the floor. Do as many as possible.

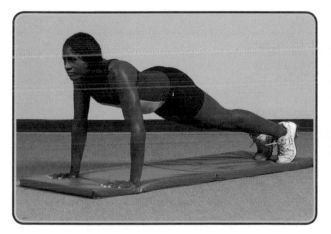
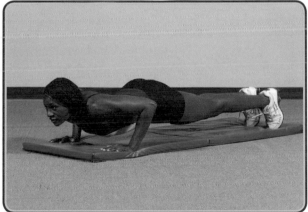

Chair Dip

The chair dip is an advanced exercise. Make sure that the chair you use is stationary. Grasp the sides of the chair and slide your feet forward while supporting your weight on your arms. Lower your body and return. Do as many as possible. You can also use parallel bars if available.

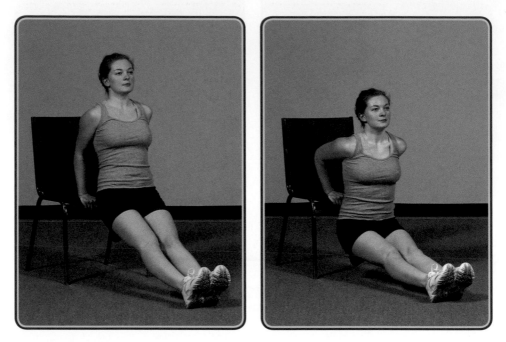

Modified Chin-Up

A good biceps and back exercise for beginners is the modified chin-up. Stand with the bar about chest height. With an underhand grasp, hang from the bar with the body straight and feet on the ground. Pull up and return. Do as many as possible.

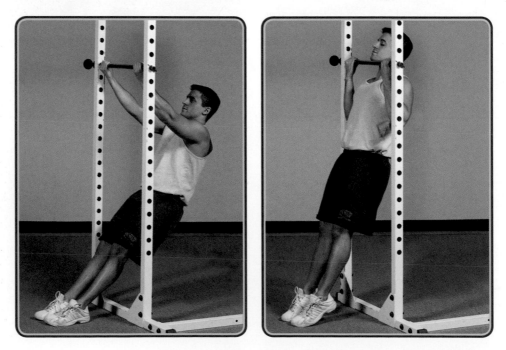

Chin-Up

The standard chin-up is the intermediate version of the exercise. With the underhand grasp, pull up until your chin is over the bar and return. Do as many as possible. Variations include using an overhand grip or climbing a rope.

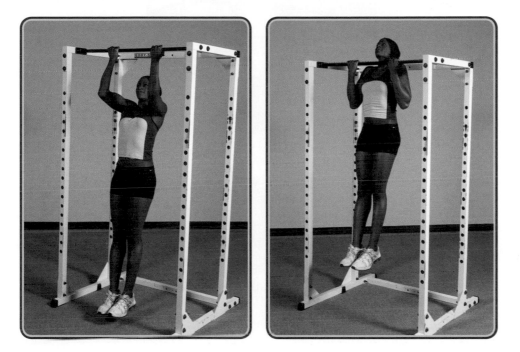

Pike Chin-Up

The pike chin-up is an advanced exercise. Perform the chin-up from the bar with legs in a pike position.

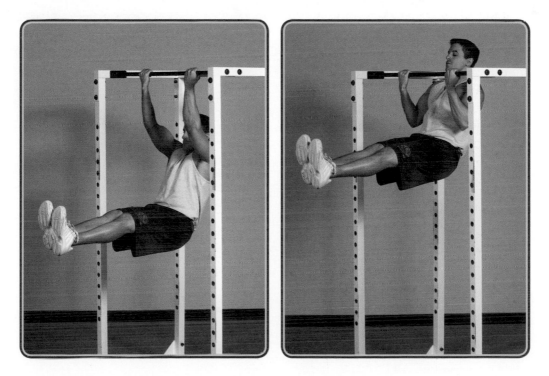

Basket Hang

The basket hang is an advanced abdominal exercise. Hang from the bar with an underhand grasp. Pull your knees up toward your chest and return. Do as many as possible.

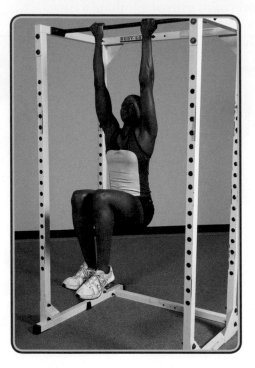

Sit-Up With Arms Crossed

A good exercise for abdominal strength and endurance is the sit-up with arms crossed. On your back with arms crossed over the chest and knees bent, curl up to a semisitting position and return. Do 10 to 15 times. Variations include doing repetitions very fast, doing the exercise on an inclined board, and holding a weight on your chest.

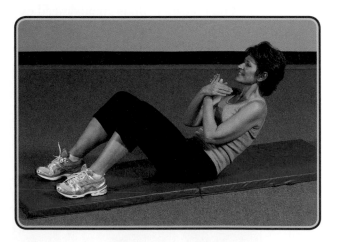

Leg Lift

The leg lift is a good exercise for back strength and endurance. Lying facedown on the floor with a partner holding your trunk down, raise your legs 5 to 10 times. Avoid hyperextension.

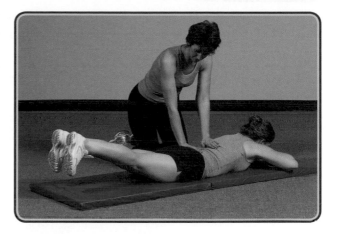

Hills

Power walk up a steep hill, stadium steps, or office stairs. For a variation, use ski poles for balance, to aid the downhill trip, or to exercise arms. Wear a weighted pack for added resistance.

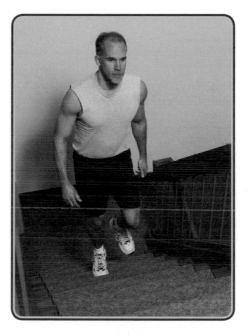

Trunk Lift

Lying facedown on the floor with fingers laced behind your head and ankles anchored to the ground, raise your trunk 5 to 10 times. Don't overextend.

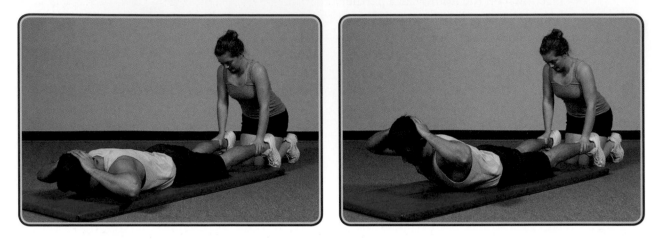

Bench Stepping

Step up and down on a bench as fast as possible for 30 seconds. Switch to lead with the other leg and repeat. You can also do bench stepping with a loaded pack.

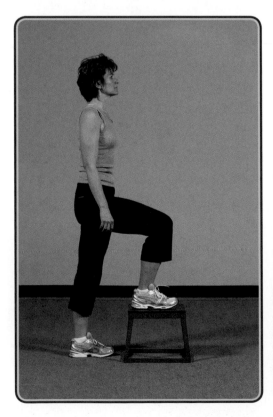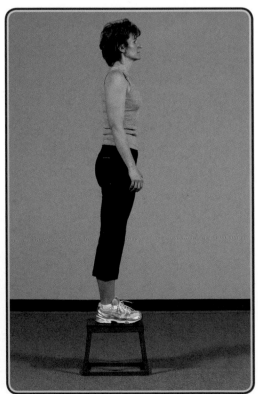

Half-Knee Bend

The half-knee bend is good for leg strength and endurance. With feet apart and hands on hips, squat until your thighs are parallel to the ground and return. Do as many as possible. Try a 2-inch (5 cm) block under the heels to aid balance. For variety, do this exercise with a weight on your back (e.g., a backpack).

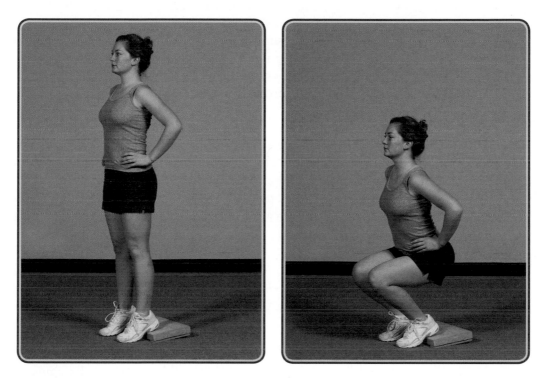

Heel Raise

Stand erect, hands at sides or on hips, feet close together. Rise up on your toes 20 to 40 times. You can do heel raises with your toes on a 2-inch (5 cm) platform or with a loaded pack.

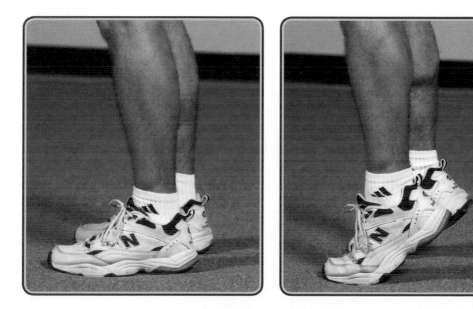

Resistance Training

Resistance training, sometimes called weight training, has emerged as an essential part of the program to improve performance, fitness, and even health. Use a weight-training apparatus (stack weights) or free weights (bar and weights). Although machines are expensive, they have several advantages over free weights: They are safer and more versatile, they save time, and they eliminate equipment theft. Using a machine also makes it much easier to change resistance as you move from one exercise to another. On the negative side, a machine restricts you to a set series of lifts and movements, and you don't learn to balance the load as well. But for general training, and especially for groups, machines are probably the best bet. Try the weight-training exercises that follow the descriptions of the apparatus in this section. Use the exercise prescriptions found in table 11.1 on page 228.

Weight-Training Machines

A number of companies manufacture weight machines. Some devices use a cam to adjust resistance throughout the lift. Most clubs have stations for triceps, chest exercises, leg press, leg flexion and extension, abdomen and trunk, military press and curls, lat pulldown, leg flexion and extension, biceps curl, bench press, and much more. A variety of variable-resistance devices are specifically designed for sports such as football, basketball, volleyball, and swimming.

Free Weights

Advanced programs often use free weights to isolate and overload specific muscles. Use the appropriate prescription to achieve your goal (e.g., 6 to 10RM for strength, more repetitions for endurance).

Isokinetics

Isokinetic devices, as well as accommodating or variable-resistance machines, are available in health and fitness clubs, in recreation centers, in schools and colleges, and even in private homes. The good ones allow you to exert near maximum force as the device moves through a full range of motion. You can vary the speed and resistance to suit specific training needs. You can use low-cost home devices in a variety of ways. Least expensive of all is isokinetic exercise with a friend (counterforce). Your partner provides resistance throughout the range of motion. For example, as you attempt forearm flexion, your partner provides resistance. You can do fast, medium, or slow isokinetics, depending on the goal of your training. But studies indicate that moderately fast training against resistance is more likely to develop strength and power.

Alternate days as you follow the program. Select the program to suit your needs, not those of the club. If you need medium or fast contractions for your sport, do them. Also, if the club recommends that you do 1 set, follow that advice for the first few weeks. But when your strength levels off, as it will with 1 set, progress to 2 and then 3 sets. Fitness clubs like lifters to use slow contractions that save wear and tear on the machines, and they advise 1 set because it eliminates long waits to use the apparatus.

Pull-Down

The pull-down works the lats. Kneel on one or both knees, or sit on a bench if one is available, and grasp the handles. Pull the bar down and return to the starting position.

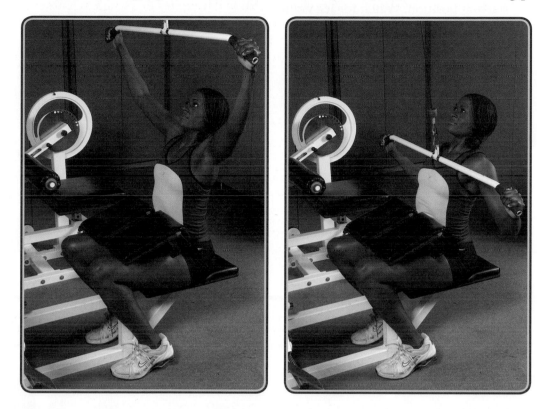

Leg Press

Leg presses work the quadriceps. Place your feet on the pedals and grasp the handles of the seat. Press your feet forward to elevate the weight and return. Inhale while lowering the weight and exhale while lifting it.

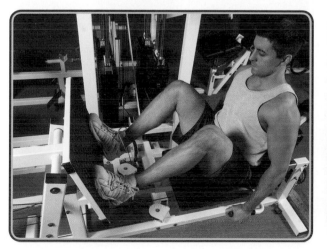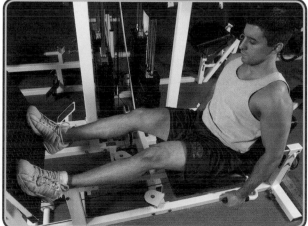

Leg Flexion

The leg flexion exercise works the hamstrings. Lie facedown on the table with your heels positioned behind the padded bar. Flex your legs to elevate the weight. Return to the starting position. Watch for leg cramps.

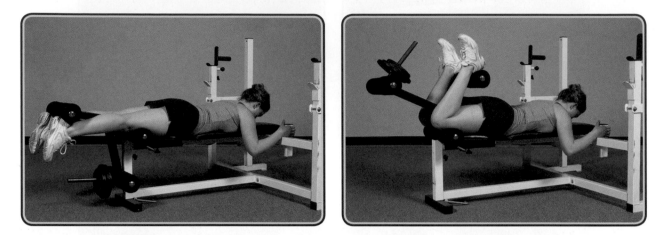

Leg Extension

The leg extension works the quadriceps. Sit on the bench with your instep under the padded bar. Extend your legs to elevate the weight. Return to the starting position.

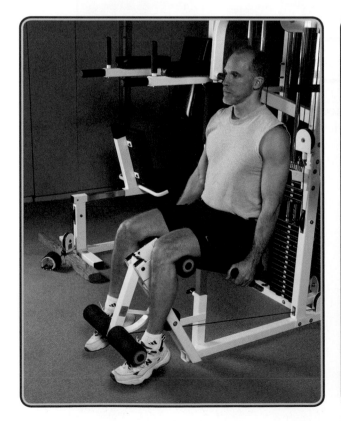
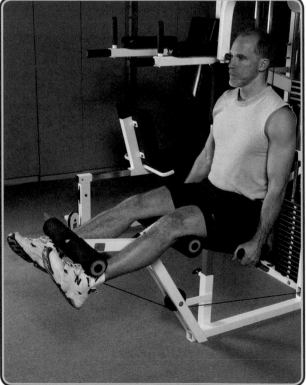

Bench Press

Bench presses exercise the chest and arm extensor muscles. Lie flat on your back with your feet on the floor astride the bench. Grasp the bar wider than shoulder-width, with arms extended. Lower the bar to your chest and then press it back up to the starting position. Inhale while lowering the weight and exhale while pressing it. A partner should assist with weights before and after the exercise.

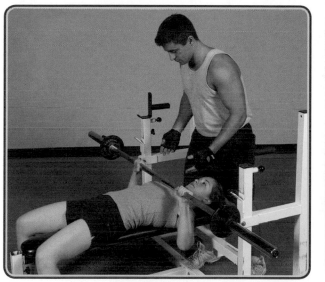 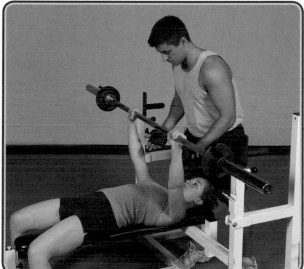

Triceps Extension

Sit astride a bench with your back straight. Grasp the bar with your hands about 2 inches (5 cm) apart, using an overhand grip. Move the bar to full arm extension above your head. Lower the bar behind your head, keeping the elbows stationary.

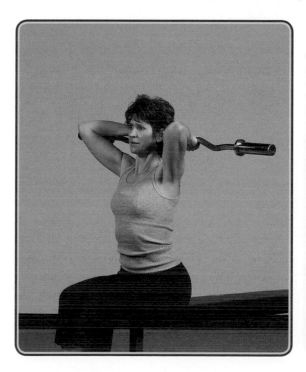 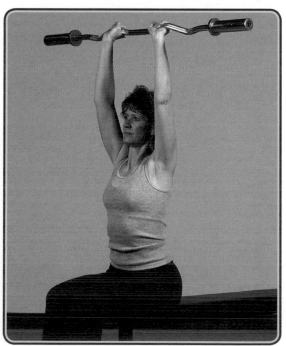

Bent Rowing

Work the back muscles with bent rowing. Stand in a bent-over position; your back is flat and slightly above parallel with the floor. Spread your feet shoulder-width apart, with your knees comfortably bent. Grasp a barbell with an overhand grip. Your hands should be slightly wider than shoulder-width. Keep your buttocks lower than your shoulders. Pull the bar to your chest and then lower it to the starting position. Keep your upper body stationary.

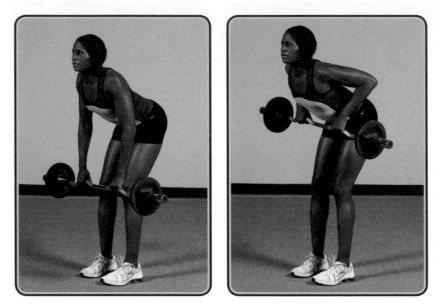

Military Press

The military press works the arm and shoulder muscles. Stand erect with feet comfortably apart. Grasp a barbell with an overhand grip and raise it to your upper chest. Then press the bar overhead until your elbows are fully extended. Lower the bar to chest position and repeat.

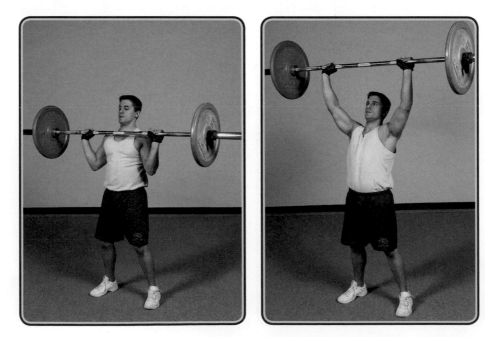

Biceps Curls

For the biceps curl, stand erect with your feet comfortably apart and knees slightly flexed. Hold the bar in front of your thighs with an underhand grip. Keep the hands shoulder-width apart and the arms straight. Flex your elbows fully, lifting the bar toward your chest. Keep your elbows close to your sides and avoid raising your shoulders. Don't lean backward or bounce the bar with your leg motion. Repeat.

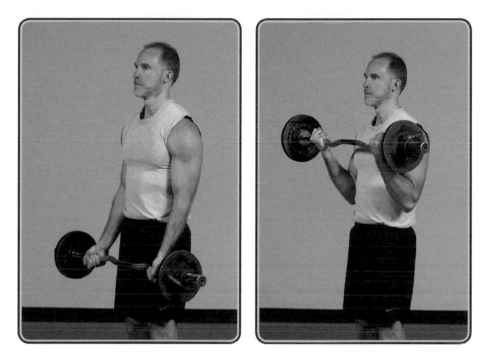

Arm Flexion

As you try to lift your arms, a partner resists the movement. Your partner should allow movement to progress slowly (through range of motion in 3 sec). Do 3 sets of 8 repetitions.

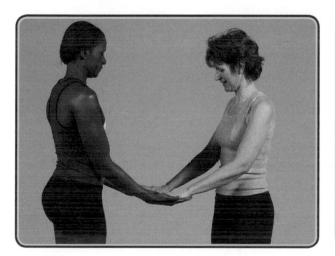
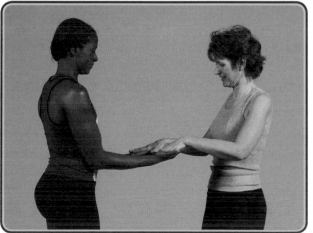

Arm Extension

As you try to extend your arms down, a partner resists the movement. Your partner should allow movement to progress slowly (through range of motion in 3 sec). Do 3 sets of 8 repetitions.

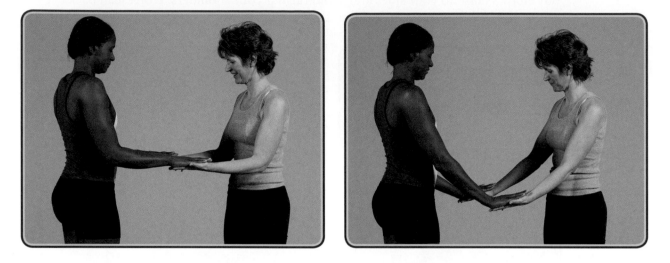

Push-Up

As you do a conventional push-up, a partner provides resistance. Do 3 sets of 8 repetitions. Switch places between sets to allow time to rest.

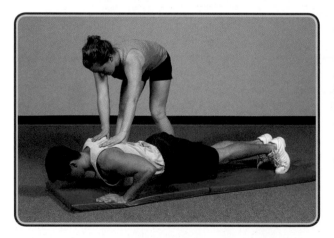
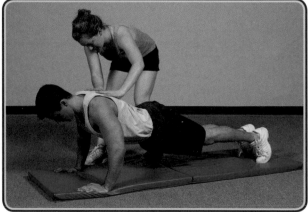

Leg Flexion

As you try to flex your leg, a partner resists the movement. Your partner should allow movement to progress slowly (through range of motion in 3 sec). Switch legs and repeat. Do 3 sets of 8 repetitions each. Switch positions between sets. Watch out for leg cramps.

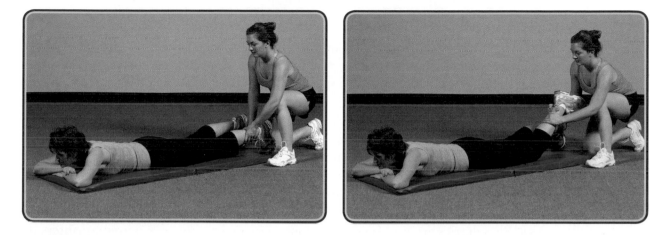

Leg Extension

As you try to extend your leg, a partner resists the movement. Your partner should allow movement to progress slowly (through range of motion in 3 sec). Switch legs and repeat. Do 3 sets of 8 repetitions each. Switch positions between sets.

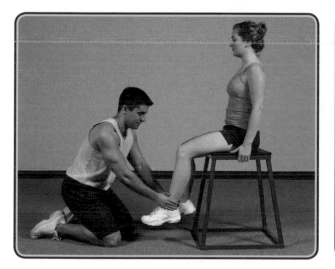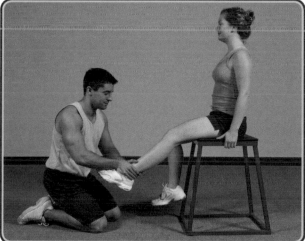

Speed and Power Training

As with other types of training, the key to speed and power training is specificity. Try to pattern the training after the intended use. To throw a baseball faster, train with a weighted ball or simulate the motion with pulley weights or an isokinetic device. To improve jumping ability, do half squats with weights, jump while wearing a weighted vest, or use an isokinetic jumping device. When in doubt, be specific. Here are some ideas on speed and power training.

• *Speed (velocity).* Do high-speed contractions with low resistance. Sprinters have gained speed by running down slight grades, running against resistance, and performing assisted running (being towed). For more on speed training, consult a good book on the subject (e.g., Dintiman and Ward 2003).

• ***Power*** *(force times velocity).* Do 3 sets of 15 to 25 high-speed contractions with 30 to 60 percent of maximal resistance. You can use accommodating resistance devices to do power training, but free weights are not well suited for high-speed training. Athletes use sport-specific devices, higher resistance (e.g., 8RM), and explosive contractions to improve power for brief, intense efforts (e.g., football).

Another approach, a popular technique borrowed from European coaches, is plyometrics. Plyometrics are explosive movements designed to improve power. Sprinters do one- and two-leg hops to gain power. High jumpers, broad jumpers, volleyball and basketball athletes, and even cross-country skiers use plyometrics to improve performance. Proponents have said that plyometrics train the capacity for preload and elastic recoil, and build strength and explosive power (Radcliffe and Farentinos 1985). Unfortunately, the research concerning the value of plyometrics for various sports and for athletes at different levels of development is not extensive. Moreover, excessive use or poor technique can lead to painful knee problems.

We recommend that you try plyometrics, if only because of the effect on skill and economy of movement. Start with a modest number, on a soft surface, and quit at the first sign of discomfort in the knees. Even if you don't gain additional power, you may become more effective in using the power that you possess. (Chapter 9 describes the phenomenon called preload and elastic recoil, and explains how it contributes to power and performance.) When training for speed or power, or doing plyometrics, consider the following precautions. Before you do speed or power training, establish a strength and endurance base to avoid injury.

- Warm up and stretch before fast or explosive efforts.
- Start relaxed and gradually increase the intensity and speed of movement.
- Start with light resistance and increase gradually.
- Do not use free weights.
- Use machines and devices designed for high speed.
- Start slowly with plyometrics. Use easy jumps and few repetitions. Increase repetitions and intensity gradually. When overdone, plyometrics can cause joint pain and delayed-onset muscle soreness.

Squat Jumps

Stand with one foot a step ahead of the other. Squat (drop quickly) until your front thigh is at a 90-degree angle to the lower leg. Then immediately jump as high as possible, extending the knees. Switch the position of your feet on the way down. Land, squat, and jump again. Perform 15 to 25 repetitions. Start gently and increase numbers and intensity slowly.

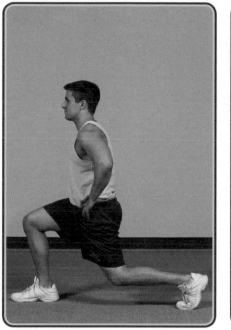
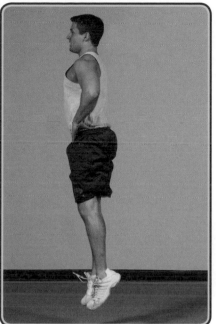

Two-Leg Jumps

Jump as high as possible with both legs. Do 10 to 20 explosive two-leg jumps.

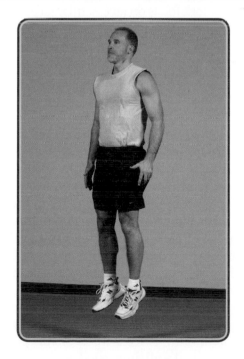

Hops

Do one-leg hops, alternating legs with a balance step between hops. Do 10 with each leg. Work up to 2 sets of 20.

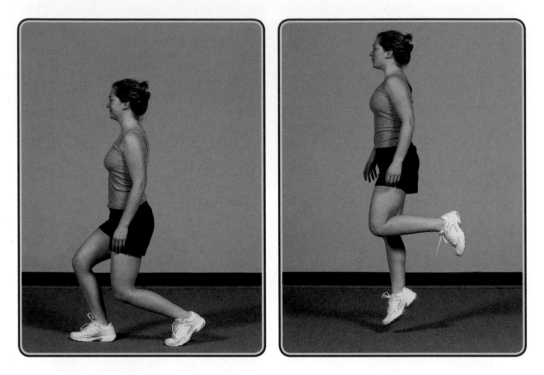

Core Training

Now let's focus on an essential facet of muscular fitness, core training. Core exercises focus on core muscles that anchor and stabilize the arms and legs involved in work, sport, and recreational activities. Core exercises recruit one or more large muscle areas (abdominal, back, trunk, chest, shoulders, hip) and involve two or more primary joints (multi-joint). They are a high priority in terms of health and performance. The core musculature consists of many different muscles that, when contracted, stabilize the spine, pelvis and shoulder girdle to create a solid base of support. Many of these run the entire length of the torso. When your core is stabilized, you can generate powerful movements of the extremities. Core training focuses on the central portion of the body, an area that provides the foundation for performance and health. A moderate amount of core training is important for lower back health. Strong and balanced muscles of the trunk allow for better transfer of power from large core muscles to the extremities, thereby reducing the risk of injury.

You can train the core in a number of ways, ranging from old fashioned calisthenics and medicine balls, to Swiss balls, yoga, and Pilates. Current studies have shown Pilates to be as effective as traditional core exercises. A study that compared Pilates and general core exercises in subjects with low back pain showed that the Pilates program produced beneficial effects similar to that of a general exercise program in regards to self-reported disability, pain, function, and health-related quality of life (Wajswlner, Metcalf, and Bennell 2012). Another study using magnetic resonance imaging (MRI) before and after a nine month, twice a week Pilates program showed muscle growth (hypertrophy) of the abdominal wall, improved core strength, and muscle balance (Dorado et al. 2012). A few popular core exercises are shown in the following figures. Additionally, a number of books and websites do an excellent job describing core training.

Push-Ups

Push-ups are a wonderful total body exercise using both upper body and core strength. Properly performed, they use muscles in the chest, shoulders, triceps, back, abs, and legs. Get on the floor and position your hands slightly wider than your shoulders. Rise up, balancing on your hands and toes. Keep your body in a straight line from head to toe without sagging in the middle or

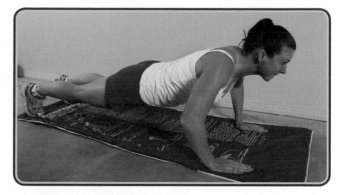

arching your back. Your feet can be close together or a bit wider, depending on what is most comfortable for you. Contract your abs and tighten your core by pulling your belly button toward your spine. Inhale as you slowly bend your elbows and lower yourself until your elbows are at a 90-degree angle. Exhale as you begin pushing back up to the start position. At the end of the upright position, your elbows should be slightly bent.

Bridge

Done correctly, this is a great method for strengthening the gluteus, hamstring, abdominal, and lower back muscles. Lie on your back with your hands by your sides, your knees bent, and your feet flat on the floor. Make sure your feet are under your knees. Tighten your abdominal and buttock muscles. Raise your hips up to

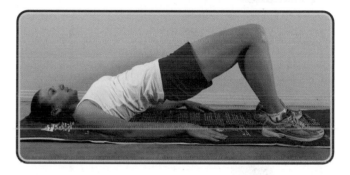

create a straight line from your knees to shoulders. Squeeze your core and try to pull your belly button back toward your spine. The goal is to hold your shoulders and your knees in alignment for 20 to 30 seconds. You may need to begin by holding the bridge position for a few seconds at a time as you build your strength. It's better to hold the correct position for a shorter time than to go longer in the incorrect position.

Plank

This simple (but hard to hold) position improves your core strength. Begin in the plank position, as shown in the photo, with your forearms and toes on the floor. Keep your torso straight and rigid and your body in a straight line from ears to toes. Do not sag or bend. Hold this position for 10 to 20 seconds to start. Over time, work up to

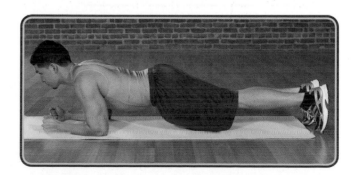

30, 60, or even 120 seconds. A variation is to slowly lift one leg off the floor 3 to 8 inches (8–20 cm) for 2 or 3 seconds. Repeat with the other leg.

Side Plank (Right and Left)

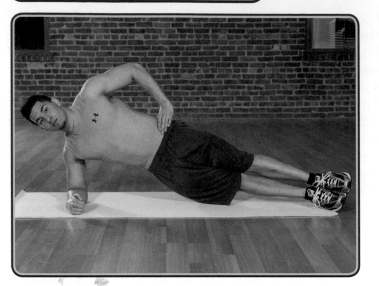

Lie on your side on the floor. Position your elbow on the floor just under your shoulder. Lift your body up, supporting your weight with that elbow. Keep your body stiff from head to toe. Hold this position for a count of 10, and then lower your hip to the floor. Rest and repeat three times. Switch sides and repeat the exercise on the other arm. As you get stronger, you can do these for 20 seconds or longer.

Hip Lift

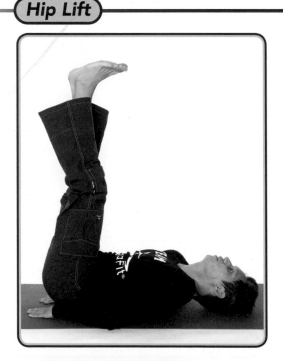

This exercise strengthens the rectus abdominis and oblique muscles. Start with a few, and gradually work up to 2 or 3 sets of 8 to 12 repetitions. Begin by lying on your back with your arms by your sides, palms facing up. Raise your legs so they are pointing straight up toward the ceiling and are perpendicular to your torso. Pull your navel toward your spine and lift your hips a few inches off the floor, keeping your legs pointed straight up. Slowly lower your hips back to the floor.

V-Sit Exercise

This is an effective abdominal and core exercise that works the rectus abdominis, external oblique, and internal oblique muscles, as well as the hip flexors. Begin in a seated position, contract your abdominal muscles and core, and lift your legs up to a 45-degree angle. Reach your arms straight forward or reach up toward your shins as you are able. Hold this *V* position for several seconds. As you get stronger, hold the position longer. Return to your starting position slowly. Start with a few and gradually increase until you can do 8 to 15 repetitions.

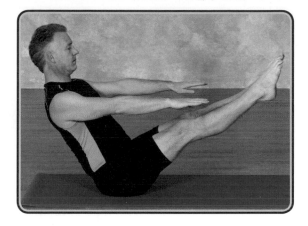

You don't need to spend a lot of time or money to achieve the benefits of core training. Abdominal and trunk exercises and Swiss balls are inexpensive. Use videos, books, and magazine articles to expand your use of core training.

Lower Back Fitness Training

More than 30 million Americans are afflicted with lower back pain, and an estimated 24 million (80%) of these problems are due to improper posture, weak muscles, or inadequate flexibility. Weak abdominal muscles cannot counter the forward tilt of the pelvis, which can displace the vertebrae and cause pain. Lack of flexibility in back and hamstring muscles has also been associated with lower back pain, which is a **hypokinetic** disease, one that results from a lack (*hypo*) of movement (*kinetic*).

Back-care specialists continue to explore new approaches, including greater use of back exercises to strengthen extensor muscles and maintain trunk flexibility. Sophisticated back-testing devices allow measurement of flexion and extension strength and range of motion. In one study using specialized equipment, isolated lumbar extension exercise with the pelvis stabilized led to increases in strength and vertebral bone mineral density, reductions in pain and symptoms, and less reutilization of the health care system. Achieved with low-volume training, the results were long lasting and independent of initial diagnosis (Carpenter and Nelson 1999).

Now, many health clubs have back-extension devices. If you have a lower back problem, ask your physician or physical therapist about these and other approaches to the prevention, diagnosis, and treatment of lower back disorders. If you decide to improve back-extension strength, avoid hyperextension. When you do have a problem, consider the results of a study of patients with acute lower back pain. The outcomes of treatment, recovery from pain, and return to function and work were similar whether the care came from primary care physicians, chiropractors, or surgeons. Care by the primary care physician, however, was the least expensive (Carey et al. 1995). Prevention is even cheaper, so begin your back health program today.

Lower Back Fitness Tests

The simple tests that follow, developed at the Sun Valley Health Institute, will help identify areas that need additional attention. Take the tests again after several months to monitor your progress.

Curl-Up

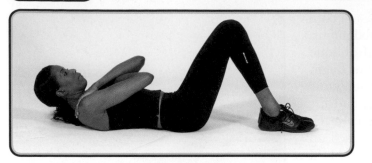

Lie on your back and bend your knees to a 90-degree angle, with your feet on the floor. Using one of the following arm positions, slowly curl up to a sitting position. Don't swing your arms or allow your feet to come off the floor. If successful, try a more difficult position (higher number). If not, try an easier one (lower number). Your score is the highest number achieved.

1. Arms at side, unable to curl up without aid of partner
2. Arms at side, hands pull back of thighs
3. Arms at side
4. Arms folded across chest
5. Hands behind neck
6. Arms extended overhead, fingers intertwined, with arms pressing against ears

This test indicates abdominal muscle strength and flexibility of back muscles. If you can't do number 5, you need more than a maintenance program. Do repetitions of number 3 and number 4 so that you can achieve number 5.

Leg Lift

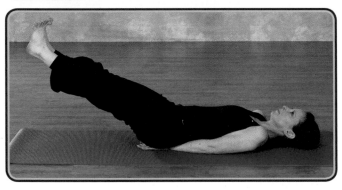

The leg lift test evaluates the strength of the lower abdominal muscles. Lie on your back with head on floor, legs straight, and hands under the hollow of your back. Flatten your back and then attempt to raise both feet 10 inches (25 cm). Hold the position for 10 seconds.

1. Unable to lift both legs
2. Back rises immediately
3. Back rises after several seconds
4. Able to hold back flat

If you can't do number 4, you need more abdominal tone. Use the basket hang and other exercises to improve abdominal tone.

Sit and Reach

The sit-and-reach test evaluates lower back and hamstring flexibility. Sit with your legs flat on the floor. Place one hand over the other and point the toes to the ceiling. Reach forward and try to touch your toes or beyond. Hold for several counts. Score as follows after several warm-up trials.

1. Well short of toes (more than 3 in., or 7.6 cm, short)
2. Touch toes (or come within 2 in., or 5 cm)
3. Touch well beyond toes (more than 3 in., or 7.6 cm, beyond)

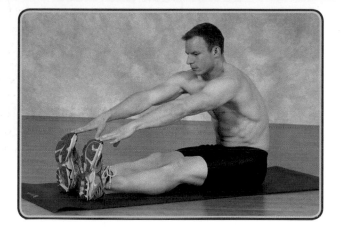

Although extreme flexibility isn't necessary for a healthy back, the lower back and leg muscles need adequate flexibility. A score of 2 is adequate. With practice, you may be able to score a 3.

Hip Flexion

Lie on your back with your legs held straight and flat. Keep your head on the floor throughout the test. Bend your right leg and pull your knee to your chest. Test both sides and score as follows.

1. Knee comes to chest, but left leg comes completely off the floor
2. Knee comes to chest, but left leg lifts somewhat
3. Knee completely to chest with left leg flat on the floor

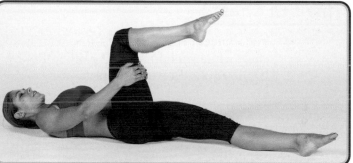

Tight hip flexors may cause an exaggerated lumbar curve, which predisposes the back to injury. Do this test and other stretching exercises to improve flexibility of the hip flexors. In time, you should be able to score a 3 with both legs.

Lower Back Exercises

Lower back pain is a huge problem for industry, responsible for numerous lost workdays and sky-high worker's compensation and medical costs. Yet in many cases, people can prevent lower back problems by assuming good posture and adhering to a regular program of flexibility, back, and abdominal exercises. Maintaining proper weight and a trim waistline also helps. To avoid injury to the lower back, use your legs instead of your back when lifting heavy objects and avoid carrying heavy objects above the level of the elbows. Other suggestions for prevention of lower back problems include the following:

- Sleep with the knees somewhat flexed. Avoid lying flat on your back or belly. Use a firm mattress or sleep with a piece of plywood under the mattress.
- Sit with one or both knees above your hips. Cross your legs or use a footrest.
- Keep your knees bent while driving. If your car seat doesn't provide lumbar support, use a cushion.
- When standing, place one foot on a stool, especially while ironing, washing dishes, or working at a counter or workbench.

Regular practice of the following exercises will help prevent or improve lower back problems and maintain lower back health (Williams 1974). Remember, when lower back pain does arise, the best treatment is not bed rest, but a return to normal activity as soon as possible (Malmivaara et al. 1995).

Knee to Chest

With knees bent and arms above your head, move one knee as far as possible toward your chest while straightening the other. Return to the starting position and repeat, switching leg positions. Relax and repeat.

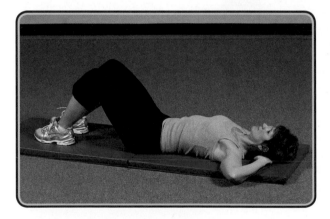 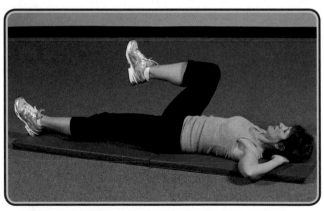

Flat Back

Bend your knees, holding your feet flat on the floor and your arms above your head. Tighten the muscles of your lower abdomen and buttocks at the same time, keeping your back flat on the floor. Hold 10 seconds, relax, and repeat.

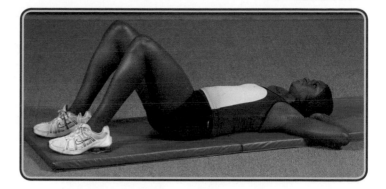

Double Knee Pull

Starting in the same position, with your arms at your sides, draw your knees to your chest and clasp your hands around your knees. Keeping your shoulders flat against the floor, pull your knees tightly against your chest. Hold 10 seconds, relax, and repeat. Repeat and touch your forehead to your knees.

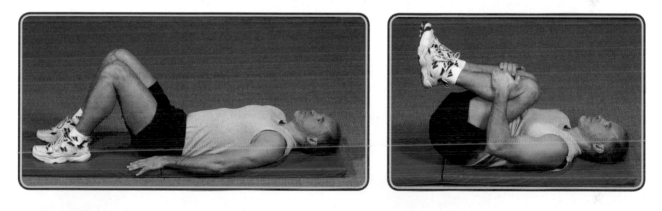

Curl-Up

Bend your knees, keeping your feet flat on the floor. Lift one leg and rest the ankle on the knee of the opposite leg. Lock your hands behind your head. Raise your head and shoulders from the floor. With chin to chest and with your back rounded, curl up as far as possible, trying to touch your elbow to the opposite knee. Be sure to pull with the abdominal muscles. Lower slowly. Do 5 to 10 repetitions, switch position, and repeat. Increase until you can do 20.

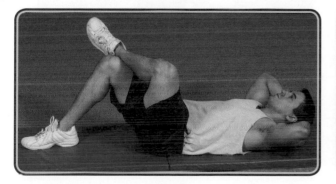
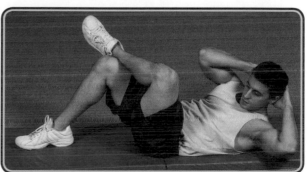

Angry Cat

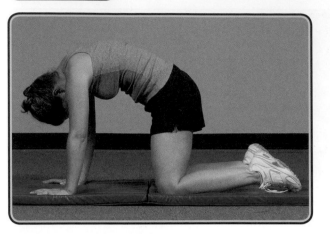

Kneel and place your hands on the floor. Lower your head and contract your abdominal and buttock muscles, arching your lower back. Hold for 5 seconds, then relax.

Seated Back Stretch

With your knees bent, bend forward at the waist to bring your head between your knees. Pull in your abdomen as you curl forward. Keep your weight back on your hips. Release your abdominal muscles and reach to stretch your lower back. Come up slowly. Relax and repeat. Move forward to involve and stretch the hamstring muscles.

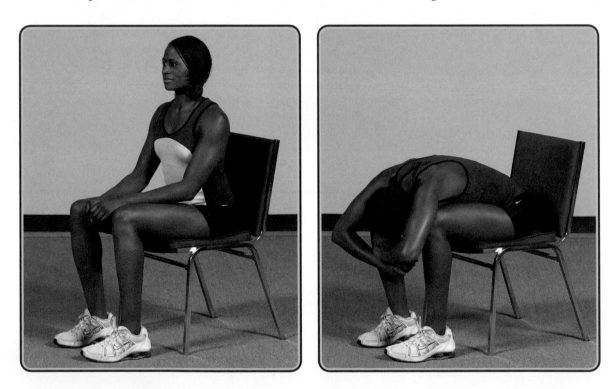

Stretching Exercises

Before stretching, warm up a bit with light exercise or calisthenics and then do your stretching. Finish the warm-up with more vigorous effort or, if you prefer, begin your run or other exercise at a modest pace. Do your warm-up and stretching before you begin to compete. You can use several different types of stretching exercises to achieve your goals.

• **Static stretching**. Here, use slow movements to reach a point in a stretch, hold the position (for 10 sec), and relax. You may repeat the stretch or perform very light bobbing.

• **Contract/relax stretch**. A variation of the static stretch is the contract and relax technique. Do a static stretch, relax, and then contract the muscle for a few seconds. Then repeat the static stretch. When performed on muscles like those in the calf, the technique seems to help the muscle relax so that you can better stretch the tendon.

• **Dynamic stretching**. This method requires moving through the range of motion, working at either end to increase the range. This technique mimics sport movements, such as the golf swing, with controlled motion. Dynamic stretches help loosen your swing before a round of golf. Use care to remain gentle in your motions.

Static stretching and the contract/relax variation are at least as effective as dynamic stretching and provide other advantages such as low risk of injury and reduction of tightness and lingering muscle soreness. When you do flexibility training correctly, the results are quite persistent. You should retain improved range of motion for at least 8 weeks. But after you have learned to enjoy stretching, you may get hooked on its subtle sensations and move on to advanced forms such as yoga. If not, just remember to do the stretches that you need to minimize soreness, reduce the risk of injury, and avoid lower back problems. You can find many resources for stretching exercises, both on the Internet and in book form.

Do your chosen stretching exercise to the point of mild discomfort, hold it for 10 seconds, and then relax. Choose exercises that help you increase the range of motion to improve performance or for joints and movements that are limited.

Shoulder and Arm Stretch

Intertwine your fingers above your head with your palms facing up. Push your arms upward and slightly to the rear. Feel a stretch in your arms, shoulders, and upper back.

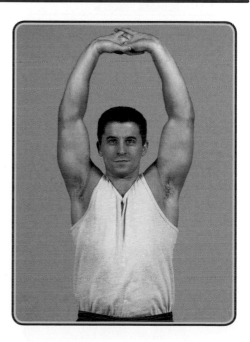

Hand Stretches

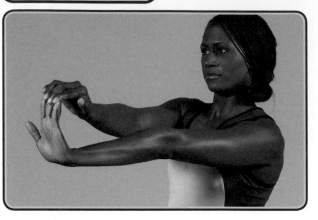

With the wrist and fingers of one hand extended, use your other hand to gently increase the extension of the fingers. Repeat with the opposite hand. Other options for stretching the hands include extending the wrist and flexing your fingers at the same time or extending your wrists while simultaneously abducting (spreading out) the fingers as far as possible.

Neck Stretch

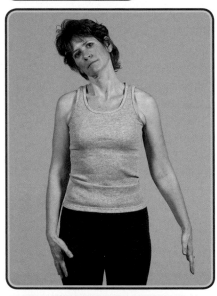

Lean your head sideways toward the right shoulder while reaching down with your left arm. To increase the stretch, use your right hand to pull your left arm downward behind your back. Repeat on the opposite side.

Shoulder Stretch

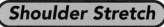

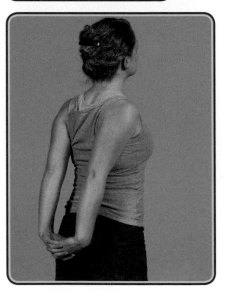

Intertwine your fingers behind your back, with palms facing inward. Start the stretch by turning your elbow while maintaining straight arms. For a second stretch, maintain an erect posture and raise your arms up behind you until you feel a mild stretch.

Upper Chest Stretch

Stand in front of a doorjamb or a similar structure. Place your hands about shoulder height on the doorjamb and gently lean forward, feeling a stretch across the front of your shoulders and chest. If you need a little more stretch, step back farther from the doorjamb and relax your shoulders, letting gravity increase the stretch.

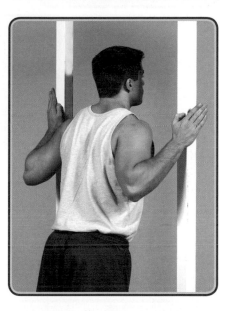

Trunk Stretch

Standing upright, look over your right shoulder and turn your upper torso as far as possible. Try to keep your hips facing forward. Repeat to the left. As an alternative, stand about 18 inches (46 cm) from a wall and face away from it. Keeping your hips facing forward, rotate both hands and shoulders and touch the wall. Go only as far as is comfortable.

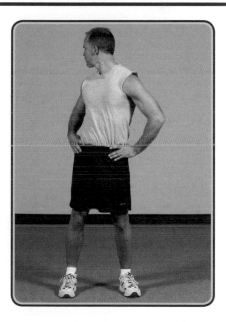

Back Stretch

Place both hands shoulder-width apart on a bar or other solid support that is at about chest height. With slightly bent knees, let your torso drop forward. Keep your hips directly above your feet. Try bending your knees a little more to increase the stretch. Experiment with holding objects at different heights.

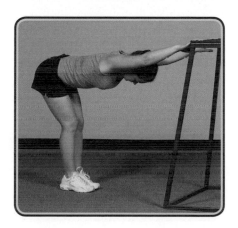

Side-Bend Stretch

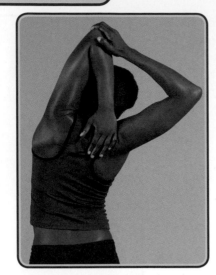

Stretch your left arm up and behind your head. Grasp the left elbow with your right hand as you bend to the right, simultaneously pulling your left arm. Feel the stretch from the elbow down through the upper arm and upper torso. Repeat on the right side.

Lower Back and Shoulder Stretch

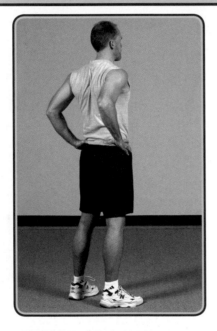

While standing or sitting, place your hands on your lower back. Bring your shoulders back and your elbows toward one another while pushing your back forward.

Spine Stretch

This stretch may be felt across the entire back, outside of the hips, and in the ribs. Sit upright on the floor with the right leg out in front. Bend the left leg and place the foot on the floor across the extended right leg. Bend your right elbow and place it on the outside of the left thigh near the knee. Use the left arm for balance as shown and twist, looking over your left shoulder while maintaining pressure with the right arm on the left knee. Repeat on the other side.

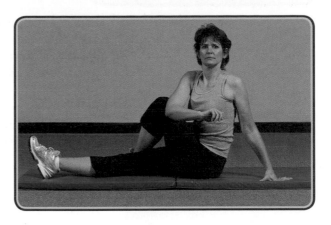

Upper Hamstring and Hip Stretch

Sitting on the floor (if necessary, sit with your back to a wall), hold the outside of your ankle (or knee) and foot as shown. Gently pull the entire leg toward your torso until you feel a slight stretch in the back of your upper leg. Repeat on the other side. For an additional stretch from this position, use your hand to gently rotate the foot through its full range of motion to exercise tight ligaments.

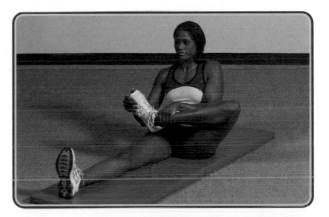

Outer Hip Stretch

Sitting on the floor as shown, with one leg extended and the other bent and placed over the extended leg, gently pull the knee across your torso toward the opposite shoulder. Repeat on the other side.

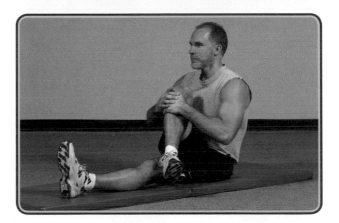

Standing Groin Stretch

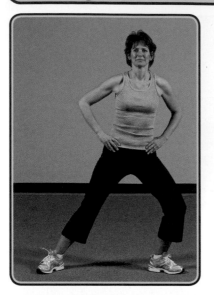

With feet spread, bend your left knee while keeping your right leg straight. Push your hip down and toward the left foot until you feel a modest stretch along the inner thigh of the right leg. Repeat on the other side.

Groin, Hamstring, and Hip Stretch

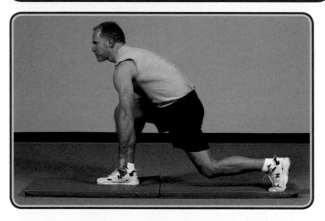

Place your right knee directly above the ankle and extend your rear leg behind you as shown. Your weight should be on the toes and ball of the rear foot. Hold an easy stretch by letting your torso relax forward, past the front knee. Use your hands for balance. Repeat on the other side.

Groin, Hamstring, and Front of Hip Stretch

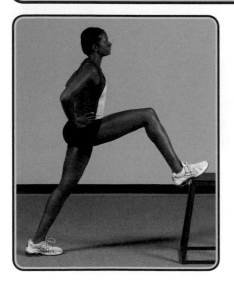

Place the ball of your foot on a secure support, such as a table. Keep the support leg pointed forward. Push your hips toward the front foot while bending the front knee. Feel the stretch in the groin and hamstring of the elevated leg and in the front of the hip on the side of the support leg. Repeat on the opposite side.

Squat Stretch

You will feel this stretch in the lower legs, knees, back, ankles, Achilles tendons, and groin. Squat down, with your feet flat, knees above the toes, and toes pointing out slightly. Changing the width of your feet and knees will change the areas being stretched.

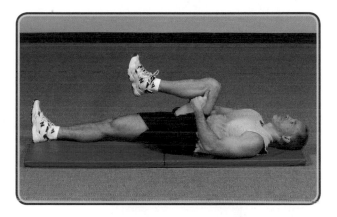

Quad and Gluteus Stretch

Lie on your back, with your head and shoulders touching the floor, one leg extended, and the other knee and hip flexed. Use both hands to hold the lower thigh behind your knee. Gently pull your knee toward your chest. Repeat on the other side.

Knee and Quad Stretch

While balancing against a wall, hold the top of your right foot with your left hand and gently pull your foot upward and toward your buttocks. Repeat on the opposite side.

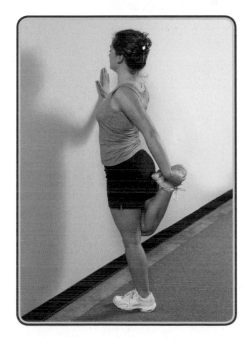

Ankle and Quad Stretch

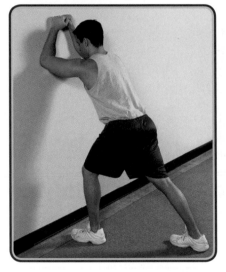

Lie on one side, supporting your head with the lower arm. Hold the top of the upper foot with the free hand, as shown. First, gently pull your heel toward your buttocks to stretch your ankle and quadriceps. Second, push the top of your foot into your hand and upward by contracting the gluteus (buttocks) muscles. This movement should further stretch the quadriceps. Repeat on the other side.

Calf Stretches

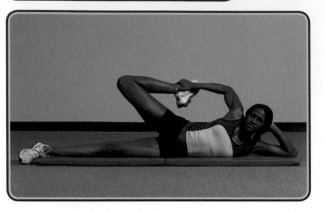

Leaning against a wall or solid support, place most of the weight on the rear foot and push your hips down and forward, keeping the rear leg straight and the heel on the ground. This causes a stretch in your upper calf. From this position, you can also stretch the lower calf. Relax the hips and focus on pushing the rear knee forward and down while keeping the heel on the ground. Repeat on the other leg.

SUMMARY

This chapter provides prescriptions and guidelines for the development of muscular strength and endurance. It suggests ways to train, shows what progress you can expect, explains how to maintain muscular fitness, and describes what happens when training stops. It also provides prescriptions for speed and power. Be certain to precede vigorous speed or power training with at least 8 weeks of a sport-specific buildup (strength and progressively faster running, throwing, and jumping) to avoid excessive soreness or injury. This chapter also deals with the important issue of lower back health and the essential contributions of muscular fitness. Chapter 14 provides more specific programs for strength and power.

Besides the obvious benefits of strength and endurance to appearance and performance, other important reasons for muscular fitness include avoiding crippling osteoporosis and lifelong maintenance of mobility. Preventing osteoporosis, the weakening of bone through loss of bone minerals, requires regular weight-bearing activity, such as walking or jogging, as well as moderate resistance exercises for the upper body. Performing normal household tasks, such as lifting, vacuuming, mowing grass, shoveling snow, and others, will help you avoid the problem. Research shows, however, that people achieve the best results with a combination of weight-bearing and resistance exercise, along with a diet that includes adequate calcium and vitamin D (exposure to sunlight is a natural way to form vitamin D). Postmenopausal women may need strength training to slow the loss of bone density and improve muscle strength and balance (Nelson et al. 1994).

Finally, living the active life, which includes engaging in aerobic and muscular activities, preserves mobility and independence. Anyone, regardless of age, can restore mobility and independence by becoming active. Studies of older adults and frail older people indicate that resistance training improves both strength and the performance of activities of daily living. These activities include getting out of a chair, walking, climbing stairs, and carrying groceries. If you can't perform these activities, you will be relegated to family care or a nursing home. Start now to maintain or improve your muscular fitness.

Activity and Weight Control

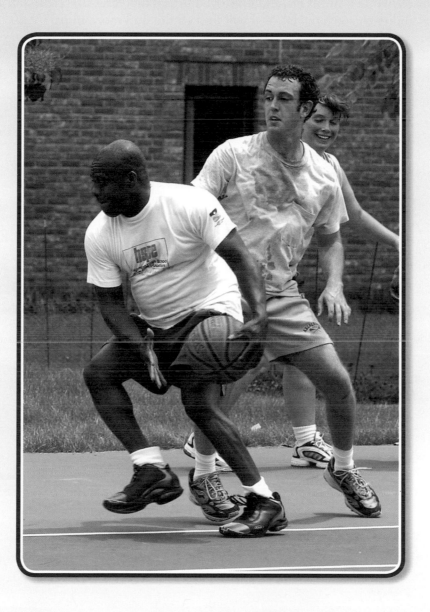

Our nation is one of paradoxes. We boast more dieters, diet books, diet foods, and diet centers than any other country on earth, yet we have become the fattest nation on earth. The reason for this is simple: dieting. What a paradox—the more we diet, the fatter we get! Part V reviews the basics of good nutrition, deals with the importance of activity in weight control, and discusses the contributions of fitness to fat metabolism and weight control. We illustrate how diet alone is a recipe for failure and how the active life provides a positive approach to weight control while allowing enjoyment of your favorite foods. These ideas are not new; they appeared in Brian's first book, published in 1974. However, in the years that followed, overweight and obesity—and their consequences—have been, so to speak, expanding.

This section provides a plan to help you gain control of your weight and then illustrates how the active life will keep you there. Of course, you don't just want to lose weight, you want to lose fat. The active life and fitness help you attain that goal by making muscle cells efficient users of fat. Diet leads to the loss of muscle, the furnace in which fat is burned. Conversely, activity conserves muscle while it burns fat, and improved fitness increases muscle tissue while further enhancing its ability to consume fat. You will find all this and more in part V.

Energy and Nutrition

Fueling the Active Life

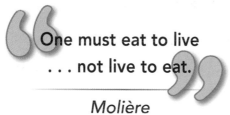

"One must eat to live
. . . not live to eat.

Molière

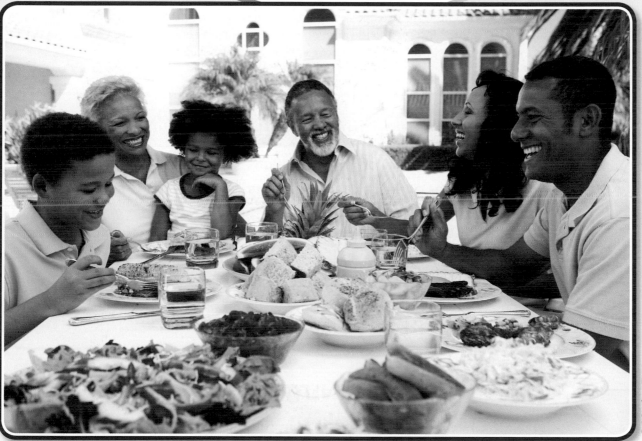

© Monkey Business

Ages ago, when the food supply was not so predictable and humans couldn't count on three meals a day plus snacks, their bodies learned how to store energy in the form of fat. Our bodies still store energy, even though the food supply now makes the practice unnecessary for most of us. This ability to store energy, coupled with both a plentiful food supply and increasingly sedentary lifestyles, has created a problem for two-thirds of the population. We put calories in the energy account, but seldom draw enough out, so our energy balance grows and grows. This chapter is about nutrition and energy (intake, energy expenditure), and the consequences of eating more energy than we expend—overweight and obesity.

As people work longer hours, less time is available for the selection and preparation of food, leading to increasing reliance on prepared food, fast food, ordering in and eating out, and loss of control over the quantity and quality of food that we eat. We select the item but have little influence over its preparation. Consequently, we eat more calories, more sugar, more saturated and hydrogenated fat, and more salt, and we run the risk of being shortchanged in other areas of nutrition.

Work once implied physical exertion, but today few of us burn many calories at work or after work. Many of us spend leisure time in front of a big screen, a computer, or a video game. Few people walk or engage in vigorous activity. Youth ride a bus, or are driven by parents, to school and stay inside after school. The convergence of these changes in eating and activity make good nutrition more important than ever before.

This chapter will help you do the following:

- Understand the basics of good nutrition
- Identify sources of energy and their contribution to performance and health
- Consider your need for vitamin and mineral supplements
- Understand the relationship between diet and health
- Select foods that are good for your health
- Calculate your energy balance, that is, your caloric intake versus caloric expenditure

NUTRIENTS

To understand nutrition and energy balance, one must first understand the components of a healthy diet. In general, the components of nutrition are broken down into macro- and micronutrients. The macronutrients are carbohydrate, fat, and protein. Vitamins and minerals are called **micronutrients** because we need only small amounts on a daily basis. They play an essential role in cell metabolism, immune function, clotting, and other important functions.

Carbohydrate

Throughout the world, carbohydrate provides the major source of energy. Carbohydrate is available in simple and complex forms. Simple sugar such as glucose, fructose, and sucrose (refined sugar, composed of molecules of glucose and fructose) contain energy but few nutrients (i.e., vitamins and minerals). Complex carbohydrate found in beans, rice, whole-grain products (bread, pasta), potatoes, and corn come with important nutrients and fiber. Unfortunately, average Americans get half of their dietary carbohydrate from concentrated or refined simple sugar, packed with so-called empty calories (empty because they lack nutrients). Fresh fruits contain simple sugar, but they also provide important nutrients. New data suggest that refined fruit juices are poor substitutes for fresh fruit and are little better than drinking sugary soda. The fructose in refined fruit juice is as likely to cause weight gain as drinking soda pop (Stanhope 2012).

Self-Evaluation for Good Nutrition

To evaluate how well you meet your nutritional needs on a daily basis, consider the following questions as you read the nutritional and energy balance sections in this chapter:

- How many servings of fruits and vegetables do you eat?
- How many calories do you consume?
- What percentage of your caloric intake comes from fat? From protein? From carbohydrate?
- What percentage of each should you get?
- What percentage of your fat intake comes from saturated fat?
- Do you meet your vitamin and mineral needs?
- How many times per week do you eat out, order in, or eat prepared foods?
- Do you regularly eat rich sauces, fatty meats, or desserts?

You can evaluate your responses later in this chapter, using information from the section on food choices.

Digestion of complex starch molecules begins in the mouth, where an enzyme (salivary amylase) reduces complex carbohydrate to simple sugar. Digestion temporarily ends in the stomach when gastric secretions inactivate the enzyme. In the small intestine, another enzyme (pancreatic amylase) helps to digest starches further. Enzymes secreted by the wall of the intestine and absorbed into the bloodstream complete the final breakdown to glucose. The absorption is rather complete; most of the sugar that you eat gets into the blood. Surprisingly, some complex carbohydrate, like potatoes, can enter the blood as quickly as table sugar does (Jenkins, Taylor, and Wolever 1982).

Because carbohydrate is important for muscular contractions and because it is not stored in large quantities, we should consume a sizable percentage of daily calories from complex carbohydrate and fruit. The performance diet recommended for active people and athletes suggests that 55 to 60 percent of calories should come from carbohydrate, which is more than the 40 to 50 percent that the average American consumes (see table 12.1).

As we've noted, carbohydrate is stored in muscles and the liver as granules of glycogen, a compound consisting of many linked molecules of glucose. We use this stored carbohydrate at the start of exercise, and its contribution to energy metabolism increases as exercise intensity increases. During prolonged exercise, when muscle glycogen stores become depleted, we are forced to use blood glucose that is supplied from the liver. When that limited supply runs out, we **bonk**—a term that cyclists coined to describe the utter

Table 12.1 Performance Diet

Component	Performance diet (% of total calories)	Typical diet (% of total calories)
Carbohydrate	55–60*	45–50
Fat	25–30**	35–40
Protein	15	10–15

*Increase before long-distance event (see Carbohydrate Loading, page 301).
**No more than one-third of fat calories from saturated fats (avoid intake of hydrogenated or trans-fatty acids).

fatigue, confusion, and lack of coordination that results when blood glucose falls below the level required by the nervous system (see figure 7.4). To avoid bonking, distance athletes consume energy bars and drink beverages containing 6 to 8 percent carbohydrate (60 to 80 g/L) at regular intervals during exercise.

Finally, be aware that chronic ingestion of a high-carbohydrate diet, especially a diet high in simple sugar, without an active lifestyle, may lead muscle to become insulin insensitive, adipose tissue to convert excess carbohydrate to fat, and the liver to increase production of very-low-density lipoprotein (VLDL) cholesterol (Graham and Adamo 1999). With regular physical activity, insulin sensitivity increases, the carbohydrate is burned, and blood lipids are lowered.

Fat

Fat is the most efficient way to store energy, with 9.3 calories per gram versus the 4.1 and 4.3 calories for carbohydrate and protein, respectively. The small intestine breaks down and absorbs dietary fat as small fat lumps, which then travel through the lymphatic system, tiny vessels and nodes that transport and filter cellular drainage. The fat clumps (chylomicrons) eventually dump into the circulation for transport to cells for energy or to adipose tissue for storage. But dietary fat intake isn't the only way to acquire this source of energy. Excess carbohydrate or protein can be converted to fat and stored in adipose tissue. We have many ways to acquire fat, but only one good way to remove it—physical activity.

Fat isn't all bad. It is an essential component of cell walls, vital insulation in the nervous system, a precursor for important compounds such as hormones, and a shock absorber for internal organs. And fat can be an efficient fuel for sustained physical activity, especially in muscles that have undergone endurance training. Furthermore, fat enhances the taste of food and helps fill us up. So we don't need to eliminate dietary fat, just limit the intake. Excess dietary fat is a major cause of overweight and obesity and a contributor to heart disease, hypertension, diabetes, some cancers, and other ills. Research indicates that high fat intake is inversely related to physical activity, suggesting a behavioral link between the two (Simoes et al. 1995).

We have many ways to acquire fat, but only one good way to remove it—physical activity.

Fat comes in several forms, including saturated and unsaturated fatty acids and triglycerides. Triglyceride fat is composed of three fatty acids and glycerol. The fatty acids can be saturated (with a hydrogen molecule filling each binding site on a carbon molecule) or unsaturated, with one or more double bonds (see figure 12.1).

Monounsaturated fatty acids have one double bond, whereas the poly-unsaturated have two or more. The double bonds of unsaturated fatty acids may be more susceptible to oxidation; therefore, unsaturated fats are recommended over saturated fats, which promote cholesterol syn-

The fatty acid may be saturated, meaning they have single bonds, such as stearic acid;

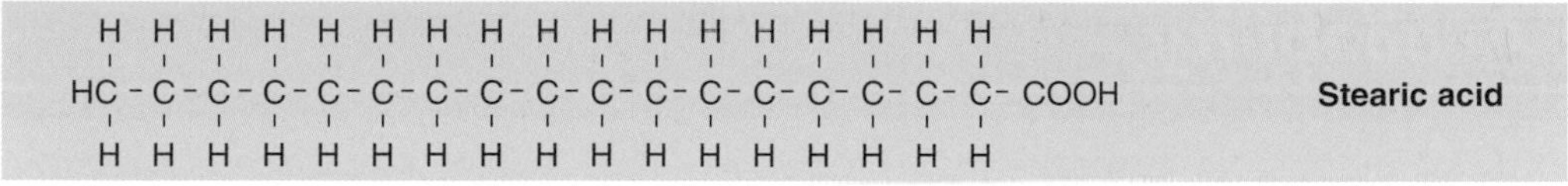

Stearic acid

they may be monounsaturated, meaning they have one double bond, such as oleic acid;

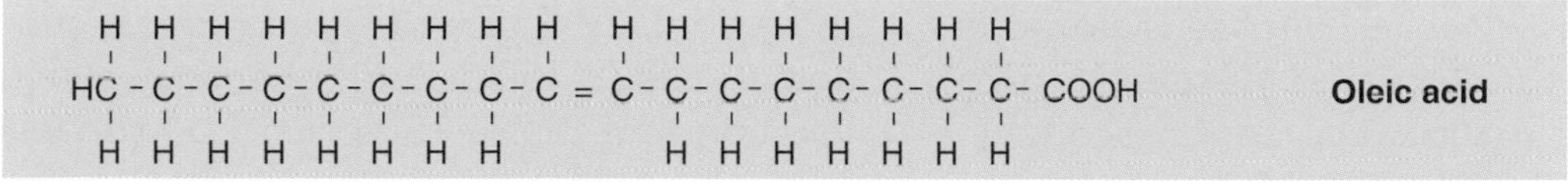

Oleic acid

or they may be polyunsaturated, meaning they have two or more double bonds, such as linoleic acid.

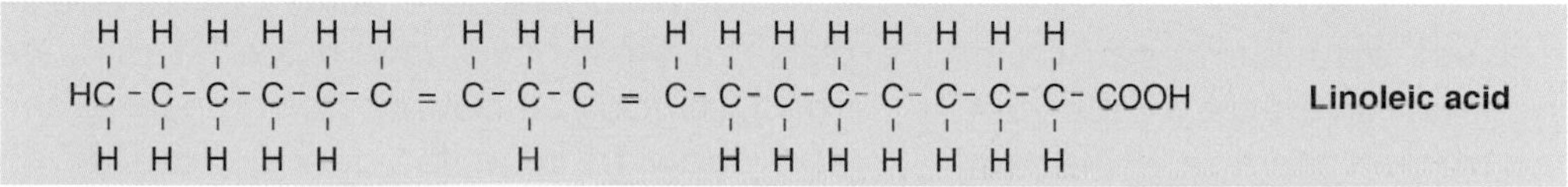

Linoleic acid

FIGURE 12.1 Fatty acids: saturated, monounsaturated, and polyunsaturated.

Adapted from Sharkey and Gaskill 2007.

thesis. Saturated fats are found in meat and dairy products. Watch out also for the tropical oils, palm and coconut, which are believed to be more atherogenic (likely to clog arteries), as are otherwise healthful oils (e.g., soybean, canola, or olive oil) when they are partially hydrogenated. Hydrogenation eliminates double bonds and creates unhealthy trans-fatty acids. These trans-fatty acids are common in snack crackers and other prepared foods, in which, to promote shelf life, otherwise healthy fats are made dangerous. Read labels and watch out for partially hydrogenated fats. The performance diet recommends that 25 percent of daily calories should come from fat, with no more than one-third of the fat or 10 percent of total calories from saturated fats, and an extremely small intake of hydrogenated or trans-fatty acids. This amount of fat is substantially less than the 30 to 40 percent that many people currently consume.

How Much Fat?

If you eat 2,000 calories a day and get 25 percent of your calories from fat, you'll get 500 fat calories. Divide 500 by 9.3 calories per gram of fat and you get 54 grams, the amount of fat that you can eat each day, far fewer than the 86 grams you'd eat if fat constituted 40 percent of your caloric intake. Labels on food packages indicate the grams of fat in each serving. Consider that a three-piece chicken dinner at Kentucky Fried Chicken contains about 55 grams of fat, a full day's serving.

Protein

When we ingest animal or plant protein, the large molecules are cleaved into amino acids and absorbed. The amino acids are building blocks used to construct cell walls, muscle tissue, hormones, enzymes, and a variety of other molecules. The blood contains several large proteins: globulin for antibody formation, albumin for buffering and osmosis, fibrinogen for clotting, and hemoglobin for oxygen transport. Training builds proteins: Aerobic training builds aerobic enzyme proteins for energy production and strength training builds

Energy Availability

A limited supply of glucose is available in the blood, but glucose is needed for brain and nerve metabolism, for which it is the sole source of energy. Glucose is stored in the liver (about 80 g) and muscle (15 g/kg of muscle, or 7 g/lb) as glycogen (see table 12.2). If you could use it all for exercise, you would have about 1,200 calories, enough to fuel a 10-mile (16 km) run.

Fat is the most abundant source of energy. Young men average 18 percent body fat; young women average 28 percent. If a male weighs 150 pounds (68 kg) and has 18 percent fat (of which 3% is essential and 15% is storage), you'll have about 22.5 pounds (10.2 kg) of fat. Because removing one pound of stored fat takes roughly 3,500 calories (through exercise or caloric reduction), 22.5 pounds of excess fat storage equals 78,750 calories of energy. When you consider that a 150-pound person will burn about 100 calories per mile (1.6 km) of walking, you'll realize that he has enough fat energy to fuel 787 miles (1,267 km) of walking! Most of us have more fat than we need, so you can benefit from teaching the body how to burn fat during exercise. In so doing, you extend your endurance dramatically, eliminate the problem of excess weight, and improve your overall health.

Table 12.2 Calorie Stores in the Human Body

Fuel-storage sites	Grams stored	Calories stored
CARBOHYDRATE STORES*		
Liver	80 g	325 cal
Muscle	408 g	1675 cal
FAT STORES**		
Adipose and muscle	10,170 g	94,581 cal

*For a 150 lb (68 kg person). Carbohydrate stores will depend on fasted state, training and other factors. The values are averages in the fed state.

**For a 150 lb male with 18% fat (3% essential fat [not listed] and 15% storage fat). The 15% fat = .15 × 150 lb = 22.5 lb = 10,170 gm fat × 9.3 kcal/gm = 94,581 cal.

contractile proteins (actin and myosin) for strength. So it should be no surprise to learn the importance of protein to the active life.

The performance diet recommends 15 percent of daily caloric intake in the form of protein. Moderately active adults can get by with 10 percent, but we recommend more for those who are very active or training. Fifteen percent of 2,000 calories is 300 calories (300 ÷ 4.3 kcal/g = 70 g, which is 1 g/kg for a person who weighs 70 kg, or 154 lb). More important than quantity, however, is the quality of protein. Quality protein is high in essential amino acids, those that the body cannot synthesize. These essential amino acids are macronutrients, major food sources that must be available for optimal function. When essential amino acids are missing, the body is unable to construct proteins that require them. Although animal protein is a better source of essential amino acids (as well as iron and vitamin B_{12}), proper combinations of plant protein can meet nutritional needs. If you are or plan to become a vegetarian, be ready to eat a variety of grains, beans, and leafy vegetables.

Protein Needs?

A review of protein needs for athletes concludes that endurance athletes will benefit from dietary intakes of 1.2 to 1.4 grams of protein per kilogram of body weight (.56–.64 g/lb), and strength athletes need 1.4 to 1.8 grams (.64–.82 g/lb) (Lemon 1995). These values are well above the RDA of .8 gram per kilogram (.36 g/lb), but they are attainable with the performance diet recommended in this chapter. If you participate in endurance and strength training, you'll need at least 1.4 grams per kilogram of body weight (.64 g/lb). Simply multiply that number times your body weight in kilograms (1 kg = 2.2 lb) to get your daily requirement.

For example, if you weigh 70 kilograms (154 lb), multiply 70 kilograms by 1.4 grams (154 lb × .64 g) to get your daily protein needs (98 g). Because each gram of protein yields 4.3 calories, you'll need about 420 calories (98 g × 4.3) of energy from protein.

Athletes usually raise total caloric intake to meet the increased energy needs of training. If your diet fails to meet the energy requirements for your type of training, increase your intake of good-quality protein (lean meats, skinned poultry, fish, beans, nuts) (see table 12.3). Evidence regarding protein utilization indicates that the timing of protein ingestion (after exercise) and the adequacy of total energy intake are important factors (Tipton and Wolfe 2004).

Table 12.3 Protein in Common Foods

Food	Portion	Protein (g)
Beans	1/2 cup (118 ml)	6–8
Beef	4 oz (113 g)	20–28
Cheese	1 oz (28 g)	7
Chicken	3 1/2 oz (99 g)	24–30
Chili	1 cup (237 ml)	20
Corn	1/2 cup (118 ml)	3
Fish	4 oz (113 g)	25–30
Hamburger	4 oz (113 g)	20
Milk	1 cup (237 ml)	9
Peanut butter	1 tablespoon (15 ml)	4
Pizza	1 slice	10

Protein isn't a major source of energy at rest or during exercise—it seldom amounts to more than 5 to 10 percent of energy needs—but when one trains hard while dieting to lose weight, the body senses starvation and begins to use tissue protein for energy. To avoid loss of muscle tissue and achieve the benefits of training, ensure adequate protein and energy intake. The best bet is to lose weight slowly or not at all during vigorous training.

Even with adequate protein, rapid weight loss while training risks the loss of the muscle and enzyme proteins that you are trying so hard to increase.

Excess protein intake accompanied by fat from animal sources (e.g., eggs, meat, fish, poultry, dairy products) leads to storage of fat. By following the performance diet, you will have the protein that you need. The recommended carbohydrate intake spares or conserves tissue protein.

Vitamins

Why are vitamins, which do not supply energy and are needed only in minute quantities, considered essential for life? In many cases, the answer lies in the structure of enzymes that are essential for cellular metabolism. Enzymes are composed of a large protein portion and a coenzyme. The shape of the protein molecule dictates the role of the enzyme, whereas the coenzyme is the active portion that performs a specific task. For example, vitamin B_1 is a coenzyme that removes carbon dioxide in a metabolic pathway. Without the vitamin coenzyme, the metabolic pathway grinds to a halt, usually with the toxic buildup of intermediary compounds. Lack of vitamin B_1 (thiamine) leads to beriberi, a vitamin deficiency disease characterized by weakness, wasting, nerve damage, and even heart failure. Fortunately, the small amount of vitamins needed is readily available from a variety of foods in a well-balanced diet. Doses far in excess of daily requirements (megadoses) do not improve function or performance, and they may be toxic.

Fortunately, the small amount of vitamins needed is readily available from a variety of foods in a well-balanced diet.

Vitamins are classified according to their solubility. The fat-soluble vitamins A, D, E, and K have widely different functions (see table 12.4). These vitamins are ingested with fats in the diet. Amounts in excess of daily needs are stored in body tissue, and megadoses can become toxic (e.g., vitamin A). Because they are stored, deficiencies are less likely, except in diets very low in fat.

The B complex vitamins and vitamin C are water soluble. Excess water-soluble vitamins are flushed away in the urine, making deficiencies more likely. Table 12.4 lists the vitamins, along with their reference daily intakes, functions, and good food sources.

Vitamins and Health

Vitamins perform many functions essential for life and health. Studies indicate that some vitamins are important to the optimal function of the immune system. To help maintain a healthy immune system, the well-balanced diet should include foods with the following micronutrients:

- Beta-carotene (carrots, sweet potatoes), which stimulates natural killer cells, immune system cells that fight infections.
- Vitamin B_6 (potatoes, nuts, spinach), which promotes proliferation of white blood cells.
- Folate (peas, salmon, romaine lettuce), which increases white blood cell activity.
- Vitamin C (citrus fruits, broccoli, peppers), an antioxidant that enhances the immune response.
- Vitamin E (whole grains, wheat germ, vegetable oils), an antioxidant that stimulates the immune response.
- The minerals selenium and zinc also aid the immune response. Selenium (tuna, eggs, whole grains) promotes action against toxic bacteria, and zinc (eggs, whole

grains, oysters) promotes wound healing. Regular, moderate physical activity bolsters the immune system, whereas exhaustion and stress impair its function, opening the door to upper respiratory and other infections.

Beta-carotene and vitamins C and E, the so-called antioxidant vitamins, may reduce muscle damage and even the risk of heart disease, cancer, and eye disease. Intense exercise produces compounds called free radicals. These highly reactive compounds can damage muscle tissue, especially in untrained people who have limited antioxidant capabilities. We have natural antioxidant protection, but the supply is limited. The antioxidant vitamins react with free radicals and reduce their ability to do microscopic damage (Kanter 1995). Regular activity and fitness training increase the body's ability to deal with free radicals.

Concerning heart disease, the antioxidant vitamins may prevent the oxidative deterioration of lipid, a step in the artery-clogging process of atherosclerosis. When oxidized, LDL turns rancid and becomes part of the growing plaque in the wall of the artery. Dietary

Table 12.4 Vitamins: Daily Intake, Functions, and Sources*

Vitamins	DRI (female/male)	Functions	Sources
FAT SOLUBLE			
Vitamin A (retinal)	700/900 µg	Vision, immune function	Milk products, liver, eggs
Vitamin D	5 µg	Bones, teeth	Sunlight, eggs, fish, milk
Vitamin E	15 mg	Antioxidant	Vegetable oils, nuts, greens
Vitamin K	90/120 µg	Blood clotting	Greens, milk, meats
WATER SOLUBLE			
Beta-carotene	3 mg	Cell growth, antioxidant	Fruits, vegetables
Vitamin B$_1$ (thiamin)	1.1/1.2 mg	Energy production	Pork, grains, legumes, nuts
Vitamin B$_2$ (riboflavin)	1.1/1.3 mg	Energy production	Milk, shellfish, meat, greens, grains
Niacin	14/16 mg	Energy production	Nuts, fish, poultry, grains, milk, eggs
Vitamin B$_6$ (pyridoxine)	1.3 mg	Energy, protein, and metabolism	Meats, grains, vegetables, fruits, fish, poultry
Folate	400 µg	Red and white blood cells, RNA, DNA, amino acids	Vegetables, grains, legumes
Vitamin B$_{12}$	2.4 µg	Blood cells, RNA, DNA, energy	Meat, fish, poultry, milk, eggs
Biotin	30 µg	Fat and amino acid metabolism, glycogen synthesis	Eggs, soybeans, fish, grains
Vitamin C (ascorbic acid)	75/90 mg	Healing, immune function, antioxidant, connective tissue	Citrus fruits, strawberries, cantaloupe, greens

*DRI = dietary reference intake; µg = micrograms/day; mg = milligrams/day; grains = whole grains; greens = dark leafy greens.

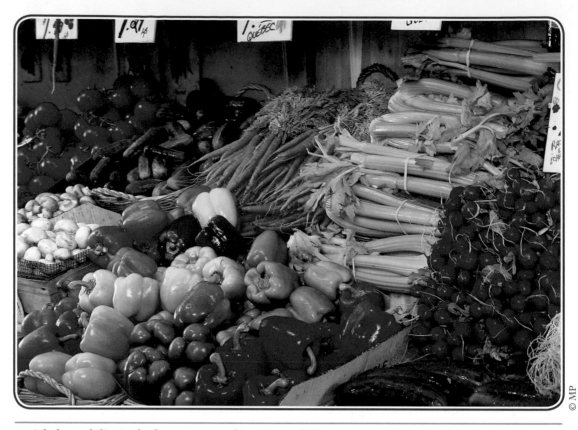

© MP

■ A balanced diet is the best way to achieve your daily vitamin needs.

antioxidants have been associated with lower risk of heart disease. Studies suggest that large doses of vitamin E may increase all-cause mortality in adults with chronic diseases (Miller et al. 2005). The American Heart Association, American Cancer Society, and the American Dietetic Association agree that scientific data do not justify the use of vitamin supplements to reduce heart disease, cancer, or other health problems.

So, you should begin consuming a diet rich in natural antioxidants now. Vitamin supplements are not as effective as the nutrients in fruits and vegetables. Vitamins in food come with other vitamins, minerals, and trace nutrients that may enhance the effect of the nutrients. Vitamin supplements are not a satisfactory replacement for a well-balanced diet. Dietary reference intake (DRI) supplements of vitamins may offer a margin of safety for those who lose considerable weight during training or will not eat nutritious food. All others should use a variety of nutritious foods as their source for micronutrients.

Vitamins and Performance

Athletes are a gullible bunch, inclined to try anything to improve performance. Plenty of snake-oil salespeople are willing to sell a food or drug guaranteed to enhance performance. Vitamin supplements are frequently marketed to this audience and to millions of others in search of health. Unfortunately, much of the money spent on vitamin megadoses washes away in the urine. Vitamin supplements will not improve the performance or health of those who consume an adequate diet.

Supplementation, however, may sometimes be prudent. Highly active people and athletes need more vitamins when they burn more energy. They should meet this increased need with a larger intake of food to satisfy energy and nutrient needs. But during periods when you combine vigorous training with weight loss, you may want to take a daily vitamin and mineral supplement that does not exceed the recommended daily intake. Because certain vitamins enhance the immune response, some believe that supplements may help reduce the risk of illness that accompanies exhaustion and overtraining (Evans 2000). Studies on endurance athletes, however, have not shown a reduction in infections with vitamin C (Nieman, Henson, and McAnulty 2002) or lipid oxidation with vitamin E (Nieman et al. 2004). Antioxidant vitamins may reduce the severity of muscle damage during intense activity. We recommend vitamins in food over those contained in pills. If you decide to take supplements, do not exceed the DRI (see table 12.4).

Minerals

Do you ever wonder why the body needs iron, zinc, magnesium, and even chromium, whereas it definitely doesn't need lead? Minerals are important for enzyme and cellular activity, some hormones, bones, muscle and nerve activity, and acid–base balance. Some are required in small daily amounts (less than 100 mg), whereas we need more of others. Minerals are available in many food sources, but concentrations are higher in animal tissues and products (see table 12.5).

Table 12.5 Minerals: Daily Intake, Functions, and Sources*

Minerals	DRI (female/male)	Functions	Sources
Calcium	1,000 mg	Bones, teeth, blood clotting, muscle–nerve function	Milk, tofu, broccoli, legumes
Chloride	2,300 mg	Digestion, fluid balance	Salt (in foods)
Chromium	25/35 µg	Energy metabolism	Grains, meats, vegetable oils
Copper	900 µg	Iron metabolism	Seafood, nuts, grains
Fluorine	3/4 mg	Bones, teeth	Water, seafood, tea
Iodine	150 µg	Thyroid hormone	Seafood, milk, iodized salt
Iron	18/8 mg	Oxygen transport	Meats, legumes, dried fruit
Magnesium	320/420 mg	Protein synthesis, muscle–nerve function	Grains, nuts, legumes, seafood, chocolate
Manganese	1.8/2.3 mg	Energy metabolism	Nuts, grains, tea, leafy vegetables
Molybdenum	45 µg	Enzymes	Organ meats, legumes, cereals
Phosphorus	700 mg	Bones, teeth, acid–base balance	Milk, meats, poultry, fish, eggs
Potassium	4,700 mg	Nerve–muscle, fluid, and acid–base balance	Meats, milk, fruits, vegetables grains, coffee
Selenium	55 µg	Antioxidant	Seafood, meats, grains
Sodium	1,500 mg	Nerve function, fluid, and acid–base balance	Salt (in food)
Sulfur	—	Liver function, hormones	Dietary protein
Zinc	8/11 mg	Enzyme activity, wound healing	Meat, poultry, fish, milk, grains, vegetables

*DRI = dietary reference intake; µg = micrograms/day; mg = milligrams/day; grains = whole grains; greens = dark leafy greens.

Minerals, like vitamins, are readily available in a well-balanced diet, one drawn from a variety of food sources. Problems arise when a person decides to eliminate a major nutrient source, such as meat.

Minerals are essential to health and performance, but supplementation beyond what the DRI calls for is unnecessary, and it could cause side effects. Excesses of some minerals pose no problems, whereas others can cause diarrhea (magnesium, zinc), high blood pressure (sodium), or cirrhosis (iron). If you are concerned that your diet may be deficient, consider a supplement that provides the recommended daily intake for vitamins and minerals, including trace minerals (see table 12.5). Supplementation may be important for those who train hard while losing weight in an effort to enhance performance. But remember that supplements are not an adequate substitute for good nutrition.

Iron

Iron is particularly important for active people, both male and female. Much of the iron absorbed in the blood goes into the production of hemoglobin, the compound in red blood cells that carries oxygen from the lungs to the working muscles. Iron is also used in muscle myoglobin to transport and store oxygen, and in important oxidative (aerobic) enzymes. People deficient in iron risk anemia and poor endurance. Because only 10 to 20 percent of the iron in food is absorbed into the bloodstream, athletes must take in 10 times the amount that they need. Lean meat is a rich source of iron, and the iron in meat is more readily absorbed than that from other sources.

Females lose blood and iron during menstruation, and all active people are subject to iron loss and reduced absorption during hard training. Meat, dates, raisins, beans, prunes, and apricots are good sources of iron. If you are concerned about your iron status, consult a physician or sports nutrition specialist before you supplement with more than the dietary reference intake (DRI).

Calcium

Calcium is a major component of bones and teeth, and it is involved in muscle contraction, nerve transmission, blood clotting, and enzyme activity. In relation to the active life,

Dehydration Weight Loss

Water constitutes 55 to 60 percent of adult body weight. Thirst, activated by excess sodium or water loss, helps us maintain body fluid levels. Several hormones, such as **antidiuretic hormone (ADH)**, assist in the maintenance of fluids and electrolytes (sodium, potassium, calcium, chloride). The kidneys get rid of excess fluid. In other words, the body knows how much water it needs, and you should not attempt to lose water as a means of weight reduction.

Because each quart of fluid weighs about 2 pounds (~1 kg), dehydration can lead to impressive, albeit short-term, weight loss. But the loss is water, not fat. You need the water, and the body will do all it can to get it back. Water and electrolyte loss during dehydration causes diminished muscular strength, and loss of blood volume reduces cardiac output and endurance. Responsible health organizations such as the American College of Sports Medicine have long cautioned against dehydration weight loss because it compromises athletic performance and health. The 1997 deaths of three collegiate wrestlers from dehydration weight loss confirmed the life-threatening effects of dehydration.

So don't exercise in a rubber suit, sauna, or steam room to lose weight. Sweat is a crucial part of the temperature-regulating mechanism. You must allow sweat to evaporate to cause evaporative heat loss and help you avoid heat stress. When you do lose weight through sweat loss, you should replace it as soon as possible. For example, if you lose 4 pounds (almost 2 kg) of weight during a run or bike ride, you'll need to replace it with more than 2 liters of fluid.

calcium is extremely important because of its relationship to osteoporosis, the loss of bone density that predisposes bones to fractures. Bone is a tissue that responds to stress. Weight-bearing exercise builds young bones, helps keep bones strong, and slows the inevitable loss of bone density with age. After menopause, when estrogen levels decline, women lose bone density at a more rapid rate than they do before menopause. Calcium, vitamin D, and weight-bearing exercise are important throughout life.

Young female athletes face a dilemma. Too much strenuous training, combined with weight loss, inadequate calcium intake, and stress, sometimes interferes with the normal menstrual cycle. These changes seem to diminish the protective effect of estrogen on bones, leading to reduced bone density and increased risk of stress fractures. Reduced training, weight gain, and increased calcium intake will stop the loss of bone, but it isn't certain that young women ever fully recover from early bone loss.

Fluids

Besides energy and nutrients, the body needs an ample supply of water. Water, found in the cells and in extracellular fluids such as blood, lymph, saliva, tears, and glands and in the gastrointestinal tract, makes up more than half of body weight. Water serves to transport energy, gases, waste products, hormones, antibodies, and heat. In the blood, it is involved in the regulation of the acid–base balance. Water lubricates surfaces and membranes and, through perspiration, serves as a main avenue for temperature regulation.

The inactive person needs about 2.5 liters daily to replace water lost in urine, feces, skin, and exhalation from the lungs. During activity in a hot environment, sweat loss can average 1 liter per hour for many hours, and can temporarily exceed a rate of 2 liters per hour. Failure to replace this fluid will lead to impaired performance, dehydration, and **heat stress** disorders ranging from muscle cramps and heat exhaustion to life-threatening heatstroke.

We'll discuss fluid replacement in chapter 15, which deals with heat stress, carbohydrate–electrolyte drinks and their effect on performance. We will also discuss fluid intake before, during, and after activity.

DIETARY GUIDELINES

The U.S. Departments of Agriculture and Health and Human Services released the policy document *Dietary Guidelines for Americans, 2010.* This revised guide to daily food choices provides science-based advice to promote health and reduce the risk for major chronic diseases (www.cnpp.usda.gov/DGAs2010-PolicyDocument.htm).

The revised guidelines are consistent with the recommendations in this chapter (table 12.1). They emphasize the need to engage in regular, moderate physical activity and weight control. The two overall concepts in the new guidelines, taken directly from the executive summary are as follows:

- **Maintain calorie balance over time to achieve and sustain a healthy weight.** People who are most successful at achieving and maintaining a healthy weight do so through continued attention to consuming only enough calories from foods and beverages to meet their needs and by being physically active. To curb the obesity epidemic and improve their health, many Americans must decrease the calories they consume and increase the calories they expend through physical activity.

- **Focus on consuming nutrient-dense foods and beverages.** Americans currently consume too much sodium and too many calories from solid fats, added sugar, and refined grains. These replace nutrient-dense foods and beverages and make it difficult for people to achieve recommended nutrient intake while controlling calorie and sodium intake. A healthy eating pattern limits intake of sodium, solid fats, added sugar, and refined grains and emphasizes nutrient-dense foods and beverages—vegetables, fruits, whole grains, fat-free or low-fat milk and milk products, seafood, lean meats and poultry, eggs, beans and peas, and nuts and seeds (USDA and USDHHS 2011).

The new dietary guidelines for Americans, found in figure 12.2, also include key recommendations in four areas (USDA and USDHHS 2011).

Whole-grain products are important as sources of energy, fiber, and micronutrients. Everyone should eat 6 servings of whole grains or enriched or whole-grain products daily. When involved in hard work or training, increase the intake of whole-grain foods to 10 servings or more. Incidentally, a serving of lean meat is several ounces, about the size of a deck of cards. If you are active, 1 serving may not be a sufficient portion for a meal. To view your personalized food guidelines, or to track your diet, you can use the government website at www.choosemyplate.gov/SuperTracker/default.aspx.

Willett's Nutrition Plan

Walter Willett is one of the most well known and respected nutritionists in the United States. He is the Fredrick John Stare professor of epidemiology and nutrition at the Harvard School of Public Health in the departments of nutrition and epidemiology. He has proposed an eating plan that is associated with daily exercise and weight control. The bottom level of his pyramid includes whole-grain foods at most meals, along with plant oils (olive, canola, soy, peanut). The next level includes vegetables in abundance and fruits two or three times per day. Next come nuts and legumes one to three times per day. The next level contains fish, poultry, and eggs zero to two times per day. Then comes dairy or calcium once or twice a day. The top level calls for sparing use of red meat, butter, white rice, white bread, potatoes, and sweets (Willett 2001).

Balancing Calories

- Improve eating and physical activity behaviors to prevent and/or reduce overweight and obesity.
- For people who are overweight or obese, consuming fewer calories from foods and beverages to control total calorie intake to manage body weight.
- Reduce time spent in sedentary behaviors and increase physical activity.
- Throughout childhood, adolescence, adulthood, pregnancy and older age, maintain calorie balance appropriate to the stage of life.

Foods and Food Components to Reduce

- Reduce salt and sodium intake to less than 2,300 milligrams and further reduce intake to 1,500 milligrams among persons who are 51 and older and those of any age who are African American or have hypertension, diabetes, or chronic kidney disease. About half of the U.S. population should be getting under 1,500 milligrams of daily sodium, including many children and the majority of adults.

- Reduce the consumption of calories from saturated fatty acids to under 10 percent of total calories by replacing them with monounsaturated and polyunsaturated fatty acids.
- Reduce dietary cholesterol to less than 300 milligrams per day.
- Eliminate or reduce as much as possible the consumption of foods that contain synthetic sources of trans fat, such as partially hydrogenated oils, and by limiting other solid fat.
- Reduce calories from solid fat and added sugar.
- Limit foods that contain refined grains, especially refined grain foods that contain solid fat, added sugar, and sodium.
- Drink alcohol in moderation—up to one drink per day for women and two drinks per day for men—at or above legal drinking ages.

Foods and Nutrients to Increase

Within their calorie needs, individuals should meet the following recommendations:
- Increase fruit and vegetable intake.
- Eat a variety of vegetables, especially dark-green and red and orange vegetables and beans and peas.
- Consume at least half of all grains as whole grains. Increase whole-grain intake by replacing refined grains with whole grains.
- Increase intake of fat-free or low-fat milk and milk products, such as milk, yogurt, cheese, or fortified soy beverages.
- Choose a variety of protein foods, including seafood, lean meat and poultry, eggs, beans and peas, soy products, and unsalted nuts and seeds.
- Increase the amount and variety of seafood consumed by choosing seafood in place of some meat and poultry.
- Replace protein foods that are higher in solid fats with choices that are lower in solid fats and calories and/or are sources of oils.
- Use oils to replace solid fats where possible.
- Choose foods that provide more potassium, dietary fiber, calcium, and vitamin D, which are nutrients of concern in American diets. These foods include vegetables, fruits, whole grains, and milk and milk products.
- If you are pregnant or nursing, you should read the specific guidelines at www.cnpp.usda.gov/Publications/DietaryGuidelines/2010/PolicyDoc/ExecSumm.pdf.
- Individuals ages 50 years and older should consume foods fortified with vitamin B_{12}, such as fortified cereals, or dietary supplements.

Building Healthy Eating Patterns

- Select an eating pattern that meets nutrient needs over time at an appropriate calorie level.
- Account for all foods and beverages consumed and assess how they fit within a total healthy eating pattern.
- Follow food safety recommendations when preparing and eating foods to reduce the risk of foodborne illnesses.

FIGURE 12.2 Dietary Guidelines for Americans.

Adapted from USDA and USDHHS 2011. Available: www.cnpp.usda.gov/DGAs2010-PolicyDocument.htm.

A new study from the Harvard School of Public Health, directed by Dr. Willett, followed more than 120,000 people over the course of as many as 20 years, to see what they ate and how it affected their weight (Mozaffarian et al. 2011). The authors reported fruits (not counting fruit juices), vegetables, high-fiber foods, nuts, and yogurt were most closely correlated with weight loss. In general, highly refined foods (sugary beverages, white bread, white rice, and potatoes) were related to greater weight gain on a diet. Since many people drink multiple servings of sugary beverages (containing high fructose corn syrup) a day, this is a major factor in weight gain.

Mediterranean Diet

A study of Mediterranean people with low rates of chronic disease and high life expectancies led researchers to recommend some variations. The Mediterranean diet emphasizes daily intake of complex carbohydrate, fruits, vegetables, olive oil, yogurt, and cheese; reduces intake of fish, poultry, eggs, and sweets to a few times per week; and limits red meat consumption to a few times per month. The diet also calls for regular physical activity and daily but moderate intake of wine. Among subjects 70 to 90 years of age from 11 European countries, adherence to the Mediterranean diet was associated with more than a 50 percent reduction in all-cause and cause-specific mortality (Knoops et al. 2004).

If your health risk is high, consider the Mediterranean diet or Willett's plan. If not, use the revised USDA food guide. If you are very active, you'll need to increase your food intake to fuel vigorous or prolonged activity and to consume somewhat more protein to meet the needs of aerobic and strength training.

High Dietary Fiber Intake

Fiber, roughage, bulk, and bran all refer to the portion of plants that is indigestible. Why consume an indigestible material? Besides its long-standing reputation for maintaining regularity, fiber has other advantages. Insoluble fiber (wheat bran, beans) holds water, increases bulk, and increases the rate at which stool and cancerous toxins are removed. Soluble fiber such as oat bran, apples, and citrus fruits forms a gel that slows absorption of carbohydrate and binds cholesterol for removal from the body. Soluble fiber may also produce a chemical that slows the rate of cholesterol production.

Epidemiologic studies show that those on a low-fiber diet

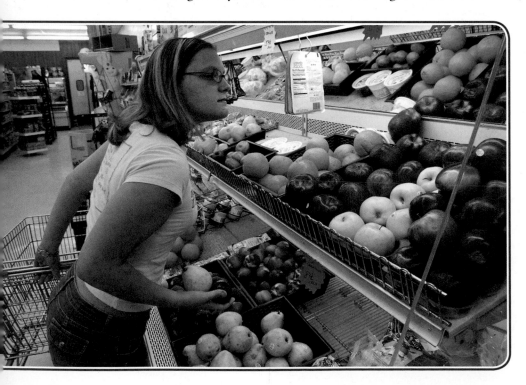

■ Citrus fruits and other foods rich in soluble fiber can help reduce cholesterol.

have a higher incidence of heart disease, cancer, and the other problems mentioned earlier. The average American consumes about one-third of the 25 to 35 grams of fiber recommended by the National Cancer Institute, and most regularly ignore fresh fruits and vegetables. If fiber isn't part of your daily regime, begin adding bran cereals, fruits, vegetables, beans, and whole-grain breads to your diet now. Read labels and try to seek a balance between soluble and insoluble fiber. Finally, consider this: When you combine fiber with a low-fat diet and activity, you'll be able to eat freely, with little concern for weight gain. Daily activity contributes to regularity and may lower risk for colon cancer by speeding the rate at which stool and toxins pass through the digestive system.

Anticancer Diet

The anticancer diet proposed by the National Academy of Sciences endorses the reduction of fat in the diet. The advice includes the following:

- Eat less fat and fewer fatty meats and dairy products.
- Eat few salt-cured, pickled, or smoked foods.
- Eat more whole-grain products, including fiber-rich foods.
- Eat more fruits and vegetables, including those in the cabbage family and those high in vitamins A and C.
- Drink alcohol in moderation, if at all.
- Keep caloric intake low.

Remember, fat is a factor in cancer, heart disease, and diabetes, and exercise is the best way to eliminate excess fat from the body.

> **R**emember, fat is a factor in cancer, heart disease, and diabetes, and exercise is the best way to eliminate excess fat from the body.

Food Concerns

Companies spend millions to convince us that we can achieve fitness and health by eating their products. Although sound nutrition is essential to health and fitness, nothing you eat will improve your fitness if you are already on an adequate diet. The only way to achieve fitness is through regular exercise. You can't get there just by eating.

Health Foods

Concerns about the quality of our food supply, such as the use of hormones, pesticides, dyes, and other chemicals, has led to wider availability of so-called health foods, also known as natural or organic foods, as an alternative source of nutrition. To the extent that these chemicals may be harmful to health, especially over extended periods, natural food sources could be safer. But the nutritional value of a food or vitamin is not related to the manner of growth. Foods grown with chemical fertilizers seem just as nutritious as those grown with organic fertilizers. What matters is the active amount of the essential ingredient, such as a vitamin, and how that contributes to the recommended daily intake. Buy more expensive health foods if you are concerned about the effects of chemicals on your health, but don't expect to get super nutrition for the extra expense.

Lite Foods

Interest in health and weight control has led to the development of so-called lite foods and beverages. The products are lower-calorie versions of the original, such as lite beer, lite or no-calorie soft drinks, low-fat crackers and meals, and so on. The products should have at least one-third fewer calories than the original. Although eating these products will not make you lose weight, they can help reduce your caloric intake, as long as you don't eat more of them. Because lite foods usually cost as much as or more than the regular versions, their popularity proves that we will pay more for less—fewer calories or less fat, sodium, or caffeine. Sometimes the products use undesirable substitutes, such as coconut, palm, or cottonseed oil or the hydrogenated form of healthy oil, such as soybean. Read the label to be certain that you are getting what you paid for.

A variation of the lite meal is the diet platter at the restaurant. People select these choices because they believe that they are more nutritious and have fewer calories and less fat. A salad isn't particularly high in nutritive value, however. If gobs of high-fat salad dressing are used, the salad could be a bad food choice, since 1 tablespoon (15 ml) of dressing can contain 100 calories and 8 grams of fat, and the ladle used to pour the dressing usually holds more than 1 tablespoon.

Responsible restaurant owners label meals to indicate better choices for those concerned with heart health and fat intake. Look for food that is nutritious but low in saturated fat. Avoid fried foods, those with cream sauces or butter, and high-calorie desserts. Ask for dressings and other sauces on the side. Request a dry muffin or toast. Eating out is difficult for those on weight-loss or low-fat diets, but the situation is improving as some restaurant owners realize what the customer wants. Of course, many fast-food outlets continue to promote high-calorie, high-fat food choices (see table 12.6). We'll talk about low-carb diets in chapter 13.

Toxic Foods

Some health activists blame the food industry for promoting the sale of toxic foods, those that are demonstrably bad for your health. These foods include tasty, high-fat fast foods that are aggressively marketed to children and teens. Although an occasional burger and fries may be safe for most consumers, a steady diet of them is not. Some schools have turned school lunch programs over to the fast-food industry. Others turn the students loose to roam nearby strip malls in search of tasty toxic foods. Schools even carry advertisements for fast food on their in-school news channel. At home, busy adults eat out, order in, or use prepared meals. Fast-food serving sizes have grown dramatically. Consequently, we have become the fattest nation in the world, and an epidemic of fat-induced adult-onset diabetes has emerged among overweight teens and adults. We eat too much and exercise too little. What can we do?

Some argue for measures similar to those imposed on the tobacco industry, including limits on advertising, no sales near schools, extra taxes on toxic foods like soda and sugary drinks, lawsuits to reclaim medical costs, and more. A better approach might involve a return to brown-bag lunches for kids and adults, limiting reliance on fast foods and meals outside the home, and selecting healthy options (when eating out). If we don't do something, the consequence will be a further explosion of disabling diseases such as obesity, diabetes, and heart disease, and enormous health care costs. Of course, regular, moderate physical activity is the other part of the solution.

The next sections look at energy balance, starting with energy intake and then expenditure. When the two are equal, we are said to be in energy balance.

ENERGY INTAKE

Energy from the sun grows plants that animals eat. Our sources of energy—carbohydrate, fat, and protein—originate from plant and animal sources. We ingest the food, digest it, and absorb it into the bloodstream for transport to cells. Carbohydrate is stored in the liver

Table 12.6 Caloric Values for Fast Foods

Food item	Energy (cal)	Protein (g)	Fat (g)	Carbohydrate (g)
MCDONALD'S				
Two hamburgers, fries, shake	1,030	40	37	135
Big Mac, fries, shake	1,100	40	41	143
Big Mac	550	21	32	45
Quarter pounder	420	25	19	37
Hamburger	260	14	9	30
French fries	180	3	10	20
Chocolate shake	315	9	8	51
BURGER KING				
Whopper, fries, shake	1,200	40	47	147
Whopper	630	29	35	50
Whopper Jr.	285	16	15	21
Double hamburger	325	24	15	24
Hamburger	230	14	10	21
French fries	220	2	12	10
Chocolate shake	365	8	8	65
HARDEE'S				
2/3 lb bacon cheese Thickboy	1,340	56	96	60
Large fries	480	5	19	72
PIZZA HUT				
10 in. Supreme (cheese, tomato sauce, sausage, pepperoni, mushrooms, and so on)	1,200	72	35	152
10 in. pizza (cheese)	1,025	65	23	140
KENTUCKY FRIED CHICKEN				
Three-piece dinner (chicken, potatoes, roll, slaw)	1,000	55	55	71
DAIRY QUEEN				
4 oz serving soft ice cream	180	5	6	27
ARBY'S				
Sliced beef sandwich, two potato patties, slaw, shake	1,200	27	40	166

To convert grams to calories, multiply protein (g) by 4.3, fat (g) by 9.3, and carbohydrate (g) by 4.1.

and muscles in clumps of glucose molecules known as glycogen. Fat is stored in adipose tissue, around organs (**visceral fat**), and in the muscles.

Using enzyme catalysts aligned in metabolic pathways, we convert these energy sources into molecules of ATP (adenosine triphosphate), the high-energy compound that fuels muscular contractions and many other cellular functions. The liver glycogen supply is a reserve that helps maintain the blood glucose level, which is the essential energy source for the brain and nervous tissue. Muscle glycogen is the major fuel that you use to power high-intensity contractions. When you deplete the supply, you are unable to sustain those contractions. You use intramuscular fat as energy for contractions, especially in lower-intensity, long-duration effort. Moreover, fat can be mobilized from adipose tissue storage and transported through the circulation to fuel working muscles. The amino acids from the protein that you eat are used to construct proteins in your body. A small portion of the energy used for activity (5%–10%) comes from tissue protein.

Alcohol, or ethanol, is another energy source, but it is not stored in the body or generally believed to be used for metabolism. However, it is quickly absorbed by freely diffusing across plasma membranes without protein-mediated transport. While chronic, excessive consumption of ethanol leads to disease, low to moderate consumption has been shown to reduce risk of certain high-incidence diseases. Numerous epidemiological studies have documented that a reduced risk of coronary heart disease usually accompanies regular consumption of a moderate level of ethanol. It has also been reported that ethanol consumption reduces the risk of development of adult-onset or non-insulin-dependent diabetes mellitus (NIDDM), often called type 2 diabetes (Bisson, Butzke, and Ebeler 1995).

The metabolic pathways control the combustion of the fuels that we burn. We measure energy needs with a unit for measuring heat, the calorie.

How is the energy or caloric value of food determined? Nutrition researchers use a **calorimeter** to measure the energy content of foods. A small amount of food is placed in a chamber and burned in the presence of oxygen. The heat liberated in the process indicates the energy content of the food (1 kilocalorie is the heat required to raise 1 kilogram of water 1 degree Celsius). When a gram of carbohydrate is ignited, the energy yield is 4.1 kilocalories, and when protein is burned, the energy yield is 4.3 kilocalories per gram. More than twice as much energy is released when fat is tested, 9.3 kilocalories per gram (see table 12.7). It takes more oxygen to burn a gram of fat, yielding less energy per liter of oxygen consumed.

Table 12.7 Caloric Equivalents of Foods

Food	Energy (cal/g)*	Oxygen (L/g)**	Caloric equivalent (cal/L)***
Fat	9.3	1.98	4.696
Carbohydrate	4.1	0.81	5.061
Protein	4.3	0.97	4.432

The alcohol in alcoholic beverages has a high caloric value, 7.1 cal/g. The calories are empty, providing little nutritional value. Moreover, because alcohol diminishes appetite and interferes with digestion by inflaming the stomach, pancreas, and intestine, alcohol consumption often leads to malnutrition. It also interferes with vitamin activation by the liver and causes liver damage (Lieber 1976).

*Cal (kilocalories) released when 1 gram of this food is oxidized.

**Liters of oxygen required to oxidize 1 gram of this food.

***The calories produced per liter of oxygen when this food is burned.

Sources: Ainsworth et al. 1993; Consolazio, Johnson, and Pecora 1963; Passmore and Durnin 1955; Roth 1968; Unpublished data from the Human Performance Laboratory, University of Montana 1964–2005.

The kilocalorie is 1,000 calories, or the heat required to raise 1 kilogram of water 1 degree Celsius. In this book, we use the term calorie as nutritionists use it: 1 calorie in nutrition refers to the kilocalorie, the standard of measurement in nutrition and exercise. For example, you take in 100 calories with one light beer, and burn 100 calories when you jog 1 mile (1.6 km).

You always expend some energy, even when you're asleep. If you stay in bed for 24 hours and do nothing at all, you will expend about 1,600 calories (for a 154 lb, or 70 kg person). This energy is used by heart and respiratory muscles, for normal cellular metabolism, and for maintenance of body temperature. Heavy thinking does little to raise energy requirements, but

> *Foods that are digested rapidly and that cause a pronounced rise in blood sugar have a high glycemic index.*

Glycemic Index

The glycemic index describes the rate of carbohydrate digestion and its effect on the rise of blood glucose. Foods that are digested rapidly and that cause a pronounced rise in blood sugar have a high glycemic index, whereas those digested and absorbed more slowly, because of fiber or other factors, have a low index. As you might expect, foods with a high glycemic index include sugar and honey, as well as corn, white bread, refined cereals, and baked potatoes. Foods with a moderate glycemic index include pasta, whole-grain breads, rice, oatmeal, bran, and peas. Foods with a low glycemic index include beans, lentils, and fruits (apples, peaches, and grapefruit). High-index foods lead to a rapid rise in blood sugar and a greater rise in insulin, the hormone responsible for lowering blood glucose (Foster-Powell and Miller 1995).

People with insulin resistance, a condition often associated with overweight, hypertension, low HDL cholesterol, and elevated triglycerides and blood glucose, are wise to select low-index foods. High-index foods prompt an insulin surge from the pancreas, stimulating body cells to store glucose. Over time, the cells become less sensitive to insulin, eventually contributing to adult-onset (type 2) diabetes. Insulin resistance is linked to heart disease, obesity, age, and inactivity. Weight loss and regular, moderate activity reduce insulin resistance.

High glycemic	Moderate glycemic	Low glycemic
White breads including bagels	Whole-grain breads	Milk products and yogurt
Cornflakes and most cold cereals	Oatmeal	Nuts including peanuts
Cane, maple, and corn syrup	Spaghetti	Legumes (peas and beans)
Honey	Corn	Apples and peaches
Glucose	Oranges	
Sucrose		
Potatoes		
White rice		
Raisins and bananas		

(continued)

Glycemic Index   *(continued)*

Should you avoid foods with a high glycemic index? No, they are useful when you want to speed glucose into cells to replace muscle glycogen after prolonged exertion. Also, when you consume a high-glycemic carbohydrate, such as potatoes, in a mixed meal along with fat and protein, you slow the entry of glucose into the bloodstream.

After a meal, absorbed sugar is taken up by the blood and by cells in the heart, skeletal muscle, and liver, in that order. After blood sugar levels are restored, heart and skeletal muscles accept glucose. The constantly working heart uses it for energy, and the skeletal muscle can store glucose for use when energy is needed. Granules

of stored glucose are called muscle glycogen. The liver accepts glucose and stores it as glycogen. When sufficient glucose has been stored in the liver (about 80–100 g), the leftover glucose suppresses fat oxidation. It is itself used for energy. Thus, an excess intake of carbohydrate does not become a supply of quick energy; it is oxidized, thereby conserving fat (Swinburn and Ravussin 1993). The glucose stored in the liver is readily available when needed, but muscle glycogen can be used directly only by the muscle in which it is stored. Nerves, muscles, or other tissues in need of energy also use blood glucose.

as soon as you begin to move, energy expenditure increases dramatically. Caloric expenditure can go from 1.2 calories per minute at rest to more than 20 calories per minute during vigorous effort. Physical activity has the greatest effect on energy needs. Walking burns about 5 calories per minute, jogging about 10, and running more than 15 calories per minute.

ENERGY EXPENDITURE

Energy intake and expenditure refer to a comparison between the calories consumed in the diet and the calories burned in the course of all daily activities (see figure 12.3). If intake exceeds expenditure, the excess will be stored as fat. Since the 1960s, Americans have reduced total dietary fat intake from 40 percent to about 35 percent of daily calories. Unfortunately, they have increased total caloric intake by about 250 calories each day and decreased physical activity. Americans eat about the same number of calories per day as they did in 1900, but they burn far fewer calories in physical activity, whether at work or play (Booth et al. 2000). The result is an epidemic of overweight and obesity, leading to a host of health and economic consequences (Thompson et al. 1999).

One pound (.45 kg) of body fat has the energy equivalent of 3,500 calories. Therefore, a person must expend (oxidize or burn) about 3,500 calories to remove 1 pound of stored fat. Conversely, 3,500 calories of excess dietary intake will lead to an additional pound of body weight. For example, suppose that the daily activity of a young man whose body weight is around 70 kilograms (154 lb) consists of

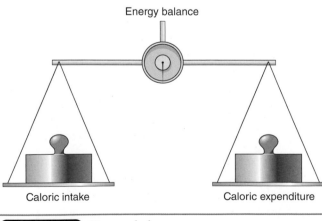

Energy balance
Caloric intake   Caloric expenditure

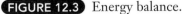

FIGURE 12.3 Energy balance.

light office work. He does not engage in any physical activity, so his daily caloric needs to maintain a constant weight are about 2,400 calories. If he eats a donut for an additional 250 calories each day, what will happen to him over the course of a year?

$$250 \text{ calories} \times 30 \text{ days per month}$$
$$= 7,500 \text{ calories} \times 12 \text{ months} = 90,000 \text{ calories per year}$$

The 90,000 calories he has gained, divided by 3,500 calories per pound, equates to 25.7 pounds (11.7 kg) of added weight. Our friend has upset his energy balance to the tune of more than 2 pounds (.9 kg) per month, or 25.7 pounds per year. If he does nothing about his diet or exercise, he could gain 257 pounds (116.5 kg) in 10 years! Of course, the reverse is also true. If he gives up (or burns) 250 calories each day, he could lose more than 25 pounds a year.

The miracle of the human body is that our metabolism will make an effort to increase our metabolic rate to burn off some of these extra calories, but there is a limit. Some of the excess calories will be stored as fat. However, for every extra 10 calories of fat that we do store daily, we will gain about one pound a year! No wonder that 66 percent of the population is overweight or obese. One purpose of this book is to teach you how to have your cake and eat it too—how to use diet and exercise to achieve control of your weight.

The human body is always expending energy, even when asleep. But when you begin to move, energy needs increase dramatically. As stated earlier, energy expenditure can go from 1.2 calories per minute during rest to more than 20 calories per minute during vigorous activity. You also need energy when you eat to power the processes of digestion and absorption. But physical activity has the greatest effect on energy expenditure. Walking involves an expenditure of about 5 calories per minute, while jogging and running can expend even more. Figure 7.5 illustrates the sources of energy at three levels of exercise.

In the fasted state (12 hours after last meal), fat, including plasma free fatty acids (plasma FFA) and muscle triglyceride, is the predominant source of energy for light (such as slow walking) and moderate (such as brisk walking) levels of exercise intensity. At higher exercise intensity levels, such as jogging and running, carbohydrate becomes the major fuel in the form of muscle glycogen and blood glucose. The contribution of carbohydrate would be somewhat higher during moderate exercise following a high-carbohydrate meal. The relative contribution of each fuel changes throughout several hours of continuous exercise. For example, during extended high-intensity exercise at 75 percent of $\dot{V}O_2max$, the contribution of muscle glycogen drops from 45 percent to near zero on depletion of muscle glycogen stores, while energy derived from muscle triglyceride declines from 25 to 10 percent. The role of blood glucose increases from 5 to 40 percent as muscle glycogen is depleted and the intensity of exercise will decrease as fats become the primary fuel source. The contribution of fat from adipose tissue (plasma FFA) increases throughout prolonged exercise, rising from 25 to 50 percent after several hours. But when the liver glycogen supply declines, blood glucose falls precipitously and the athlete will be forced to slow further to a walk, or even to stop (Coyle 1995).

Your energy expenditure depends on the size of your body. The greater your body weight, the higher your caloric expenditure for any activity. The caloric expenditure tables at the end of this chapter (form 12.2, page 298) are based on a body weight of about 70 kilograms (154 lb). If you weigh 7 kilograms (about 15 lb) more, add 10 percent. If you weigh 7 kilograms less, subtract 10 percent, and so forth. For example, if you weigh 124 pounds (56.2 kg), and the caloric cost of slow jogging is listed at 10 calories per minute, subtract 20 percent, or 2 calories, to find the calories burned when you jog (8 cal/min).

Your energy expenditure depends on the size of your body.

Measuring Energy Expenditure

In the early 1900s, scientists found a way to measure human energy expenditure. They placed subjects in a double-walled chamber very much like a food calorimeter. Heat generated in physical activity eventually increased the temperature of the water layer surrounding the chamber, indicating the caloric (heat) expenditure. But this method was far too expensive, time consuming, and cumbersome for measurement of vigorous activity. Drawing on their knowledge about the oxygen requirements of metabolism, researchers developed indirect methods of calorimetry. Because each liter of oxygen consumed is equivalent to about 5 calories, they simply measured the oxygen used during exercise. The subject breathes readily available atmospheric air, and researchers collect the exhaled air for analysis. The oxygen consumed and carbon dioxide produced during the activity are measured, along with the total volume of exhaled air. After adjusting for temperature, barometric pressure and humidity, oxygen consumption per minute is simply calculated as follows:

$$(\text{atmospheric oxygen} - \text{exhaled oxygen}) \times \text{volume exhaled air}$$

For moderate exercise, values look like this:

$$(20.93\% - 17.93\%) \times 33.3 \text{ liters exhaled} = 1.0 \text{ liter oxygen per minute.}$$

This method of **indirect calorimetry** is still used in hospitals and labs to measure resting or basal metabolic rates, physical activity, and aerobic athlete performance.

One liter of oxygen equals about 5 calories per minute, the energy cost of a brisk walk. Jogging requires about 2 liters per minute, or about 10 calories. Exercise tables often refer to the cost of physical activity in terms of oxygen use or metabolic equivalents of resting metabolism (METs). Regardless of the units that a source gives for the oxygen or caloric demands of an **exercise mode**, it is easy to do metabolic conversions to estimate your total caloric expenditure for an exercise session. Figure 12.4 can help you convert values among several units of measure, including total calories, calories per minute, oxygen use in liters and adjusted for body weight, and METs of resting energy use.

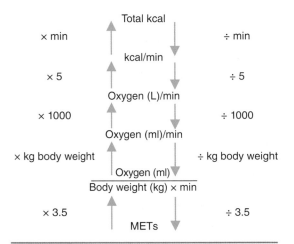

FIGURE 12.4 Metabolic conversion chart. To convert from one unit to another, simply carry out the calculation in the direction indicated by the arrow. For example, if you use 1 liter of oxygen per minute (1 L/min) in a brisk walk, you'll burn 5 calories per minute (1 L × 5 = 5 cal/min), or 300 calories per hour (5 × 60).

Set Point

The set-point theory has been around for many years. New research has validated the theory, but with some caveats (Farias, Cuevas, and Rodriguez 2011). Data supporting this theory show that our metabolism attempts to maintain our current weight within a fairly tight range. In order to maintain a current stable weight, when we overeat (take in more calories than we expend), our metabolism increases slightly, and when we undereat, our metabolism slows down slightly (Flodmark et al. 2004). Each of us has a different ability to adjust, but the range seems to be about plus or minus .02 to .15 calorie per minute. While this is a small change in resting metabolism, over a day of 1440 minutes, this range becomes 48 to 410 calories per day.

The body's effort to maintain the set point counters any attempt to gain or lose weight. For example, if you eat less, the body lowers your metabolism, making it harder to lose weight, especially if your metabolism adjusts on the high side of this range. Remember the young man from the previous section who eats an extra doughnut (250 calories) every day. Depending on the efficiency of his body to compensate, he may or may not gain weight. If his body is only able to compensate about 200 calories a day, he will store the extra 50 calories as fat. Fifty stored calories a day will end up being about 5 pounds (2 kg) of stored fat annually.

$$50 \text{ cal/day} \times 365 \text{ days/year} = 18{,}250 \text{ cal} \div 3500 \text{ cal/lb} = 5.2 \text{ lb fat}$$

The set point seems to change slowly, which may explain why gradual weight-loss programs are more successful than rapid weight-loss programs in keeping weight off (Dokken and Tsao 2007). If the weight is lost rapidly, your metabolism will remain low and you will feel hungry, making it difficult to maintain the weight loss.

Exercise has a dramatic method of working with the **set-point theory** to enhance weight-loss programs. As we have said, a low-calorie diet without exercise causes a slight lowering of the metabolic rate along with loss of muscle, which further lowers resting and exercise metabolic rates. When exercise is added to a gradual weight-loss program, muscle mass is maintained or increased, and resting metabolic rate is slightly elevated for several to many hours after the physical activity, counteracting the influence of the set point.

The set-point theory may discourage people from embarking on a weight-loss program or give them an excuse to quit. It shouldn't. The set point, if it exists, may make weight loss more difficult for some, but it can still happen, so long as exercise is part of the weight-loss program.

CALCULATING CALORIC INTAKE

Determining your caloric intake is the first step in calculating your energy balance. Many online calculators or personal computer software programs include comprehensive calorie charts organized according to general categories (e.g., vegetables, meat). We recommend using the excellent resource from the U.S. Department of Agriculture, which can be used to evaluate your diet as well as your physical activity. Set up your profile at www.choosemyplate.gov/SuperTracker/default.aspx.

To use the dietary analysis program, the main skill that you will need to develop is how to accurately estimate your serving sizes. It is very helpful to become comfortable with the size of a cup, one-half cup, tablespoon, teaspoon, pound, ounce (oz), and other units of measure. Periodically look at samples to help correctly visualize these volumes and weights. We have included a few of these conversions below to help you (English to metric conversions are listed after the English conversions):

3 teaspoons	= 1 tablespoon
2 tablespoons	= 1 fluid ounce
16 tablespoons	= 1 cup
1 cup	= 8 fluid ounces, or 1/2 pint
4 cups	= 1 quart
1 pound	= 16 ounces
1 tablespoon	= 14.8 milliliters
1 fluid ounce	= 29.6 milliliters
1 cup	= 237 milliliters, or .24 liter
1 quart	= .95 liter
1 pound	= 453.6 grams, or .45 kilogram

Determine your daily caloric intake by keeping an accurate account of everything that you eat and drink. The most accurate picture comes when you keep records for several days. Record the food or drink and the amount that you actually consume using a small pocket notebook or a recording sheet, such as that provided in form 12.1. Then, go to www.choosemyplate.gov/SuperTracker/default.aspx to determine your caloric intake. For example, breakfast consists of 1 cup of cornflakes (100 cal) with one-half cup nonfat milk (40 cal), sugar (25 cal), and a sliced banana (94 cal), plus two pieces of toast (110 cal) with butter (20 cal) and jelly (50 cal), and black coffee (1 cal). Total caloric intake is 440 calories. Do the same for all meals, snacks, beverages—everything.

Carry your notebook or recording log with you at all times and be sure to carefully record all your snacks and meals with accurate amounts. If you do this for a week, you will have a good snapshot of your eating habits. At the end of each day, record your foods and amounts at www.choosemyplate.gov/SuperTracker/default.aspx. During the days that you record your food intake, it is important to keep your normal dietary habits so that you will have a good starting point for future change.

Add up the total for each day and average across the days that you recorded accurately to find your average caloric intake. In the next section, you will learn how to calculate your energy expenditure. If it regularly exceeds your daily caloric expenditure, you will gain weight.

As you are analyzing your diet, pay attention to high-fat foods if you decide to pursue a low-fat diet, which helps to reduce body weight and blood lipids. Each gram of fat contains 9.3 calories. If your goal is to reduce fat intake, try to lower your daily fat to less than 30 percent of your total calories.

For example, if your goal is a daily caloric intake of 2,000 calories, the fat percentage is as follows:

30 percent fat = 65 grams

(30% × 2,000 cal = 600 cal; 600 cal ÷ 9.3 cal/g fat = 65 g fat)

20 percent fat = 43 grams

10 percent fat = 22 grams

ESTIMATING CALORIC EXPENDITURE

For the next few days, keep an inventory of your physical activity. Simply list your activity (exercise, work, household chores) and the time spent for each (see form 5.3 on p. 99). Don't omit anything, even sleeping. This activity inventory is educational, because it shows you when you burn calories and provides insight about how you can increase caloric expenditures in your normal routine.

Then use the caloric expenditure tables and log (form 12.2) or www.choosemyplate.gov/SuperTracker/default.aspx to estimate your expenditures. The method requires that you keep records of your daily activities: sleep, dressing, cooking, work, and all physical activity, including walking, stair climbing, fitness, and recreation. Review table 13.2 on page 331 to have an idea of all of the activities and how to record them.

Begin by making a list of your daily activities and the time spent in each. Then determine the cost of each activity in calories per minute from table 13.2 or by using www.choosemyplate.gov/SuperTracker/default.aspx. Finally, get the total for each activity and the total for the day. Form 12.2 leads you through the steps to do this. The web calculator adjusts the caloric expenditure for your weight. You should do this for several days. Best practice is to do keep an activity diary for the same days you are keeping your food diary.

Use www.choosemyplate.gov/SuperTracker/default.aspx or other dietary analysis program to analyze your diet.

Date_____ Weight _____

	Food and drinks	Portion size
Morning snacks		
Breakfast		
Lunch		
Afternoon snacks		
Dinner		
Desserts		
Evening snacks		

Form 12.2 Caloric Expenditure Log and Assessment

Time	Activities	Minutes*	Cal/min**	Calories***
Midnight–6 a.m. (360 available min)				
6 a.m.–9 a.m. (180 available min)				
9 a.m.–noon (180 available min)				
Noon–3 p.m. (180 available min)				

Time	Activities	Minutes*	Cal/min**	Calories***
3 p.m.–6 p.m. (180 available min)				
6 p.m.–9 p.m. (180 available min)				
9 p.m.–midnight (180 available min)				

Total minutes_____ Calories/day_____

Now, adjust your total calories per day for your body weight:

_____cal/day × _____lb (your weight) ÷ 150 = _____cal/day

or

_____cal/day × _____kg (your weight) ÷ 68 = _____cal/day

* The minutes in each section should equal the time for that section.

** Calories per minute for each activity are determined using table 13.2.

*** Calories for the activity are the product of [min× cal/min] for that activity.

Note: If it is easier, just list each activity and the minutes as they occur chronologically. Be sure that the total equals 1440 minutes for the day.

From B.J. Sharkey and S.E. Gaskill, 2013, *Fitness and health, seventh edition* (Champaign, IL: Human Kinetics).

Table 13.2, which shows caloric expenditure, is a brief guide to exercise intensity. Intensity is directly related to calories expended per minute. The caloric expenditure charts can guide you to appropriate weight-control activities. You can readily see that walking burns more calories than recreational volleyball and that running burns more calories than doing calisthenics. The charts will allow you to determine how long you should exercise to burn a specific number of calories (e.g., 10 cal/min for 10 min will burn 100 cal).

Be sure to adjust the totals for your body weight: Add 10 percent for each 15 pounds (6.8 kilograms) above 150 pounds (68 kilograms), and subtract 10 percent for each 15 pounds below 150 pounds.

If you have kept both a food and an activity diary and have completed the calculations to determine energy intake and output, you can now calculate your energy balance as follows using your daily averages:

Caloric intake (_____ calories) – caloric expenditure (_____ calories) = _____ calories

An Alternative Method to Estimate Total Daily Energy Expenditure

Here is another way to calculate energy expenditure that illustrates the effects of body size and age on energy expenditure. Follow steps 1 through 4:

1. Calculate basal energy expenditure using table 12.8.
2. Add increases in caloric expenditure using your main daily occupation listed below.

Bed rest (eating and reading):	Add 10%
Quiet sitting (reading, knitting):	Add 30%
Light activity (office work):	Add 40%–60%
Moderate activity (housekeeping):	Add 60%–80%
Heavy occupational activity (construction):	Add 100%

3. Adjust total for age: Subtract 4% of caloric expenditure for each decade (10 years) over 25 years of age.
4. Add calories expended in nonwork (recreational) activities.

Use the caloric expenditure charts in tables 12.8 and 13.2 to calculate minutes of activity and cost in calories per minute.

For example, consider a 45-year-old construction worker, 5 feet 10 inches tall (178 cm), weighing 200 pounds (91 kg) who plays 30 minutes of table tennis with his son:

1. Basal metabolic rate	= 1,815 cal
2. Add 100% for heavy construction work	1,815 + 1,815 = 3,630 cal
3. Subtract 8% for age	3,630 – (3,630 × .08) = 3,340 cal
4. + 30 min of table tennis with son	3,340 + (30 min × 5 cal per min) = 3,490 cal/day

If intake regularly exceeds expenditure, you have a positive energy balance, and the excess energy will be stored as fat. If caloric intake regularly falls short of expenditure, you will lose weight. Note that in all of these equations, we assume that resting and basal metabolic rates remain constant and that we all have the same metabolic rates. While it is true that we all have similar rates of energy expenditure, even small differences, or errors in the estimates that you have made, will result in some measurement and estimation error. However, the final result of calculating your energy balance will give you a pretty good picture of how you are doing. The simplest way to evaluate your energy balance is check your weight gain over a year. For every pound of fat you gain, you have stored 3,500 calories. This averages out to only about 10 stored calories a day for each stored pound of fat.

When you know your energy balance, you'll have a clear idea of what you can do to reduce caloric intake and increase caloric expenditure. Table 12.8 indicates basal

Table 12.8 Basal Energy Expenditure for Men and Women

MEN		WOMEN	
Weight	Energy expenditure* (cal)	Weight	Energy expenditure** (cal)
140 lb (64 kg)	1,550	100 lb (45 kg)	1,225
160 lb (73 kg)	1,640	120 lb (54 kg)	1,320
180 lb (82 kg)	1,730	160 lb (73 kg)	1,485
220 lb (100 kg)	1,900	180 lb (82 kg)	1,575

*5 ft 10 in. (178 cm) tall: Add 20 cal for each in. taller; if shorter, subtract 20 cal for each in.

**5 ft 6 in. (168 cm) tall: Add 20 cal for each in. taller; if shorter, subtract 20 cal for each in.

Basal energy = calories expended in 24 hr of complete bed rest

energy needs for 24 hours of complete bed rest, averaging 1.2 calories per minute. Because of fluctuations and differences based on a number of factors, the average may vary as much as ± .15 calories per minute (Flodmark et al. 2004). Evidence shows that the sleeping metabolic rate is lower than the resting metabolic rate (RMR) in obese people who are metabolically efficient, and higher than RMR in nonobese subjects (Zhang et al. 2002).

DIET AND PERFORMANCE

This section presents a few basic facts concerning diet and performance. One fact is that athletes use the same sources of energy and nutrients as everyone else does. They need more calories to fuel hard training and may need additional nutrients, but those usually come with an increase in nutritious foods (see chapter 13). Here are some ways to ensure adequate energy for performance.

Carbohydrate Loading

Years before it became popular, researchers observed that the best endurance performances occurred when athletes were on a high-carbohydrate diet, such as the performance diet discussed at the beginning of this chapter. That diet provides sufficient energy for continuous events lasting up to 1 hour. Carbo-loading goes a step further, raising muscle glycogen levels for high-intensity performances lasting more than 1 hour. Using a needle to get a sample of muscle tissue (see muscle biopsy photo in chapter 8, page 157), researchers studied how performance depends on muscle glycogen levels and how glycogen levels depend on carbohydrate intake.

Here is what you can do to ensure proper glycogen levels for competition. For events lasting 1 to 2 hours, do a long, hard workout several days before the event to deplete muscle glycogen stores. This activates an enzyme responsible for packing glycogen into muscle fibers. Next, begin immediately to raise your carbohydrate intake for the next few days by adding extra carbohydrate to the diet. Be sure to drink lots of water, because carbohydrate is stored with water (hydrated). This scheme will double muscle glycogen stores as long as you reduce (taper) training before the event.

For events longer than 2 hours, start your depletion effort 6 days before the event. Do another hard workout the next day to deplete muscle glycogen stores further. Keep carbohydrate intake down for those 2 days. Then, after the second depletion effort, return to a high-carbohydrate intake with water. Taper your training to allow maximum carbohydrate loading. This scheme has raised muscle glycogen levels three to four times, enough to fuel an entire marathon.

Be aware that carbo-loading takes place only in the muscles that you deplete with exercise. Other muscles can't easily use the glycogen, so the effect is specific. If you plan to carbo-load for an important race, be certain to try it first in a less important event. Some people feel bloated and heavy when they carbo-load, but the best performances take place when muscle glycogen levels are highest. One study has shown that inactivity combined with high intake of carbohydrate (up to 10 g of carbohydrate per kg of body weight, with emphasis on foods with a high glycemic index) enables trained athletes to attain maximal muscle glycogen levels within 1 day (Bussau et al. 2002).

Women tend to use more fat and less carbohydrate during submaximal endurance events. Their preference for fat utilization appears to be hormonally controlled, and it diminishes as training progresses (Ruby and Robergs 1994). A study shows that aerobically trained women increase muscle glycogen in response to high carbohydrate intake (78% carbohydrate), but the magnitude was smaller than that previously observed in men. The increase in muscle glycogen from the high-carbohydrate diet was associated with increased cycling performance to exhaustion (8.4%) when compared with the moderate-carbohydrate intake (48% carbohydrate diet) (Walker et al. 2000).

Pre-, During, and Postevent Feeding

Generally speaking, you should eat the precompetition meal that works for you. Eat at least 3 hours before the event to ensure an empty stomach at race time. Emphasize carbohydrate and avoid difficult-to-digest fats and excess protein. Especially nervous people may want to use a liquid meal before competition. A peanut butter and honey sandwich works for shorter events, and pancakes plus an egg (to slow entry of glucose) works for long events, such as a 50-kilometer (31 mile) ski race.

• *Pre-event.* Drink 1 to 2 cups (237 to 473 ml) of water before an event, but avoid high carbohydrate intake that might raise insulin levels, lower blood glucose, cause hypoglycemia, reduce free fatty acid availability, and increase reliance on muscle glycogen.

• *During the event.* Drink a cup (237 ml) or more of water every 15 to 20 minutes. In longer events, drink a sport drink with 6 to 8 percent (60 to 80 g/L) carbohydrate every 15 to 20 minutes to maintain blood glucose levels. Cyclists and skiers are able to tolerate more carbohydrate in drinks or solid food (bananas, energy bars, gels) during competition. The carbohydrate provides energy for muscles and the nervous system and helps to enhance the immune system and cognitive function. Studies suggest that some protein intake during the event may improve endurance performance.

• *Postevent.* Immediately after the event, begin to consume carbohydrate and some protein (a ratio of 4 g carbs to 1 g protein) to maximize replacement of muscle glycogen and speed muscle recovery (Ivy et al. 2002). The maximal rate of replacement occurs in the first 2 hours after the event. Select foods with a high glycemic index to maximize replacement of muscle glycogen. Drink lots of juices and water to ensure fluid replacement, but avoid alcoholic beverages, which function as a diuretic.

Blood Sugar

We have noted how endurance training improves the ability to mobilize and metabolize fat, thereby conserving blood sugar. Nerve tissue depends on the blood sugar (glucose) as its source of energy. This means that the brain and nervous system require a constant supply of glucose. Blood glucose rises after a meal and then drops until it reaches a normal resting level (about 80 mg). Thereafter, the liver strives to maintain that level, at least until its supply is depleted. The symptoms of hypoglycemia indicate the influence of low blood sugar on behavior and performance. Pay attention to the following symptoms, but be aware that hypoglycemia symptoms are individual. They may occur as any of the following or a grouping of several.

Nervousness	Anxiety	Irritability
Confusion	Exhaustion	Rapid pulse
Faintness	Dizziness	Muscle pains
Tremor	Cold sweat	Indecisiveness
Depression	Lack of coordination	Vertigo
Lack of concentration	Drowsiness	Blurred vision
Headaches		

Muscles can use blood sugar as an energy source, so long runs, bike rides, or hikes certainly can lead to hypoglycemia. High-energy snacks such as energy bars lead to a big boost of blood sugar, but they also call forth a large secretion of insulin. The insulin speeds the sugar into the muscle. Within a couple of hours, one begins to sag again (reactive hypoglycemia). To avoid the problem, simply eat at regular intervals and use energy snacks and carbohydrate drinks to maintain blood sugar levels.

SUMMARY

This chapter provides a thumbnail sketch of nutrition as well as suggestions for improving health and performance. Although we could write much more on the subject, the basics provided here form the framework for a safe and sensible eating plan. Minor dietary adjustments will lower your daily intake of fat. Reduce fat further if your family history or risk factors indicate the need. Select foods from a variety of sources to ensure the availability of essential amino acids, vitamins, and minerals. Use a daily vitamin and mineral supplement with the recommended dietary intake (RDI) during heavy training or weight loss, or if you are concerned about your diet. It's that simple.

Overweight and obesity clearly have a genetic link, and people who inherit the tendency are more metabolically efficient (they use less energy), even when sleeping. These people can become overweight even though they eat little more than those who remain thin. The set-point theory can explain much of this and why it is difficult to lose weight. But how much of the problem of obesity and overweight can we attribute to heredity and how much can we attribute to a positive energy balance, to intake of calories exceeding expenditure? Obesity researcher Claude Bouchard has estimated that 40 percent of the variance in body weight among people of similar stature can be attributed to genetic causes, leaving 60 percent as one's personal responsibility (Malina and Bouchard 1991). Immigrants come to the United States with a low rate of obesity, but after 15 years, they resemble U.S. born adults in BMI and obesity (Sanghavi et al. 2004).

According to the National Health and Nutrition Examination Surveys (NHANES), between 1971 and 2000, U.S. men increased caloric intake 168 calories per day, while women increased their intake 335 calories per day. With that positive energy balance, a man could gain 17.5 pounds (7.9 kg) in one year, while a woman could gain 34.8 pounds (15.8 kg)! The percentage of calories from fat decreased, although absolute fat consumption increased. The percentage of daily calories from carbohydrate increased 277.6 calories for men and 255.8 calories for women (Wright et al. 2004). Apparently, we are eating more calories while burning far fewer in work or recreational activity.

Calorie-burning exercise is the positive side of the fat balance equation. Moderate-intensity exercise burns fat while preserving lean tissue, something that dieting alone cannot do. Chapter 13 will tell you how to incorporate activity into a sensible program of weight control and will show you how improved aerobic and muscular fitness magnify the benefits of regular, moderate activity.

Before we move on, we want to make a confession. We've been using a daily vitamin and mineral supplement for many years. We exercise regularly, train often, and strive to maintain or even lose weight, in spite of prodigious appetites. At times, we engage in strenuous or even exhausting activities, such as long-duration hiking, biking, or cross-country ski trips, for which we may be inadequately prepared. The RDI supplement is a hedge against less-than-perfect nutrition. For several years, one of us also supplemented his diet with modest amounts of antioxidant vitamins C, E, and beta-carotene. He added these in response to studies suggesting that antioxidants contributed to lower risk of heart, eye, and other problems, and reduced muscle damage from oxidative stress. Our physician friends did the same, until studies cast doubt on their effectiveness.

So, now we say eat a variety of foods, fruits and vegetables, and whole-grain products. We take steps to minimize inherited risks of heart disease or other potential problems and engage in regular, moderate physical activity. One bonus of this behavior is a healthy immune system. Over the years, we have enjoyed consistent good health and effortless weight control. In the next chapter, you'll learn how to gain lifelong control of your weight.

Weight Control

More Than Calories

"When the stomach is full,
it is easy to talk of fasting."

St. Jerome

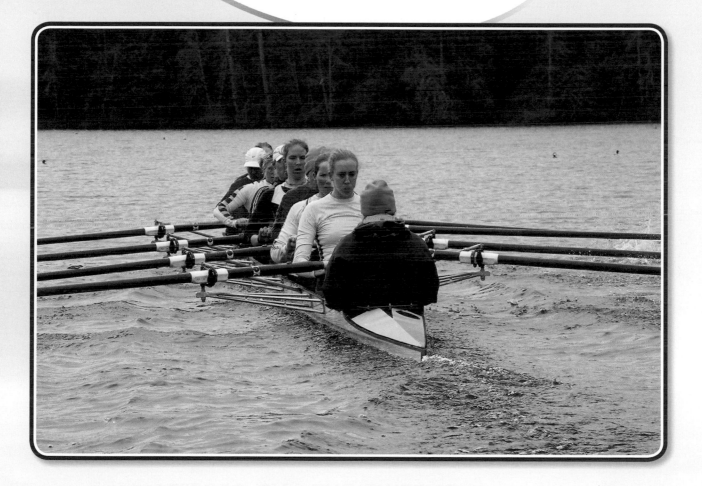

Weight control is a lifelong journey. The best time to start is when you are young; the next best time is today. Physical activity is the positive approach to weight control. When you decide to do something about your weight, you are committing to a course of action. No other approach is so physiologically sound, so definite, so enjoyable. Action is more psychologically rewarding than avoidance. When you take a walk after dinner, you relax, improve your digestion, enhance your vitality, and burn fat and calories. After the walk, you feel better both physically and emotionally. Problems loom large when you sit and brood, but how quickly they shrink when you undertake a plan of action!

Dieting carries negative connotations of avoidance, deprivation, and punishment. It creates false hopes, contributes to stress, ruins the disposition, causes fatigue, and often leads to increases in body weight and fat. The ups and downs of frequent dieting (weight cycling, or yo-yo dieting) increase the risk of psychopathology, dissatisfaction with life, binge eating, morbidity, and mortality (Brownell and Rodin 1994). This is also true in young women who are dieting for body image, with the additional problem that weight cycling may promote the onset of atherosclerosis (Montani et al. 2006).

The most exciting part of this chapter deals with the extra benefits that you obtain with improved fitness, benefits that exceed the effects of activity. This material, although not new, is finally coming to the attention of public health and fitness professionals. In our estimation, these extra benefits provide the most convincing case for activity and fitness and their relationship to weight control and health.

Finally, we outline activity, food choices (diet), and a lifelong approach to rational weight control.

This chapter will help you do the following:

- Understand the causes and consequences of overweight and obesity
- Establish sensible body weight and body fat goals
- Understand why activity is superior to dieting as a means of weight control
- Determine the effects of activity on the appetite
- Understand the extra weight-control and fat-metabolism benefits associated with improved fitness
- Implement the weight-control program best suited to your needs: to lose, maintain, or gain weight

OVERWEIGHT AND OBESITY

In horse racing, the favorite often is handicapped to provide a better contest. If a few pounds are added, the favorite may become an also-ran. Excess weight can affect performance in humans as well; few of us realize how much. Excess weight proves a burden physically, socially, psychologically, and economically. It may be the most significant health problem for most people. Yet it is a symptom, not a disease, and it is among the least complicated of all health problems.

What are the medical consequences of overweight and obesity? Disease risks and costs increase substantially with increased body weight. A common measure of proper weight is the body mass index (BMI). Body mass index relates weight to height, and is calculated as weight in kilograms divided by the square of height in meters (kg/m^2). It can also be calculated in pounds and inches as $lb/in.^2 \times 703$. The death rate rises gradually as BMI increases above $25 \ kg/m^2$ and rises more rapidly above $30 \ kg/m^2$, especially in the younger age groups. The National Heart, Lung, and Blood Institute classifies BMI values of <19.5 kg/m^2 as underweight, 19.6 to 24.9 kg/m^2 as normal, 25 to 29.9 kg/m^2 as overweight, 30 to 39.9 kg/m^2 as obese, and >40 kg/m^2 as morbidly obese. Those with a high BMI have a higher incidence of atherosclerotic heart disease, hypertension, some cancers, diabetes, and cirrhosis of the liver. Accidents and surgical complications are more prevalent, as are complications of pregnancy. When a person removes the excess weight through diet and exercise, these problems diminish or disappear. The body mass index provides a simple way for you to assess body composition. All you need is your body weight in pounds (or kg) and your height in inches (or cm). Then use figure 13.1 to get your score.

You should strive to remain in the desirable category because heavier men and women in all age groups have increased risk of death from all causes (Calle et al. 1999). You should also realize that low fitness is an independent predictor of mortality in all body mass index groups, and the risk of death from being overweight is much lower in those who maintain a higher level of aerobic fitness (Wei et al. 1999). Incidentally, health risks associated with having a BMI above 25 are somewhat lower if waist measurement is less than 35 inches (88.9 cm) for women or 40 inches (101.6 cm) for men, a condition common in athletes who engage in significant training.

You may say, "I'm not overweight; I weigh the same as I did in my senior year of high school." True, your weight may be the same, but what about your ratio of lean to fat tissue? Isn't it possible that you have lost muscle and gained fat? Has your waist measurement remained the same? Overweight is defined as a BMI of 25 to 29. An alternative to the BMI for determining overweight is comparison with desirable body weight (see table 13.1). Desirable weights are associated with the longest life span. A large body of evidence suggests that fitness reduces the risks of being overweight and that fit but overweight men have lower all-cause mortality than do unfit men of normal weight (Lee, Jackson, and Blair 1998, Katzmarzyk et al. 2001).

> You should strive to remain in the desirable category because heavier men and women in all age groups have an increased risk of death from all causes.

Getting Fat

Excess caloric intake starts the process. Fat intake poses more of a problem, though, because it has 9.3 calories per gram, whereas carbohydrate and protein have 4.1 and 4.3 calories per gram, respectively. Moreover, fat is similar to the composition of our adipose tissue and is easier to store. Obese people eat more fat and engage in less physical activity (Rising et al. 1994), thereby contributing to the problem. Some researchers believe fat cells may continue to increase in size and number in severely obese individuals with increasing food intake, creating an even greater urge to eat. Rising obesity increases levels of the enzyme lipoprotein lipase (LPL), which helps fat cells take on more fat. Changes in a large number of other enzymes and hormones are also associated with increased obesity, including acyl-coenzyme A, diacylglycerol transferase (DGAT), fatty acid synthase (FAS), and **leptin**. Excess fat seems to inhibit the action of insulin, the hormone that helps glucose get into cells, leading to feelings of weakness and hunger that cause one to eat more. This also creates high levels of blood glucose (type 2 diabetes, or non-insulin-dependent diabetes mellitus), leading to artery damage and high blood pressure. And the cycle continues.

Height (in) / Weight (lb)	49	51	53	55	57	59	61	63	65	67	69	71	73	75	77	79	81	83
66	19	18	16	15	14	13	12	12	11	10	10	9	9	8	8	8	7	7
70	20	19	18	16	15	14	13	13	12	11	10	10	9	9	8	8	8	7
75	22	20	19	17	16	15	14	13	12	12	11	10	10	9	9	9	8	8
79	23	21	20	18	17	16	15	14	13	12	12	11	11	10	9	9	9	8
84	24	22	21	19	18	17	16	15	14	13	12	12	11	11	10	10	9	9
88	26	24	22	20	19	18	17	16	15	14	13	12	12	11	11	10	10	9
92	27	25	23	21	20	19	17	16	15	15	14	13	12	12	11	11	10	10
97	28	26	24	22	21	20	18	17	16	15	14	14	13	12	12	11	10	10
101	29	27	25	23	22	20	19	18	17	16	15	14	13	13	12	12	11	10
106	31	28	26	24	23	21	20	19	18	17	16	15	14	13	13	12	11	11
110	32	30	27	26	24	22	21	20	18	17	16	15	15	14	13	13	11	11
114	33	31	29	27	25	23	22	20	19	18	17	16	15	14	14	13	12	12
119	35	32	30	28	26	24	22	21	20	19	18	17	16	15	14	14	13	12
123	36	33	31	29	27	25	23	22	21	19	18	17	16	16	15	14	13	13
128	37	34	32	30	28	26	24	23	21	20	19	18	17	16	15	15	14	13
132	38	36	33	31	29	27	25	23	22	21	20	19	18	17	16	15	14	14
136	40	37	34	32	29	28	26	24	23	21	20	19	18	17	16	16	15	14
141	41	38	35	33	30	28	27	25	24	22	21	20	19	18	17	16	15	15
145	42	39	36	34	31	29	27	26	24	23	22	20	19	18	17	17	16	15
150	44	40	37	35	32	30	28	27	25	24	22	21	20	19	18	17	16	15
154	45	41	38	36	33	31	29	27	26	24	23	22	20	19	18	18	17	16
158	46	43	40	37	34	32	30	28	26	25	24	22	21	20	19	18	17	16
163	47	44	41	38	35	33	31	29	27	26	24	23	22	20	19	19	18	17
167	49	45	42	39	36	34	32	30	28	26	25	23	22	21	20	19	18	17
172	50	46	43	40	37	35	32	30	29	27	25	24	23	22	21	20	19	18
176	51	47	44	41	38	36	33	31	29	28	26	25	23	22	21	20	19	18
180	52	49	45	42	39	36	34	32	30	28	27	25	24	23	22	21	20	19
185	54	50	46	43	40	37	35	33	31	29	27	26	25	23	22	21	20	19
189	55	51	47	44	41	38	36	34	32	30	28	27	25	24	23	22	20	20
194	56	52	48	45	42	39	37	34	32	30	29	27	26	24	23	22	21	20
198	58	53	49	46	43	40	37	35	33	31	29	28	26	25	24	23	21	20
202	59	54	50	47	44	41	38	36	34	32	30	28	27	25	24	23	22	21
207	60	56	52	48	45	42	39	37	35	33	31	29	27	26	25	24	22	21
211	61	57	53	49	46	43	40	38	35	33	31	30	28	27	25	24	23	22
216	63	58	54	50	47	44	41	38	36	34	32	30	29	27	26	25	23	22
220	64	59	55	51	48	44	42	39	37	35	33	31	29	28	26	25	24	23
224	65	60	56	52	49	45	42	40	37	35	33	31	30	28	27	26	24	23
229	67	62	57	53	49	46	43	41	38	36	34	32	30	29	27	26	25	24
233	68	63	58	54	50	47	44	41	39	37	35	33	31	29	28	27	25	24
238	69	64	59	55	51	48	45	42	40	37	35	33	32	30	28	27	26	24
242	70	65	60	56	52	49	46	43	40	38	36	34	32	30	29	28	26	25
246	72	66	61	57	53	50	47	44	41	39	37	35	33	31	29	28	27	25
251	73	67	63	58	54	51	47	45	42	39	37	35	33	32	30	29	27	26
255	74	69	64	59	55	52	48	45	43	40	38	36	34	32	31	29	28	26
260	76	70	65	60	56	52	49	46	43	41	39	36	34	33	31	30	28	27
264	77	71	66	61	57	53	50	47	44	42	39	37	35	33	32	30	29	27
268	78	72	67	62	58	54	51	48	45	42	40	38	36	34	32	31	29	28
273	79	73	68	63	59	55	52	48	46	43	40	38	36	34	33	31	30	28
277	81	75	69	64	60	56	52	49	46	44	41	39	37	35	33	32	30	29
282	82	76	70	65	61	57	53	50	47	44	42	40	37	35	34	32	30	29
286	83	77	71	66	62	58	54	51	48	45	42	40	38	36	34	33	31	29
290	84	78	72	67	63	59	55	52	48	46	43	41	39	37	35	33	31	30
295	86	79	74	68	64	60	56	52	49	46	44	41	39	37	35	34	32	30
299	87	80	75	69	65	60	57	53	50	47	44	42	40	38	36	34	32	31
304	88	82	76	70	66	61	57	54	51	48	45	43	40	38	36	35	33	31
308	90	83	77	71	67	62	58	55	51	48	46	43	41	39	37	35	33	32
312	91	84	78	72	68	63	59	55	52	49	46	44	41	39	37	36	34	32

Underweight (<19)

Desirable (19-25)

Increased health risks (25-30)

Obese (30-40)

Extremely obese (>40)

FIGURE 13.1 Body mass index chart.

From National Heart, Lung, and Blood Institute 1998.

Table 13.1 Desirable Weights for Men and Women*

Height (without shoes) in ft and in. (cm)	Weight (without clothes) in lb (kg)	
	Women	Men
5 ft 0 in. (152.4)	103–115 (46.7–52.2)	—
5 ft 1 in. (154.9)	106–118 (48.0–53.5)	111–122 (50.3–55.3)
5 ft 2 in. (157.5)	109–122 (49.4–55.3)	114–126 (51.7–57.2)
5 ft 3 in. (160.0)	112–126 (50.8–57.2)	117–129 (53.1–58.5)
5 ft 4 in. (162.5)	116–131 (52.6–59.4)	120–132 (54.4–59.9)
5 ft 5 in. (165.1)	120–135 (54.4–61.2)	123–136 (55.8–61.7)
5 ft 6 in. (167.6)	124–139 (56.2–63.0)	127–140 (57.6–63.5)
5 ft 7 in. (170.2)	128–143 (58.0–64.9)	131–145 (59.4–65.8)
5 ft 8 in. (172.7)	132–147 (59.9–66.7)	135–149 (61.2–67.6)
5 ft 9 in. (175.3)	136–151 (61.7–68.5)	139–153 (63.0–69.4)
5 ft 10 in. (177.8)	140–155 (63.5–70.3)	143–158 (64.9–71.7)
5 ft 11 in. (180.3)	144-159 (65.3-72.1)	147–163 (66.7–73.9)
6 ft 0 in. (182.9)	148-163 (67.1-73.9)	151–168 (68.5–76.2)
6 ft 1 in. (185.4)	152-167 (68.9-75.7)	155 173 (70.3–78.5)
6 ft 2 in. (188.0)	157-172 (71.2-78.0)	160–178 (72.6–80.7)
6 ft 3 in. (190.5)	162-177 (73.5-80.3)	165 183 (74.8–83.0)

*Age 25 and above. Weight ranges for women 6 ft and taller added by the authors.

These guidelines, issued by the Metropolitan Life Insurance Company in 1959, are recommended over more recent editions, which provide false reassurance to a large fraction of people who are not defined as overweight but who are at substantially increased risk of heart disease.

Reprinted with permission of the Metropolitan Life Insurance Company.

This is also true for youth and adolescents (Eisenmann 2007, Bouziotas 2004). Incidentally, because overweight and low fitness are associated with heart disease, diabetes, and hypertension, some insurance companies charge a higher premium for people judged to be 20 percent or more above desirable weight, or physically inactive, or both.

Excess fat or muscle can make you overweight, although extra fat poses more of a burden because the muscles can do useful work and take less space for equal weight (muscle is denser than fat). But even excess muscle seems unnecessary for adults, unless they need it for sport or occupational reasons. Muscular men with excess fat, such as inactive former football players, seem to have increased risk of high blood pressure and heart disease.

Obesity is defined as an excessive accumulation of fat beyond what is considered normal for one's age, sex, and body type. Obesity is a case of being overfat, not just overweight. A person can be underweight and still be obese, by having excess fat along with poorly developed muscles. Obesity is defined as having more than 20 percent fat for men or more than 30 percent fat for women (or as being more than 20 percent above desirable weight, or having a BMI of 30 or greater). These levels were determined by noting thresholds where chronic disease, morbidity, and death increase more rapidly. Some experts prefer lower or higher levels, but when using the BMI standard of 30kg/m², one-third of the

American adult population is obese. Using the BMI standard of 25 to 29.9 kg/m², 85 percent of American adults are overweight or obese (CDC 2011a). Sadly, we note that we now have a new category, morbid obesity, defined as a percent body fat or BMI score of 40 kg/m² or more. People in the morbid obese category have a greatly increased risk of morbidity and mortality.

Why are more than 100 million Americans overweight to the point of obesity? Is it merely because their caloric intake exceeds expenditure? To a large extent, the answer is yes! Although Americans have lowered the proportion of fat in their diet, they have simultaneously increased carbohydrate and total caloric intake and decreased their level of physical activity, thus decreasing caloric output. Even so, scientists continue to study other possible contributions to the epidemic of obesity.

Heredity Versus Environment

When we see obese parents with obese offspring, we are likely to think that the problem runs in the family. When both parents are obese, a child has an 80 percent risk of obesity. Studies of identical twins reared in different environments also indicate that obesity has a genetic root. But the pattern and extent of that relationship have not been well defined.

Much of the obesity that we see in families could be due as much to the environment as to a genetic cause. Overweight people eat more and exercise less, and the same may be true of their children. But in a study of identical and fraternal twins (Stunkard, Foch, and Hrubec 1986), the authors found a high heritability for weight and body mass index. They concluded that body weight and obesity are under strong genetic control and that childhood family environment by itself has little effect. The same author, in a different study of adopted children found a strong relationship between natural parents of adopted children in body fatness, but no relation of the adopted youth to their adoptive parents. They reported "We conclude that genetic influences have an important role in determining human fatness in adults, whereas the family environment alone has no apparent effect" (Stunkard et al. 1986). The discovery of genes partially responsible for obesity supports this reasoning.

Leptin, a genetically influenced hormone that governs how efficiently we burn fat, is released by fat cells. Higher levels of fat reduce the sensitivity of the body to leptin, making it possible to gain more weight. Conversely, leptin levels have been found to be low in restrained eaters, those with the eating disorder anorexia nervosa (Matejek et al. 1999). Clearly, behavior modulates genetic expression.

Do genetic influences on body weight mean that energy balance doesn't apply? No, it doesn't. In spite of genetic influence, the basic cause of overweight and obesity remains a positive energy balance because of excess caloric intake, inadequate caloric expenditure, or both. Further proof is the fact that our current epidemic of overweight and obesity has emerged in

Genetics?

To see whether physical activity protects susceptible populations from developing obesity and type 2, or adult-onset, diabetes, a study compared physical activity levels of two groups of genetically similar Pima Indians, one group living in Arizona and the other in Mexico. The U.S. Pima Indians had a high incidence of obesity and diabetes, whereas the Mexican Indians did not. Physical activity was higher in the Mexican Pimas, with an average total energy expenditure of 3,289 calories per day versus 2,671 for the Arizona Indians. The authors concluded that physical activity played a significant role in the prevention of obesity in a genetically susceptible population (Esparza et al. 2000). The authors also noted the contribution of high-fat fast-food diets on the development of obesity and diabetes in the U.S. Pimas.

the last several decades, far faster than it could occur because of the influence of heredity. What else influences this tendency to store fat?

Glandular Causes

One authority has said, "With the exception of diabetes, glandular disease is associated with obesity in less than one case out of a thousand. Even in the presence of the disease, the individual is obese because energy acquisition has exceeded energy expenditure" (Gwinup 1970). The many social and societal causes of obesity remain difficult to pinpoint, but all are related to more energy intake than expenditure. Crothers and colleagues (2009) report that glandular and metabolic diseases are more a result of obesity than a cause, and that very few children have illness that directly lead to obesity. It seems that overeating, particularly on a high-fat diet, may lead to obesity and non-insulin-dependent diabetes (Ivy, Zderic, and Fogt 1999). Obese people have a significantly higher incidence of diabetes than do people of normal or desirable weight, and obesity is a major risk factor for developing type 2 diabetes. After modest weight reduction, all of the risk factors for diabetes and heart disease improve, and fasting blood glucose is reduced (Wing et al. 2011). After major weight loss, such as from bariatric surgery, the diabetes may improve tremendously (Schauer et al. 2012).

Diabetes is characterized by problems associated with the hormone insulin, which is needed to get blood sugar into cells, including fat cells. Normally, soon after eating, the increase in macronutrients stimulates the pancreas to secrete the hormone insulin, which then initiates the rapid transport of sugar out of blood and into cells. Increased body fat increases insulin resistance, thereby requiring more insulin to do the same job. Eventually, insulin resistance inhibits glucose uptake into muscle and other cells. When sugar doesn't reach the cells, blood glucose levels remain high, muscle glucose remains low, energy is low, and the appetite is often stimulated, leading to further obesity. When fasting blood glucose levels rise above 100 milligrams per deciliter, as happens when people become insulin resistant, they are considered to be prediabetic. Associated problems of high blood pressure, high triglycerides, and other health issues often occur. Once fasted blood glucose levels rise above 130 milligrams per deciliter, a person is considered to be diabetic. When diabetes mellitus is the result of insulin resistance (most diabetes cases) it is called non-insulin-dependent diabetes mellitus (NIDDM, or type 2 diabetes), since the person produces insulin, but the insulin has little effect on the cell receptors that stimulate glucose uptake into muscle cells. After a while, years perhaps, the pancreatic cells responsible for the production of insulin may fatigue, and the person may no longer produce pancreatic insulin, therefore requiring exogenous insulin (shots). People who lose the ability to produce insulin, often at an early age, are categorized as having insulin-dependent diabetes mellitus (IDDM, or type 1 diabetes).

Before the discovery of insulin in 1921, diet and exercise were the only treatments available to people with NIDDM (type 2 diabetes), and there was no treatment for people with IDDM (type 1 diabetes). Nowadays, diet, insulin, and other drugs are used to control this metabolic malfunction of insulin production and sugar utilization. Muscular activity acts much like insulin to increase the transport of glucose into muscle cells, even in the absence of insulin or failure of insulin to stimulate glucose uptake. Because muscular activity is effective in the reduction of body weight and the risk of heart disease (diabetes and heart disease are frequently associated), attention has turned again to the use of exercise in the treatment and control of type 2 diabetes. Moderate physical activity reduces insulin

"With the exception of diabetes, glandular disease is associated with obesity in less than one case out of a thousand. Even in the presence of the disease, the individual is obese because energy acquisition has exceeded energy expenditure" (Gwinup 1970).

resistance and insulin requirements for all people, including those with type 2 diabetes. Regular participation in aerobic activity, especially when coupled with fat loss, often relieves many of the symptoms of type 2 diabetes. It can lower blood glucose and pressure as long as the weight loss is maintained. Type 1 diabetics also benefit from physical activity, but they must take care to properly adjust their insulin doses both prior to and after exercise.

Larger and More Numerous Fat Cells

Researchers have studied the growth and development of fat cells. Excess calories are stored in fat cells in the form of triglycerides. Some people have more fat cells, causing them to store fat more readily. With the development of methods to determine fat cell size and number, researchers have been able to follow the development of obesity. Fat cells are apparently able to increase in size or number, and overfeeding can stimulate the increase. Traditionally, a chubby baby has been considered a healthy baby, but overfeeding during the first few years of life will stimulate the development of larger and more numerous fat cells (three times more). These cells remain for life and may influence the appetite when they are not filled. This early onset of hypercellularity generally leads to the most severe form of obesity. Another period of intense concern comes at or around

Waist-to-Hip Ratio

Unfortunately, the fat located around visceral organs can't be measured with skinfold calipers because it lies below abdominal muscles. Researchers are looking at the waist-to-hip-ratio (WHR) to determine why one fat storage location carries a greater risk of heart disease, hypertension, stroke, diabetes, and some cancers. To calculate your ratio, simply measure the waist at the level of the navel and the hips at the greatest circumference of the buttocks (measure to the nearest .25 in., or .6 cm) and divide the waist measurement by the hip measurement. Results suggest that WHR values above .9 for men or .8 for women exceed safe limits (see figure 13.2).

Why is visceral fat a risk? Abdominal fat, fat stored in and around the viscera, has a direct circulatory route to the liver. Fat cells in that region are likely to send free fatty acids directly to the liver, where they can be used to synthesize cholesterol. Whatever the reason, visceral fat is a risk, and we know that exercise is an effective way to reduce the amount of metabolically active

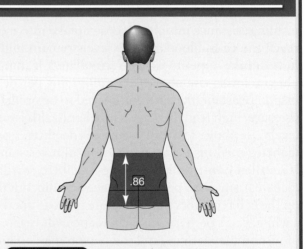

FIGURE 13.2 Waist-to-hip ratio (e.g., 32/37 = .86).

visceral fat, especially in men (Trichopoulou et al. 2001). In the normal, overweight, and obese BMI categories, those with higher waist circumference measurements are increasingly likely to have hypertension, diabetes, lipid problems, and the metabolic syndrome when compared with those with normal waist circumference values (Janssen, Katzmarzyk, and Ross 2002).

the time of puberty, when overfeeding can lead to increases in the number and size of fat cells (Malina and Bouchard 1991).

Enlarged fat cells characterize adult-onset obesity. The number of fat cells, however, does not seem subject to significant change. The pattern of obesity is a significant factor in determining health risk. Obesity that begins in childhood and continues into the adult years is a greater risk than adult-onset obesity. The location of stored fat also predicts health risk; potbellies are associated with a higher risk of heart disease, whereas pear shapes are not. The tendency of men to accumulate fat in their abdomens may be a factor in their higher risk of heart disease. Studies are now under way to determine why some cells take in more fat and why that is related to heart disease.

Lower Metabolic Rate

Studies on obese infants, adolescents, and adults agree that fat people are more fuel efficient; their bodies burn calories more sparingly than the bodies of normal-weight subjects do. Their lower metabolic rate or energy expenditure makes weight loss more difficult. This finding may explain how heredity influences overweight and obesity. Why is the metabolic rate lower? One line of reasoning points to a lethargic or less active sympathetic nervous system. This portion of the autonomic nervous system secretes epinephrine (adrenaline) to speed up the heart rate and other responses during stress or exercise. Epinephrine also prompts the release of fatty acids from fat cells. Less sympathetic activity means less epinephrine, and less epinephrine means a lower metabolic rate and less fat utilization.

Some other lines of research tend to lift some of the blame for excess fat from the shoulders of the obese.

• *Brown fat thermogenesis.* Brown fat, a form of fat that uses excess food to make heat, may be deficient in some obese people. Normally, brown fat serves to keep extra calories from being stored as fat. Studies on lean and obese humans will shed more light on this potential contributor to obesity.

• *Lipoprotein lipase.* **Lipoprotein lipase (LPL)** is an enzyme in adipose tissue (also found in muscle). Its activity has been found to increase in the fat cells of obese people who lose weight, leading researchers to wonder if it might be a reason why previously overfat people usually regain lost weight.

If one or both of these lines of research are confirmed on human subjects, we will be better able to understand why so many millions are overweight or obese. We have evidence that Americans eat a similar number of calories as our ancestors did in 1900, but that we are far less active than they were. Clearly, weight loss through dieting is associated with a reduction in 24-hour energy expenditure, and this reduction makes it more difficult to maintain a body weight that is different from the usual weight (Leibel, Rosenbaum, and Hirsch 1995). Regardless of genetic, glandular, psychological, or other complications or causes, overweight and obesity are problems of energy balance. We take in too many calories, or expend too few, or both.

Psychological Origins

Overweight can stem from an underlying emotional problem. Eating may be a defense mechanism, a retreat from reality, or a defiant gesture used to get attention or sympathy. All of us have used food as a crutch when we were bored or lonely, and all of us have eating habits that border on overfeeding—doughnuts during coffee break, chips with TV, or late-night snacks. Eating and drinking are complex social behaviors, and others may view failure to participate as a social rebuff. The psychological and social causes of overeating are beyond the scope of this book, but eating behaviors are not. We dealt with ways to alter behavior in chapter 5.

Although some obese people suffer anxiety and depression, it isn't clear whether these reactions are a consequence of excess weight, of social and psychological treatment by others, or of problems related to dieting. In other words, emotional problems associated with obesity may be a cause or a result of excess weight, and some may be a consequence of the treatment, dieting.

Lack of Activity

At a symposium devoted to the causes and treatment of obesity, researchers concluded that the most likely factor contributing to the current epidemic of obesity is a continued decline in daily energy expenditure that has not been matched by an equivalent reduction in energy intake. Because daily energy expenditure is decreasing, and because most people do not restrict intake to meet lower energy requirements, more people are becoming obese (Hill and Melanson 1999). This outcome is true for adults and children.

It is amazing that Americans are not becoming an even more obese population than they already are. According to a study published in the *New England Journal of Medicine* in March 2000, the average annual weight gain in American adults under age 25 was approximately .5 to 1.5 pounds (.2–.7 kg). Between the ages of 25 and 44, the annual increase in weight jumped to 3.4 percent in men and 5.2 percent in women. This means that if a man and a woman who each weigh 160 pounds (73 kg) both gained weight at this rate, the man would gain a little more than 5 pounds (2 kg) each year and the woman would gain a little more than 8 pounds (3.6 kg) each year. For every 10 calories a day you store as fat, you will gain 1 pound (.5 kg) per year. Based on the average weight gain, this means that the average American adult is storing about 50 to 80 extra calories as fat each day, for males and females respectively. Currently, Americans eat 250 to 300 calories more each day than we ate on average between 1900 and 1950. Therefore, there is some evidence that our set-point metabolism has increased in an attempt to maintain a healthy weight, but it is unable to counteract our consumption or does not adjust enough to compensate for our energy imbalance. Some researchers have thus proposed that simply reducing diet or increasing physical activity by 50 to 80 calories a day will help people stabilize their weight. Some early encouraging data suggest that this works. Unfortunately, for those who are overweight, this is not enough change in energy balance to lose weight, improve health, or receive exercise health benefits, which start at about 150 to 300 calories of daily exercise.

Previously, researchers found that overweight children are less active than their thinner counterparts. Trained observers plotted the movements of fat and thin children while they engaged in games such as volleyball. The thin children ranged all over the court, whereas the heavyweights literally held down their positions (Mayer and Bullen 1974).

You may be wondering which comes first, inactivity or fat? The earlier section on fat cells answers part of that question (overfeeding), but we do know that people reduce their activity and range of movement as they become larger, not wishing to call attention to their size. When adult-onset obesity follows an active childhood, the overweight person is likely to be less inhibited and more active than one who became obese as a child. This leads to an urgent call to increase youth and adolescent physical activity.

Regardless of when inactivity starts, it leads to weight gain, which leads to further inactivity, which leads to more weight gain, and so on. The problem is to break this painful cycle and restore normal levels of activity and food intake. No time is too late to start. Active youth have a better chance of becoming active adults. Active parents are more likely to have active children.

We talked about energy balance, caloric intake versus caloric expenditure. Some research suggests we may need to refine that equation and focus specifically on fat balance. Unlike carbohydrate and protein stores, fat stores are not controlled, and their capacity for expansion is enormous (Swinburn and Ravussin 1993). We can view obesity as a long-standing positive fat balance, often the consequence of a high-fat diet, but always the result of a positive energy balance including excess carbohydrates and inactivity. The message is clear. Lower your dietary intake of saturated fat and trans-fatty acids (hydrogenated oils) and total caloric intake, and use physical activity to burn excess calories.

Dieting

Are you surprised that we list dieting as a contributor to obesity? How can dieting lead to overweight or obesity? When animals or humans gain weight, go on a diet, regain weight, diet, and so on—a process called weight cycling—the body becomes more fuel efficient, and the metabolic rate declines. Thereafter, the body needs more dieting or exercise to reduce excess weight. Weight loss slows, and weight is regained three times faster during the second cycle. Eventually, the body maintains weight on a reduced caloric intake that inhibits weight loss and promotes regaining (Brownell et al. 1986). In other words, the weight cycling, or yo-yo approach to weight control, leads to weight gain, not loss.

Every time you diet to lose weight, you lose lean tissue; therefore, you must further decrease caloric intake to avoid subsequent weight gain.

The reason for this weight gain is the loss of muscle protein with each cycle of dieting. Muscle is metabolically active; it is the furnace that burns excess calories. If you lose muscle, you have less ability to burn calories, at rest or during exercise. When you diet, the body turns to protein as an energy source, thereby reducing muscle mass. Every time you diet to lose weight, you lose lean tissue; therefore, you must further decrease caloric intake to avoid subsequent weight gain. If you return to past eating habits, you increase weight and fat above previous levels. Exercise is the only way to minimize the loss of lean tissue while dieting. In fact, if you do enough exercise, you can reverse the drop in metabolic rate and increase lean tissue, thereby easing the problem of weight control.

MEASURING BODY FAT

At the University of Montana in the 1970s, college-aged men averaged 12.5 to 15 percent fat and college women averaged about 25 percent. In 2010, those averages had risen to 14 to 20 percent for males and 24 to 30 percent for females. These increases reflect what is happening across America. The standard method for determining percentage of body fat is **hydrostatic (underwater) weighing**. The subject is weighed both in air and while submerged in water. After making appropriate adjustments for air in the lungs and gas in the gastrointestinal tract, body density is determined.

$$\frac{\text{weight in air}}{\text{weight in air} - \text{weight in water}}$$

Because fat is less dense than bone or muscle, we can calculate the percentage of body fat. As the percentage of body fat goes up, the weight in water goes down, and vice versa. Thus, lean people sink and fat people float because fat weighs less than muscle per unit of volume.

A less accurate but serviceable method for the estimation of percentage body fat uses skinfold calipers. The skinfold calculation of body fat is based on the relationship of subcutaneous (under the skin) fat to total body fat. About one-third of the fat in the body may be located just under the skin, and the rest is around internal organs, around nerves as insulation, and in all cells, including muscle. To perform the skinfold measurements, grasp skinfolds between the thumb and forefinger and then apply calipers about .5 inch (1.3 cm) from the fingers. Take the measurement, release, repeat the measurement, and continue until your measurement is consistent. Use chest, abdomen, and thigh skinfolds for males, and use triceps, thigh, and suprailium skinfolds for females (see figure 13.3).

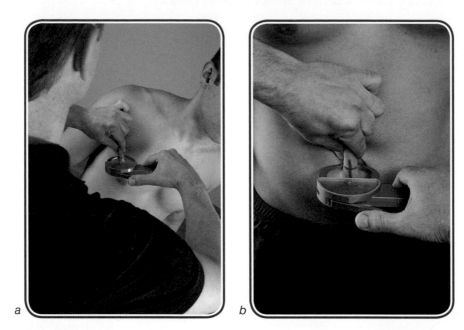

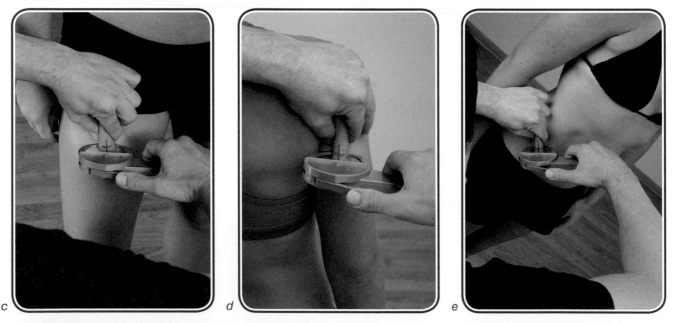

FIGURE 13.3 Sites for estimation of body fat: *(a)* chest: a diagonal fold taken halfway between the shoulder crease and the nipple, *(b)* abdomen: a vertical fold taken 1 inch (2.5 cm) to the right of the umbilicus, *(c)* thigh: a vertical fold taken on the front of the thigh halfway between the knee and the hip crease, *(d)* triceps: a vertical fold taken on the back medial aspect of the triceps (back of the upper arm) midway between the shoulder and the elbow, *(e)* suprailium: a diagonal fold measured above the crest of the ilium on the side of the hip. Males use *a*, *b*, and *c*. Females use *c*, *d*, and *e*.

Several carefully selected skinfold sites provide an estimate of body fat (use figure 13.4 to calculate the percentage of fat). Inexpensive but accurate skinfold calipers are available from several sources (e.g., www.fitnessmart.com and many other locations).

Other methods used to determine body fat range from girth or other body measurements to expensive laboratory techniques. Many health clubs use a **bioelectric impedance** technique that estimates fat from body water content. The technique, based on the fixed amount of water in fat, requires strict adherence to hydration standards to achieve acceptable accuracy. Some labs now use an air displacement technique, such as the Bod Pod, to determine body fat. Scientists use the potassium-40 emitted from lean tissue, or sophisticated imaging techniques such as CAT scans and MRI to measure fat. New methods of estimating fat are often compared with underwater weighing to see whether they are

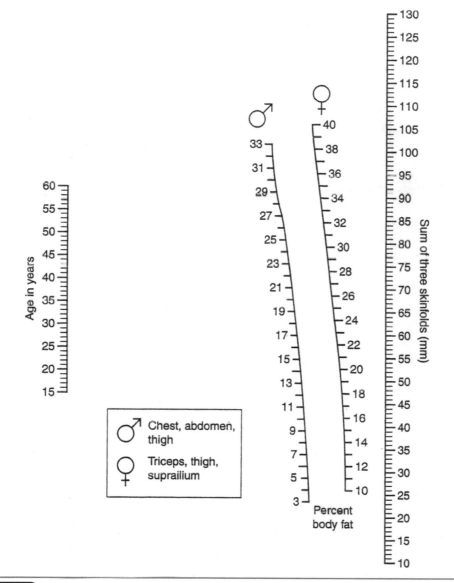

FIGURE 13.4 A nomogram for the estimate of percent body fat for both male and female populations, using age and the sum of three skinfolds. Use a straight edge to draw a line from your age to the sum of the three skinfolds, and read your percent fat from the appropriate scale.

Reprinted with permission from *Research Quarterly for Exercise and Sport*, Vol. 52, pp. 382, Copyright 1981 by the American Alliance for Health, Physical Education, Recreation and Dance, 1900 Association Drive, Reston, VA 20191.

accurate. Studies indicate, however, that underwater weighing itself is subject to errors, especially with younger and older subjects and those at the extremes of leanness and fatness (Going 1996). Age-related differences in body water and bone density can throw off this method, as can dehydration or estimating the air remaining in the lung (**residual lung volume**). However, underwater weighing, when coupled with a measurement of residual lung volume is within ± 1.5 percent of actual fat percentage in the majority of people aged 16 to 65 with BMI values of 19 to 35kg/m².

IDEAL BODY WEIGHT

Is there such a thing as an ideal body weight or an ideal amount of body fat? Should one strive to reduce body fat to the minimum? The minimum amount of fat consistent with good health and nutrition is around 6 to 7 percent for young men and 11 to 12 percent for young women. Healthy high school wrestlers and male distance runners may have a bit less than 5 percent, but only during a few days of competition. Female distance runners have had a temporary low of 7 percent. These figures do not suggest, however, that all men and women should attempt to achieve those levels. We offer them only to indicate the minimum level consistent with health and performance. Studies show that weight shouldn't regularly fall more than 10 percent below the desirable weight. The upper limit consistent with good health probably approaches 20 percent above the desirable weight.

Somewhere between the extremes (minus 10% to plus 20% of desirable weight) lies a level that is best for you. The level you choose will relate to your current activity and interests. If you are training for a long-distance race, you'll want to minimize your weight handicap. If you've been burdened with a large number of fat cells, you may be doing well to keep the level below 20 percent. Data indicate that those who weigh less than the desirable body weight for their height and frame live longer than those who weigh more. Because desirable weights are based on average values of body fat, maintaining body weight and body fat at or below desirable weight or average fat levels seem advisable. But in the absence of heart disease,

Optimal Weight: A Practical Approach

Some believe that U.S. weight guidelines are too lax, encouraging obesity in both men and women. The researchers found that 40 percent of all heart attacks in middle-aged women were due to overweight, a figure similar to that found in men. Women of average (not desirable) weight had a 50 percent higher risk of heart attack than those 15 percent below the average U.S. weight. Also, gaining more than 10 pounds (4.5 kg) in early to middle adult life increased the risk (Manson et al. 1995). Based on this study, we can estimate optimal weight as follows:

- Women—100 pounds (45.4 kg) for 5 feet (60 in., or 152.4 cm) plus 5 pounds (2.3 kg) for each additional inch (or every 2.5 cm). For example, the optimal weight for a woman 5 feet, 6 inches (167.6 cm) tall is 100 + (5 × 6), or 130 pounds (59.0 kg).

- Men—106 pounds (48.1 kg) for 5 feet, plus 6 pounds (2.7 kg) for each additional inch (2.5 cm). For example, the optimal weight for a man 5 feet, 10 inches (177.8 cm) tall is 106 + (6 × 10), or 166 pounds (75.3 kg).

Your estimated optimal weight should be within ± 10 percent of the calculated weight. For example, the 166-pound (75 kg) male range would be (166 – 16.6) to (166+16.6) or 149.4 to 182.6 pounds (68–83 kg).

hypertension, or diabetes, little health difference occurs between the extremes of 5 percent and 20 percent body fat for men, or between 12 percent and 30 percent body fat for women. Suggested desirable weights are shown in table 13.1 on page 309, and in the highlight box on this page.

Sex-Specific Fat

Some of the fat differences between males and females are due to sex-specific fat. Female hormones dictate different patterns of fat deposition, including breasts, which are largely fat. But only a portion of the difference, perhaps an extra 6 percent, is due to sex-specific fat. The rest is probably because of lack of activity or excess caloric intake or both. That circumstance is changing, however, as more women undertake the active life. Active college-age women average 18 to 22 percent fat, and female endurance athletes are often in the range of 12 to 17 percent fat (Sharkey 1984).

Age and Body Fat

With each decade above age 25, the body loses about 4 percent of its metabolically active cells. If diet remains relatively unchanged during a 10-year period, a person will gain weight because total energy expenditure declines. To maintain a desirable weight, the adult should either exercise more or eat less. People who can claim that their weight has not changed since college deserve congratulations. But they should also know that the loss of metabolically active cells with age usually means a decline in lean body weight, including muscle (Piers et al. 1998). Therefore, maintenance of body weight usually indicates an increase in the percentage of body fat.

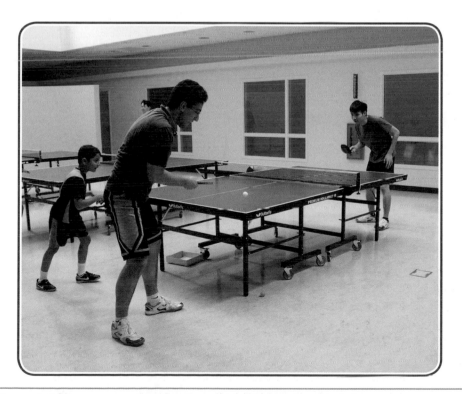

■ Regular activity can counteract a slowing metabolism and maintain lean tissue as you age.

Seasonal Fluctuation

Body weight and body fat fluctuate from season to season and year to year. Typically, lean body weight (body weight minus fat weight) does not change as rapidly. Lean body weight consists mainly of muscles, bones, and organs. Thus, seasonal changes in body weight result from differences in the amount of fat being stored in adipose tissue. Total body fat storage often is higher during winter months, when subcutaneous fat serves as insulation against the cold. In summer, weight and fat often decline in response to an increase in energy expenditure and a decrease in appetite (stimulated in part by the increase in daylight).

ACTIVITY AND WEIGHT CONTROL

The only way to remove stored fat is to burn it off. By now, you know that exercise increases caloric expenditure and that energy expenditure is related to both the intensity and the duration of activity. As exercise becomes more intense, the duration of participation must necessarily become shorter. Although we may be able to expend as many as 125 calories in a fast mile (1.6 km) run, we can walk briskly or jog at a comfortable pace for 3 miles (4.8 km) and triple the caloric expenditure without becoming exhausted. This notion explains why we recommend moderate activity instead of high-intensity effort for weight control. The relationship of exercise to caloric expenditure also helps explain why the benefits grow with improved fitness. More fitness allows more activity, and therefore more control over your weight.

The effects of exercise do not stop when the exercise ceases. The excess postexercise oxygen consumption (EPOC), the amount that exceeds the resting level after exercise, indicates a prolonged postexercise elevation in caloric expenditure. Caloric expenditure can remain elevated for 30 minutes or more after vigorous exercise. Long-duration effort such as a distance run will elevate oxygen consumption and body temperature and call forth hormones to mobilize energy and increase metabolism. When the exercise stops, caloric expenditure remains elevated above resting levels during the recovery period. The EPOC is often neglected when the caloric benefits of exercise are tabulated.

Exercise Versus Dieting

Some people believe that dieting is better than exercise for controlling weight. They point out, quite correctly, that it is easier to reduce caloric intake by refusing a piece of cake (250 cal) than it is to burn off the cake after eating it, which would require jogging more than 2 miles (3.2 km) at 110 calories per mile. But let's examine the question of whether dieting is a better method of weight control. The answer has been available for over 35 years, and the answer is no.

Is dieting a better method of weight control? The answer has been available for over 35 years, and the answer is no.

Oscai and Holloszy (1969) compared the effects of dieting and exercise on the body composition of laboratory rats. They controlled the experiment so that both groups lost the same amount of weight. Following 18 weeks of either food restriction (dieting) or swimming (exercise), they performed carcass analysis. The analysis indicated that exercise was a more effective way to lose fat (78% of the total weight loss for the exercising group versus 62% for the dieting group). Furthermore, the study provided vivid evidence of the protein-conserving effects of exercise, 5 percent protein loss for exercisers versus 11 percent for dieters. The amount of water lost through caloric restriction was 16 percent for exercisers versus 26 percent for dieters. A control group of sedentary, freely eating animals gained weight during the study. Their weight gain consisted of 87 percent fat and 10 percent water.

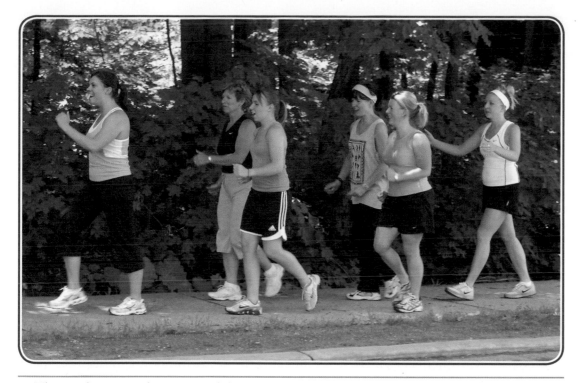

■ The combination of exercise and dieting burns more fat and retains more lean tissue than dieting alone.

The results of the previous animal study have been confirmed in a number of human studies. A famous study at the University of Minnesota, "The Semi-Starvation Study" confirmed that initial weight loss in sedentary dieters is due primarily to water loss, with loss of lean muscle and fat contributing to later weight loss when the dietary restrictions are extreme. Water loss, a common occurrence among dieters, accounts for the early success of most fad diets and the eventual failure of the overall goal, fat loss.

A study involving 16 obese patients compared a period of 6 months of dieting with a similar period of dieting and exercise. The exercise group achieved greater fat loss, and the exercise produced other benefits, including a lower resting heart rate and improved heart rate recovery after exercise (Kenrick, Ball, and Canary 1972). And when 25 women created a deficit of 500 calories per day by dieting, exercise, or a combination of the two, all the women lost the same amount of weight, but those in the dieting group lost less fat and more lean tissue. The authors of the study (Zuti and Golding 1976) recommended that those interested in losing weight combine dieting and exercise to ensure greater fat loss and conservation of lean tissue. A study of 24 obese women confirms the superiority of diet and exercise for the reduction of adipose tissue and preservation of lean tissue (skeletal muscle), as compared with diet alone (Ross, Pedwell, and Rissanen 1995).

These studies clearly indicate the need for activity in a program of weight control. Dieting or caloric restriction can lead to loss of weight, but a loss of protein (lean tissue) and water accompanies the weight loss. When the body loses lean tissue, it becomes less able to burn calories and eventually gains more fat weight. Dietary weight loss leads to a disproportionate decline in the metabolic rate and almost certain future weight gain (Leibel, Rosenbaum, and Hirsch 1995). A complication in the loss of lean tissue is a possible resetting

Exercise and dieting combine to provide a positive attack on both causes of overweight: inadequate caloric expenditure and excess caloric intake.

Metabolic Rate

Exercise has an added benefit in relation to weight control and diet. In one study, several weeks of severe caloric restriction imposed by dieting led to the usual loss of lean tissue and a decrease in metabolic rate. The drop in metabolic rate makes it difficult for dieters to maintain a lower body weight because the more efficient body burns 10 to 15 percent fewer calories daily. On the bright side, however, just 2 weeks of exercise restored the metabolic rate to predicted levels. Moreover, the exercise reduced the loss of protein and increased the use of fat as the source of energy (Móle et al. 1989).

of the metabolic thermostat, making weight gain likely with even less caloric intake. Four decades of research show that weight loss with exercise maximizes the removal of fat, minimizes the loss of protein, and helps maintain the metabolic rate. Exercise and dieting combine to provide a positive attack on both causes of overweight: inadequate caloric expenditure and excess caloric intake.

Exercise and Appetite

In the past, the use of activity to achieve energy balance and weight control received criticism. Detractors argued that exercise would increase the appetite as the body attempted to keep pace with energy needs. Many assume that the desire for food signifies a real need for nourishment, but it doesn't. Appetite is a psychological desire that is influenced by several factors. The control center for food intake, the **appestat**, is located in the hypothalamus, an area of the brain that functions like a thermostat to turn on eating behavior and then turn it off when the desire or hunger has been satisfied. Unfortunately, it takes many minutes for the food that you eat to reach the bloodstream, where the appestat can see that you've satisfied the need. You may tuck away several hundred extra calories before the appestat gets the message.

Physiological factors such as low blood sugar, hormones, hours of daylight, cold temperatures, hunger pangs from an empty stomach, and unfilled fat cells can stimulate the appestat. Physical activity also stimulates eating behavior, but the increased caloric intake serves only to maintain body weight. Sedentary people take in more calories than they need. More exercise means more food intake, but the appetite doesn't keep pace with energy output. Regular activity seems to help the appestat adjust caloric intake to energy needs. The appestat is rather imprecise at a low level of energy expenditure, but for regularly active people, appetite control is much more related to energy requirements (Mayer and Bullen 1974). An exercise study with obese women cycling at 50 percent of $\dot{V}O_2$max found that 25 of 28 participants ate less during the 12-week program and continued to eat less during a 10-week follow-up (Vailodash 2000). At the high end of the activity scale, where endurance athletes and workers burn 4,000 to 6,000 calories daily in running, cycling, swimming, or work, the appetite usually underestimates energy needs (Ruby, Schoeller, and Sharkey 2001). Conversely, when a sedentary routine is imposed on otherwise active men, no reduction in energy intake occurs, leading to a positive energy balance (Stubbs et al. 2004).

Psychological factors such as the smell, sight, or taste of food can evoke the desire to eat. Habit and emotional factors also condition eating behavior. Television and screen activities are often associated with eating. Sedentary habits often lead to snacking. Have you ever noticed the snack jars on the desks of office workers? While sitting at your computer, have you ever gotten the urge to eat? We eat to celebrate, to prolong feelings of excitement. Appetite is a complex phenomenon, subject to many influences, reflecting more than the need for nourishment. The appestat frequently overestimates energy needs. Weight

Premeal or Postmeal Exercise

Years ago, when the American diet was first implicated as a culprit in the heart disease epidemic, researchers roamed the world studying the relationship between diet and the incidence of heart disease. They found that diet alone did not account for the presence or absence of the problem; other factors such as a lack of tension and stress or physical activity confounded the relationship. Several researchers have focused on the effect of pre- or postmeal exercise on **postprandial lipemia**, the presence of fat in the blood after a meal. Studies conducted at the University of Florida have shown that exercise before or after a meal is effective in reducing the magnitude and duration of postprandial lipemia (Zauner, Burt, and Mapes 1968). Light exercise proved to be as effective as strenuous effort in this regard. A study on females confirms the ability of prior exercise to increase the utilization of dietary fat (Votruba et al. 2002). Research also indicates that the effect of exercise on postprandial lipemia is greater than and different from the effect attributable to a comparable caloric deficit. A 90-minute walk reduced postprandial lipemia 20 percent below control levels, whereas caloric restriction reduced it only 7 percent (Gill and Hardman 2000).

Lipemia has long been associated with atherosclerosis, reduced myocardial (heart) blood flow, and accelerated blood clotting. Thus, anything that reduces the level of fat in the blood seems prudent and advisable. Vigorous premeal exercise may inhibit the appetite and increase the metabolism of fat and all foods ingested after the exercise. The metabolic rate remains somewhat elevated after exercise, and the ingested foods are used quickly to restore energy burned during exercise. Mild postmeal effort, such as a walk after dinner, also serves to reduce lipemia. Both pre- and postmeal exercise increase caloric expenditure and fat metabolism, lead to improved fitness, and contribute to health and weight control.

While we're on the subject of meals and blood lipids, you should know that the number of meals that you eat influences blood fat levels. By spreading the same number of calories over more meals (three to six), you will lower your cholesterol levels. Apparently, we are able to handle fat better in smaller doses. Conversely, if you avoid meals in an effort to lose weight, your metabolic rate will decline and your cholesterol level will climb. Rapid weight gain may follow your temporary weight loss.

control becomes possible when you realize that your eyes are bigger than your stomach and that your potential for energy intake is greater than your regular energy expenditure.

Increased Caloric Expenditure

Because unfit people tire quickly during exercise, they have limited ability to expend calories. As fitness improves, caloric expenditure rises, with increases in the frequency and duration, and, as one becomes more fit, with intensity of exercise. Becoming more fit is often associated with the inevitable participation in activities that are more vigorous but no longer feel difficult. The fit person does more with less fatigue. Increased fitness undoubtedly contributes to energy expenditure and weight control.

We have studied the effects of training on the perception of effort and fatigue (Docktor and Sharkey 1971). Other studies also confirm the beneficial effects of training on one's perception of effort (Gaskill et al. 2005). As fitness improves, a person can perform more work at the same heart rate and level of perceived exertion. Work levels once perceived as difficult become less so, and once-fatiguing exertion can be managed with ease. After training, a person can accomplish a given task with a lower heart rate as well as a lower level of perceived exertion. Thus, subjects can burn more energy without experiencing a greater sense of fatigue.

A great definition of physical fitness is the ability to perform the necessary tasks of daily living and still have energy for leisure activities at the end of the day. Becoming more physically active and fit will improve your cognition. It will help you perform better during the day at work or school, stay alert, and have the energy to get out for a walk, a run, or a social engagement.

Further proof of the value of fitness to caloric expenditure is found in the relationship of caloric expenditure to heart rate. Caloric expenditure is related directly to heart rate, but level of fitness also influences the relationship. For people in low-fitness categories, a high heart rate does not indicate extremely high caloric expenditure (see figure 13.5). For those in high-fitness categories, the same heart rate (HR) indicates much higher energy expenditure:

140 HR for very poor fitness level = 6 to 7 calories per minute expended

140 HR for very good fitness level = 12 calories per minute expended

You can use figure 13.5 to estimate your caloric expenditure in any activity. After several minutes of participation, stop and immediately take your pulse at the wrist or throat (use

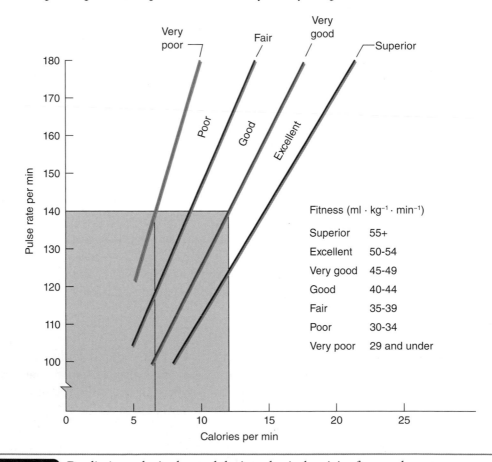

FIGURE 13.5 Predicting calories burned during physical activity from pulse rate.

Reprinted from B.J. Sharkey, 1974, *Physiological fitness and weight control* (Missoula, MT: Mountain Press), 130. By permission of B.J. Sharkey.

gentle contact) for 15 seconds. Multiply by 4 to get your rate per minute. Then use the line corresponding to your fitness level to estimate your caloric expenditure per minute. Notice how caloric expenditure improves (at the same heart rate) as your fitness improves. This finding should convince you that fitness provides extra benefits to those who persevere.

Increased Fat Mobilization

Fat is stored in fat cells in the form of triglycerides (3 molecules of fatty acid and 1 molecule of glycerol). A triglyceride molecule is too large to pass through the wall of the fat cell into the circulation, so when energy is needed, the triglyceride is broken down. The fatty-acid molecules pass into the blood for transport to the working muscles. The hormone epinephrine stimulates a receptor in the fat cell membrane and activates the enzyme **lipase**. Lipase splits the triglyceride molecule, and the fatty acids are free to enter the circulation.

As exercise becomes more intense, we produce lactic acid. The point at which lactic acid begins to accumulate in the blood, the second lactate threshold, indicates when lactate production exceeds removal. At this intensity, a significant portion of energy for metabolism is derived from carbohydrate. You will recall that the second lactate threshold is related to activity and fitness. It may be below 50 percent of the maximal oxygen uptake for the unfit and above 80 percent for the highly trained. But what does that have to do with fat?

Years ago, researchers discovered that lactic acid seemed to inhibit the mobilization of free fatty acids (FFAs) from adipose tissue (see figure 8.4, page 163). The lactic acid blocked the action of epinephrine, thereby reducing the availability of fat for muscle metabolism (Issekutz and Miller 1962). One of the best-documented effects of training is that more work can be accomplished before lactic acid levels rise. After improving fitness, a person who formerly produced lactic acid at a given workload can accomplish the same workload with little increase in lactic acid. This result may be because of a decrease in lactic acid production or an increase in lactic acid clearance. Whatever the case, improved aerobic fitness allows a person to accomplish more work aerobically. The lactate threshold increases, and more fat is available for use as an energy source.

A study of trained subjects illustrates that moderate levels of lactic acid do not affect FFA mobilization and utilization (Vega deJesus and Siconolfi 1988). The fit subjects were able to mobilize fat at the second lactate threshold (4 millimoles lactic acid), which defines the highest

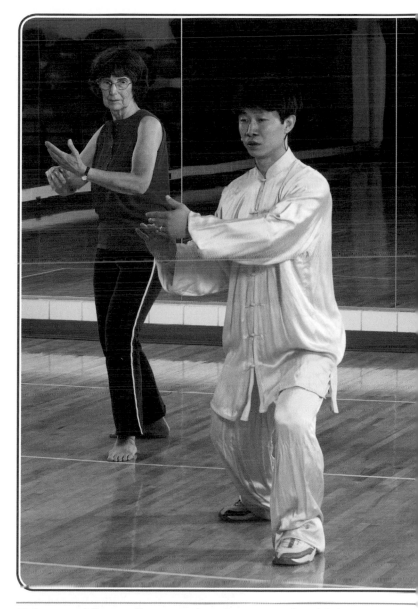

■ Improved fitness allows people to burn more fat with less perceived exertion.

level of exercise intensity that a person can sustain during prolonged exertion. These findings help explain the tremendous increase in endurance associated with training. Fat is the most abundant energy source (50 times more abundant than carbohydrate). Improved fitness allows greater access to that immense storehouse of energy.

Greater Fat Utilization

The mobilization of fat does not ensure its metabolism. How does training influence the utilization of FFA as a source of energy for muscular contractions? Studies have shown that trained animals and humans are capable of extracting a greater percentage of their energy from FFA during submaximal exercise. How, then, does fitness influence fat utilization?

Móle, Oscai, and Holloszy (1971) provided convincing proof of the effect of training on FFA utilization. They found that the ability of rat muscle to oxidize the fatty acid palmitate doubled following 12 weeks of treadmill training. The authors suggested that the shift to fat metabolism was a key factor in the development of endurance fitness and an important mechanism serving to spare carbohydrate stores and prevent low blood sugar during prolonged exertion. Thus, the physically fit person can derive a greater percentage of energy requirements from fat than the unfit subject can. At a given workload, fit subjects may obtain as much as 90 percent of their energy from fat. Free fatty acids are used during all forms of muscular activity, except for all-out bursts of effort, such as the 100-yard dash. Training even seems to improve the ability of the heart muscle to oxidize fat (Keul 1971).

When exercise begins, the initial source of energy from fat is from intramuscular fat, a supply that is enhanced with training. When prolonged activity depletes intramuscular fat, the body uses fat that comes from adipose tissue by way of the blood (Coggan and Williams 1995). Improved fitness increases the availability of fat through mobilization of FFAs, as well as from an increase in enzyme activity. Both contribute to the rate of FFA utilization.

Lactic Acid

Lactic acid is produced when the breakdown of muscle glycogen to pyruvic acid exceeds the ability of the mitochondria to process the pyruvate. So, the pyruvic acid picks up hydrogen, becomes lactic acid, and begins to accumulate in the muscle and blood. The heart and skeletal muscle can use lactate as a source of energy, and the liver can oxidize it. But when the production of lactate exceeds its removal, the acid level in muscle and blood increases. The rising level of acid in the muscle reduces force production by interfering with muscle contractions and decreases endurance by lowering the efficiency of aerobic enzymes.

Reduced Blood Lipids

Blood lipids—cholesterol and triglycerides—have been associated with the incidence and severity of coronary heart disease. They are related to other risk factors, including diet, overweight, and lack of exercise. Findings suggest that fitness training also influences the lipids.

Triglycerides

Dietary fat intake shows up in the blood as chylomicrons, large clumps of triglycerides. Most of the triglycerides are removed from the plasma in the capillaries adjacent to muscle and adipose tissue. The liver clears any remains from the circulation. Chylomicrons are responsible for the milky appearance of blood plasma following a meal (postprandial lipemia). Besides containing 80 to 95 percent triglyceride, chylomicrons contain 2 to 7 percent cholesterol, 3 to 6 percent phospholipid, and 1 to 2 percent protein.

Dieting or participation in regular physical activity can reduce fasting serum triglyceride levels. The exercise-induced reduction occurs several hours afterward and lasts for about 2 days. With regular exercise, further reductions occur until subjects reach a lower level consistent with their exercise, diet, and other factors, including inherited blood lipid patterns.

Earlier in this chapter, we established the influence of

Maximal Fat Oxidation

To determine when **maximal fat oxidation** occurred during exercise, moderately trained subjects were exercised on a progressive laboratory bicycle test. Fat oxidation peaked at 55 to 72 percent of VO_2max, or 68 to 79 percent of maximal heart rate, values higher than those previously noted (Achten, Gleeson, and Jeukendrup 2002). This study, performed after subjects fasted for 10 hours, shows that fat can be a significant source of energy for rather vigorous exercise. Ingesting carbohydrate before performing exercise lowers the contribution of fat to energy expenditure. So, if your goal is oxidation of fat, exercise before breakfast or other meals. However, as mentioned earlier, if your goal is to burn more calories, you will need to find an intensity that you can sustain for a long period of time. As you become more fit, you may find joy in being able to jog or run at your second lactate threshold for an hour or more.

exercise on postmeal fat in blood. The research supports the hypothesis that regular exercise enhances the removal and utilization of triglyceride by muscle cells, rather than allowing their deposit in adipose tissue or processing by the liver, possibly to synthesize more cholesterol.

A researcher trained sedentary rats for 12 weeks on a treadmill. Following the training, the muscles were analyzed for the activity of lipoprotein lipase (LPL), the enzyme responsible for the uptake of plasma triglyceride fatty acids (TGFA) from plasma chylomicrons and other sources in the blood. The researcher reasoned that an increase in LPL activity would accompany any increase in the uptake of TGFA by skeletal muscle during exercise. The results of the study confirmed the hypothesis. Regular endurance training led to a two- to fourfold increase in LPL activity, indicating that training increases the capacity of muscle fibers to take up and oxidize fatty acids originating in plasma triglycerides (Borensztajn 1975).

Because the fat is used before it can be deposited in adipose tissue, these findings have tremendous significance in the area of weight control. The implications for cardiovascular health are even more exciting, as is the realization that these benefits are associated with an entirely natural, enjoyable, and satisfying experience—aerobic training.

Cholesterol

Cholesterol ingested in the diet is absorbed in the small intestine, finds its way into the lymph system, and then is dumped into the blood. There it joins cholesterol produced by the body in the chylomicrons and in very-low-density lipoprotein particles (VLDL). Once in the plasma, the same enzymes that act on the chylomicrons attack the VLDL. Much of the triglyceride is removed (within 2 to 6 hours). The VLDL is degraded to low-density lipoprotein (LDL), which the liver removes over a period of 2 to 5 days. Because of the smaller size of the LDL particle and its high concentration of cholesterol, the LDL particle seems to be involved directly in the development of coronary artery disease (CAD). The LDL particles find their way into coronary arteries and contribute to the growth of atherosclerotic plaques. Thus, LDL is believed to be a major culprit in the development of coronary artery disease.

Until the mid-1970s, diet, weight loss, and drugs were believed to be the major weapons in the fight against cholesterol. Studies on the effect of exercise on cholesterol typically reported a modest reduction, but only when the exercise was vigorous and of long duration; for example, 3 or more miles (4.8 km or more) of running per day. But remember that the blood transports cholesterol in several ways. A single measure of serum cholesterol does not indicate how the cholesterol is distributed among the several lipoprotein fractions, nor does it indicate the effects of exercise.

Dr. Wood (1975) of the Stanford Heart Disease Prevention Program compared the lipoprotein patterns of sedentary and active middle-aged men (35 to 59 years old). The active group consisted of joggers who averaged at least 15 miles (24.1 km) per week for the preceding year. As expected, the triglycerides were "strikingly" lower for the active group, while total cholesterol was only "modestly" lower. But when the lipoprotein pattern was analyzed, the joggers exhibited a significantly lower level of dangerous LDL and an elevated level of high-density lipoprotein (HDL). These findings were significant, because there is a direct relationship between LDL and heart disease and an inverse relationship between HDL and heart disease (as HDL goes up, the incidence of heart disease goes down). HDL seems to carry cholesterol away from the tissues for removal by the liver. Dr. Wood noted that the lipoprotein pattern of the active men was similar to that of young women, who have the lowest risk of heart disease in the adult population. Evidence on raising HDL with drug therapy shows that this process also fails to reduce CAD risk. This suggests that physical activity and diet related to increased HDL levels may cause the reduced risk of heart disease, not the increase in HDL cholesterol (Voight et al. 2012).

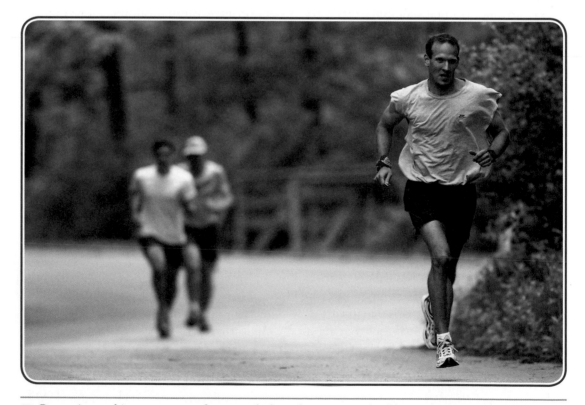

■ Get active and improve your fitness to help reduce your risk of heart disease.

When researchers studied the effects of 7 weeks of training on the serum lipids and lipoproteins of medical students, triglycerides fell by 27 percent. Furthermore, they found a marked reduction of LDL and VLDL cholesterol, an increase in HDL cholesterol, and no changes in body weight to confuse the results (Lopez et al. 1974). Studies in our lab (Sharkey et al. 1980) agree with those reported by Dr. Wood and many others (Leon et al. 2002). They indicate how training helps shift cholesterol from the dangerous LDL to the favorable HDL and how activity and fitness help reduce the risk of coronary artery disease.

Leptin

Leptin, a hormone produced by fat cells, helps regulate body weight and metabolism. Named after the Greek word *leptos*, which means thin, leptin influences hunger, feeding behavior, body temperature, and energy expenditure. Leptin stimulates lipid metabolism and increases energy expenditure, and it may limit excess energy storage. Leptin levels are correlated to the amount of fat stored in the body, although not all obese people have increased levels. Studies indicate that exercise lasting 1 hour or more reduces serum-leptin concentrations (Hulver and Houmar 2003). Exercise, diet, and sleep influence leptin levels. High-fat diets reduce the stimulatory effect of leptin on fatty-acid metabolism in skeletal muscle (Steinberg 2003). Sleep restriction is associated with decreased leptin levels, increased hunger, and greater appetite (Spiegel et al. 2004). Over the past 40 years, self-reported sleep duration in the United States has decreased 2 hours per night. Does lack of sleep contribute to overweight?

How's that for an extra benefit of fitness? Fitness not only allows increased caloric expenditure and enhanced fat utilization, but also directly affects the blood lipids and reduces risk of heart disease. In our view, this effect is one of the most important benefits of exercise and fitness. If all this doesn't convince you to become active and improve your aerobic fitness, well, we'll just have to keep trying. For example, evidence indicates that it may be possible to lower serum cholesterol levels enough to reverse the process of atherosclerosis, removing fatty buildup from the lining of the coronary arteries (Ornish 1993). If it proves to be true that diet and exercise, perhaps with the help of drug therapy, can accomplish this reversal, it will be possible to prevent or cure, not just treat, many cases of the nation's number-one killer.

Increased Lean Tissue

Finally, let us remind you that muscle is the furnace that burns fat. Whereas dieting leads to loss of muscle, a lower metabolic rate, and reduced ability to exercise and burn fat, fitness training has the capacity to maintain or increase muscle mass and to burn more calories and more fat. Aerobic training such as running leads to a small increase in lean body weight. Training with more resistance, such as in cycling, can cause more noticeable changes in muscle. And, of course, muscular fitness (resistance) training leads to impressive changes in muscle mass. Fortunately, activity and training can rapidly reclaim muscle lost in dieting.

Whereas aerobic exercise doesn't have a great effect on the resting metabolic rate, resistance training has been shown to increase strength and metabolic rate and maintain metabolically active tissue in older adults (Campbell et al. 1994). It has been established that for every pound (.45 kg) of muscle that is added, basal metabolic rate increases by about 10 calories a day, which is about the equivalent of 1 pound of fat per year. Moreover, resistance training lowers visceral fat, the fat associated with a higher risk of heart disease (Treuth, Hunter, and Kekes-Szabo 1995).

The National Weight Control Registry

The National Weight Control Registry (NWCR), established in 1994 by Rena Wing, PhD from Brown Medical School, and James O. Hill, PhD from the University of Colorado, is the largest prospective investigation of long-term successful weight-loss maintenance. The NWCR identifies and investigates the characteristics of people who have succeeded at long-term weight loss. It is tracking more than 10,000 people who have lost significant amounts of weight and have kept it off for long periods of time. Detailed questionnaires and annual follow-up surveys examine the behavioral and psychological characteristics of these subjects, as well as the strategies they use to maintain their weight losses. The NWCR website is a wonderful source of information about what real people are doing for weight loss. We encourage you to visit the site to read individual stories and review their data summaries at www.nwcr.ws/default.htm. Some of their findings include the following:

- Registry members have lost an average of 66 pounds (30 kg) and have kept it off for 5.5 years.
- Weight losses have ranged from 30 to 300 pounds (13.6–136 kg).

- Some have lost the weight rapidly, while others have lost weight very slowly, over as many as 14 years.
- 45 percent of registry participants lost the weight on their own, and the other 55 percent lost weight with the help of some type of program.
- 98 percent of registry participants report that they modified their food intake in some way to lose weight.
- 94 percent increased their physical activity, and walking is the most frequently reported form of activity.
- Most registry participants report continuing to maintain a low-calorie, low-fat diet and doing high levels of activity.
- 90 percent exercise, on average, about 1 hour per day.
- 62 percent watch less than 10 hours of TV per week.
- 78 percent eat breakfast every day.
- 75 percent weigh themselves at least once a week.

If you have lost significant weight and kept it off, we encourage you to join the registry.

EXERCISE PRESCRIPTION FOR WEIGHT CONTROL

Some types of exercise are better than others for weight control. As you know, we gradually shift from fat to carbohydrate metabolism as exercise becomes more vigorous. If you want to burn excess fat, consider light to moderate exercise (see table 13.2). Because you cannot sustain extremely vigorous activity for long, total caloric expenditure may not be great. In addition, fat utilization increases over time, with more fat being burned after 30 minutes of exercise. You can continue light to moderate activity for hours without undue fatigue, thereby allowing significant fat metabolism and caloric expenditure.

Incidentally, while we are on the subject of fat metabolism, the best time to exercise for weight control may be in the morning, before breakfast, when you are more likely to burn fat after an overnight fast. So, if you are interested in fat metabolism and weight control, try morning exercise. If that approach doesn't suit your biological clock, don't despair. Exercise always burns calories, so it always contributes to weight control.

Table 13.2 Physical Activity and Caloric Expenditure

Work intensity	Pulse rate (beats/min)	Expenditure (cal/min)	Examples
Light*	Below 90	2–3	Slow walking (<3 mph)
Moderate*	90–130	3–5	Golf, bowling, brisk walking, volleyball, most light physical work
Vigorous	130–150	5–10	Jogging, tennis, bike riding, basketball, racquetball, strenuous physical work
Heavy	Above 150	Above 10	Running; fast swimming; other brief, intense efforts

*Light to moderate activity is preferred for weight control, so long as it is continued for a sufficient time (e.g., 300 or more calories).

Adapted from B.J. Sharkey, 1974, *Physiological fitness and weight control* (Missoula, MT: Mountain Press), 28. By permission of B.J. Sharkey.

Sources: Ainsworth et al. 1993; Consolazio, Johnson, and Pecora 1963; Passmore and Durnin 1955; Roth 1968; Unpublished data from the Human Performance Laboratory, University of Montana 1964-2005.

Your weight-control program should include both aerobic training and muscular fitness training. The aerobic fitness prescription for weight loss or weight control maximizes caloric expenditure (duration) at the expense of exercise intensity. You should extend exercise duration to increase caloric expenditure, and you should increase both duration and frequency of exercise to achieve the maximal benefit of exercise. Thus, if your fitness prescription suggests 100 to 200 calories of exercise several days per week, you should try to work at the low edge of your training zone (intensity) and increase the caloric expenditure (duration). Also, increase the frequency to daily or twice daily, if possible, and add supplemental activities. The addition of moderate exercise to a caloric restriction (diet) program provides advantages in fat utilization, fat loss, and caloric expenditure, even for obese people (Kempen, Saris, and Westerterp 1995).

The muscular fitness portion of the weight-control program is aimed at maintaining or increasing lean body weight (muscle) and maintaining or increasing the resting metabolic rate (Ryan et al. 1995). Unless you are interested in gaining strength for a particular reason, our recommendation is to engage in muscular endurance training, performing at least one set of 15 to 25 repetitions with moderate resistance. Do this for 8 to 10 exercises, 2 or 3

Vigorous Physical Activity Increases Metabolic Rate For Up to 14 Hours!

In one study (Knab et al. 2011), researchers using a metabolic chamber found that 45 minutes of vigorous exercise caused 190 additional calories to be burned later in the day while the participant was at rest, with the increased metabolic rate lasting up to 14 hours.

Subjects completed two experimental trials. During the first session, they were mostly inactive, but they performed everyday tasks of living as needed. During the second session, participants followed the same routine, but they cycled vigorously (73% of maximal oxygen uptake) for 45 minutes. The subjects were matched for diet and other factors during the two trials. The 190 extra calories burned after exercise, compared to the resting trial, represented a 37 percent increase in net energy expended. 190 calories is the equivalent of walking an extra 1.9 miles (3 km) for an average person. Thus the exercise, burned calories not only during the exercise, but also throughout the rest of the day!

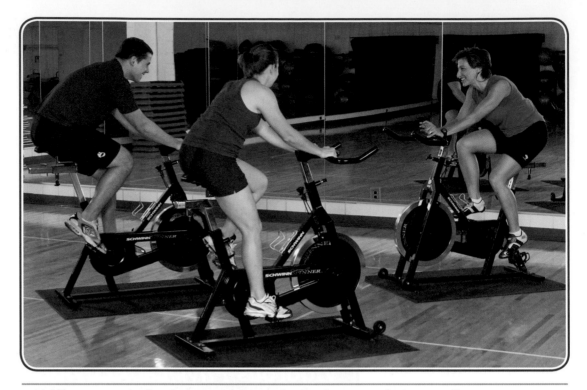

■ Adding an exercise break to your daily routine can increase caloric expenditure.

times per week, and you will maintain muscle mass and resting metabolic rate, both of which are important to the long-term success of your weight-control program.

Your daily exercise session is only one of the many ways to increase caloric expenditure. Walk to work, during work, to lunch, during coffee breaks, or after dinner. Take an exercise break during the day. Climb stairs, jump rope, or do calisthenics. Do anything that increases caloric expenditure. If you expend 200 calories in your training session and another 100 walking or climbing stairs, you have accelerated your exercise weight loss by 50 percent. When you become more fit and capable of burning 500 calories daily through exercise, you will be able to lose 1 pound (.45 kg) per week (500 cal × 7 days = 3,500 cal) through exercise alone.

The best way to achieve permanent weight loss is to make a change in lifestyle. The change could be to return to old ways of doing things. Avoid using unnecessary labor-saving devices (remote control, power mower, snow thrower). Seek out and employ energy-using devices such as the snow shovel, the bicycle, or your own two feet. The best advice is never to use a machine when you can do the job yourself. You will be doing yourself a favor, saving energy (electricity, gas, oil, coal) and reducing pollution, all at the same time.

Perhaps the best idea is to find an active hobby or sport and make it an essential part of your life. Try woodworking, racquetball, golf, or dancing. Get a canoe or cross-country skis, or start a garden. Dig out the tennis racket and try it. Go ice-skating in winter or roller-skating any time of year. You'll enrich your life and lower your weight at the same time. Of course, you'll look better too!

When you combine exercise with a modest diet, you combine the benefits of physical activity with the convenience of caloric reduction, and you can easily lose 1 to 2 pounds

(.45 to .9 kg) per week. A program with a caloric deficit of 500 calories per day results in a 3,500-calorie deficit per week, which is the equivalent of 1 pound (.45 kg) of fat.

Chapter 12 talks about the set point. When people attempt a weight-loss program without exercise, their resting metabolic rate may adjust downward in an attempt to maintain body fat by up to 400 kcal a day (.2 cal/min to .25 cal/min). If you combine this with the information that storing 10 calories a day as fat will become about 1 pound each year, it quickly becomes apparent that in order to start losing weight by diet alone, people who have been gaining weight need to overcome both the calories they have been storing every day and their change in basal metabolic rate. For example, imagine someone has been gaining 4 pounds (1.8 kg) a year and would now like to start losing weight. In

Caloric Cost

You may be encouraged to know that energy expenditure values based on the oxygen cost and caloric expenditure of various activities sometimes underestimate your actual caloric expenditure. For example, when we study the energy cost of running by having highly trained endurance runners run on a treadmill, the values underestimate your cost of running for the following reasons:

- The treadmill is perfectly flat (unlike the road or trail that you may use).
- The air in the lab is still (whereas outside, even on a calm day, the moving body must overcome some wind resistance).
- Trained runners are up to 10 percent more efficient than untrained runners are.
- The lab values don't consider the postexercise period, when your body uses energy to replace stores of energy consumed during the run. The excess postexercise oxygen consumption (EPOC) may be elevated for up to an hour after prolonged, hard exertion. Widely used values for the energy cost of running may be 10 percent too low for many joggers. Over a period of weeks, an error of that size renders a serious disservice to exercise and its role in weight control.

order to start to lose weight, this person will need to reduce diet by 40 calories a day to overcome the weight gain, and then will further have to reduce the diet by 400 kcal, for a total reduction of about 440 calories per day. Now, if the goal is to lose 20 pounds (9 kg) during the next year, this person needs to cut an additional 200 calories per day (a daily deficit of 10 cal/day for 1 year is about 1 pound lost). So, the total daily diet needs to be reduced by 40 + 400 + 200 (reverse weight gain + set point + weight loss) = 640 calories. This is in line with most diets.

A great benefit for those who add an exercise program including resistance training two or more times a week is that the set-point reductions in metabolic rate are somewhat reversed by the effects of exercise and excess post-exercise oxygen consumption (EPOC), reducing the metabolic rate loss to about 200 kcal per day. Thus, in the previous example, if the subject increases physical exercise an average of 250 calories a day (walking about 2 mi for a 185 lb [84 kg] person), the total energy deficit will be reduced from 640 calories to 440 calories, with 250 calories already metabolized through physical activity. The diet will only need to be adjusted downward by about 190 calories (440–250). This can easily be done by reducing dietary fat. The great aspect of adding aerobic and resistance training is that muscle mass is maintained and resting metabolism remains higher than through changing diet alone. Exercise also makes it much easier to maintain weight loss.

Here is a real program that one of the authors set up for a student. John was 40 pounds (18 kg) overweight and in the poor fitness category. He had been gaining 5 pounds (2 kg) a year for the past 3 years. A dietary analysis showed that his caloric intake was 2,500 calories per day. He wanted to lose 20 pounds (9 kg) in 1 year. The set-point information suggested that John was storing 50 calories a day as fat (remember, each 10 cal/day = 1 lb/year). Thus, his change in diet and exercise behaviors needed to equal at least 450 calories a day (50 to overcome current weight gain, 200 to overcome metabolic rate decreases, and 200 to reduce fat stores). A 14-week plan was written for John to start to lose the 20 pounds (equivalent to 70,000 fat cal) by reducing his caloric intake by 200 calories per day and by beginning a walking program. This program got him up to an average of 300 calories, for a total deficit of 500 calories (see table 13.3). John weighed 225 pounds (102 kg) and burned about 150 calories per mile walked at the start of the program. A behavior change of 500 calories was determined to account for the increased distance that he would have to walk to maintain his caloric loss as he lost weight. Note that the program in table 13.3 starts with smaller daily caloric goals and builds up to 500 calories per day. The diet and physical activity are changes from his current behavior.

John continued his program faithfully for a year, and lost 19 pounds (8.6 kg) of fat with his average loss about .5 pound per week. More importantly, during this year, he learned to love his lunchtime walks and stopped his snacking habits by replacing his high-caloric chips and soda with fruits and vegetables.

John's program was a success in many ways. A comparison of blood lipid profiles (cholesterol, LDL and HDL cholesterol, and triglycerides) from before and after his program showed great progress, with a slight decrease in total cholesterol but a 15-point decrease in LDL (135 to 120 mg/dl), a great rise in HDL (36 to 62 mg/dl), and a large drop in triglycerides. John's experience is typical of most people, in that his weight loss was slightly less than expected, but he gained great fitness and health benefits.

Table 13.3   Sample Weight-Loss Program for a 225 Pound (102 kg) Person, Creating a 500 kcal/day Deficit

		Calories	Weight loss *
Weeks 1 and 2 300 cal/day	Exercise = 1 mi = 150 cal/day** × 14 days Diet = 150 cal/day × 14 days Total for the 2 weeks:	= 2,100 = 2,100 4,200	.2 lb (.09 kg) fat
Weeks 3 and 4 400 cal/day	Exercise = 1.33 mi = 200 cal/day** × 14 days Diet = 200 cal/day × 14 days Total for the 2 weeks:	= 2,800 = 2,800 5,600	.29 lb (.13 kg) fat
Weeks 5 on 500 cal/day	Exercise = 2 mi = 300 cal/day** × 14 days Diet = 200 cal/day × 14 days Total for the 2 weeks:	= 4,200 = 2,800 7,000	1 lb (.45 kg) fat

*Only deficits over 250 calories/day (3,500 calories/2 weeks) for this person will result in weight loss, since 50 calories/day are needed to overcome his weight gain of 5 pounds (2 kg) a year. Approximately 200 calories/day are needed to overcome the metabolic rate decrease. Since each pound of fat stores about 3,500 calories, to determine weight loss, divide the excess calories metabolized by 3,500. For the first week, John creates a total deficit of 4,200, of which 700 are reducing his weight. Thus, he should lose 700/3500 = .2 pounds of fat.

**To determine how far you need to walk to burn the needed calories in this chart, use one of the following formulas:

Miles to walk = 1.5 × calories to burn / your weight (lb).

Kilometers to walk = 1.12 × calories to burn / your weight (kg).

After his yearlong program, John had a number of possible choices to maintain his new weight or to even continue to lower it until he was back to his ideal weight:

- Continue to exercise and eat as he pleases.
- Continue activity while eating less fat and fewer calories.
- Return to sedentary habits and restrict caloric intake for life.
- Return to sedentary habits, eat a high-fat diet, and regain all the weight he has lost and more.

In line with successful weight loss, as shown by the National Weight Control Registry, he made the lifestyle changes to increase his physical activity to about an hour a day. He has continued to maintain a low-fat diet and a reasonable caloric intake. He eventually lost 36 pounds (16 kg) and has remained at this weight for 6 years (at the time of this book's publication).

The following worksheet (form 13.1) will help you determine how many calories you might need to reduce in order to reach weight-loss goals. We encourage you to use a program of both diet and exercise, along with a slow rate of weight loss in the range of .5 to 1 pound (.2–.45 kg) per week.

Form 13.1   Calorie Reduction Worksheet

Use this worksheet to determine caloric deficit in an exercise and diet program needed to lose a desired amount of weight in 1 year. If you use metric values, you will need to convert kilograms to pounds (kg × 2.2 = lb).

How much weight did you gain last year? _____ pounds × 10 =_____calories/day

How many pounds do you want to lose in a year? _____ pounds × 10 =_____calories/day

Overcoming metabolism decrease when diet is combined with exercise   =__200__calories/day

Total = _____calories/day

How many calories per day will you reduce from your diet? –_____calories/day

Subtract diet calories from total.   Activity calories =_____calories/day

Now determine how many miles (km) this represents for you. Use the following formula to calculate your miles, or you can use the activity calorie charts in table 13.2 (page 331) to come up with the necessary duration for an activity that you enjoy.

Miles to walk = 1.5 × activity calories / your weight (lb) = _____miles.

Kilometers to walk = 1.12 × calories to burn / your weight (kg) =_____km.

From B.J. Sharkey and S.E. Gaskill, 2013, *Fitness and health, seventh edition* (Champaign, IL: Human Kinetics).

ADOPTING A HEALTHY DIET

If you're searching for one of those fad diets that regularly come and go, don't look here. When we say dieting, we simply mean reduced caloric intake, which most successful dieters usually accomplish by reducing high-calorie fat in the diet and little else. As we said in chapter 7, each gram of fat contains 9.3 calories, verses only 4.1 and 4.3 calories for carbohydrate and protein, respectively. Almost 40 percent of the calories in the average diet come from fat. If you've been eating 2,000 calories daily, 800 probably come from fat. We'll tell you how to reduce fat intake later in this chapter. But first let us say what we don't mean by dieting.

When you restrict calories, the daily caloric deficit should not exceed 1,000 calories regularly. Of course, you can restrict caloric intake far below energy needs. If you do that for more than a few days, however, you are on a starvation diet. Your body won't receive essential nutrients, your energy level will sag, your immune system will suffer, and your resistance to infection will decline. Furthermore, the body will interpret the starvation diet as a signal to reduce caloric expenditure. In response, your **resting energy expenditure** will decline, you'll lose lean tissue, and you'll be on your way to increased weight-loss problems.

Diet Recommendations

You do not have to change your eating habits overnight, and you don't have to reduce fat intake to 10 percent, unless your risk of coronary artery disease (CAD) is high. Otherwise, a fat intake of 25 percent is both reasonable and attainable. Begin today to reduce the fat content of your diet. Limit saturated fat (avoid hydrogenated or trans-fatty acids) to one-third of total fat calories. Try to make some of the substitutions that we've mentioned. Experiment with complex carbohydrates. Use beans and corn in a Mexican dinner. Try rice and soy for an Asian experience. Become familiar with the glycemic index, use potatoes occasionally (with fat-free sour cream), and use whole-grain products. The proper combination of these low-fat foods provides energy and meets the need for protein, fiber, and other nutrients. Avoid empty calories such as table sugar and soda pop. Substitute a carrot, celery, or fruit for your usual snacks. You can easily reduce fat intake to 25 percent as we await the final word concerning the relationship of dietary fat to health and disease.

The dietary program that we recommend emphasizes maintenance of a moderate diet, including the energy proportions of the performance diet—60 percent carbohydrate, 25 percent fat, and 15 percent protein—and adequate levels of vitamins, minerals, and water. Remember that calories do count. If you cut caloric intake, you will lose weight. If you cut caloric intake substantially, you may live longer.

Assess Food Choices

Take a good look at your caloric intake list. If patterns of behavior are not readily apparent, you should continue to count your calories for several days, as discussed in chapter 12. Besides recording what you eat, consider when, where, and why you eat (see form 12.1). Do you have a doughnut on your coffee break just because it's there? Do you have a candy bar at lunch? Do you have a drink now and then? You may be able to eliminate several hundred calories daily by eliminating or cutting back on unnecessary or ritualized eating behaviors. Years ago, one of us developed the habit of eating crackers with peanut butter and jelly as a reward for an evening's work. When he realized how quickly the fat calories added up and what could happen to his weight, he vowed to break the ritual. Sure, he still gets the urge, and sometimes he is unable to resist (an addict is never cured). But for the present, he rewards himself with a nutritious but low-calorie treat, such as an apple or orange. In this way, he has reduced both calories and fat intake.

Reduce or Eliminate Sugar-Sweetened Drinks

Soft drinks and fruit punches contain quantities of high-fructose corn syrup and other sweeteners that may contribute to overweight and adult-onset (type 2) diabetes. Data from the Nurses' Health Study showed that high consumption of sugar-sweetened beverages is associated with greater weight gain and increased risk of type 2 diabetes, probably due to the intake of excess calories and rapidly absorbable sugars (Schulze et al. 2004).

Modify Your Meals

Now that you've eliminated the extras, look at the size and content of your meals. Some think that dieting means avoiding meals, often breakfast. Skipping meals is the worst thing you can do for several reasons. People work better when they eat breakfast. When you avoid meals, you become weak and hungry; thus, you are more likely to grab a doughnut. People who are susceptible to low blood sugar may even notice poor performance in sports skills or work. Eventually, you sit down to a meal and overeat. In addition, when you eat fewer than three meals a day, triglyceride and cholesterol levels are higher than they are when you eat more frequently. By eating meals more frequently, you will avoid the feelings of hunger and fatigue often associated with diet and you will reduce blood lipid levels.

The easiest way to reduce mealtime calories is to reduce the size and number of helpings that you consume. Use a smaller plate and fill it only once. Refuse second helpings, except for salad or vegetables. And, of course, eliminate high-calorie desserts, toppings, dressings, gravies, and sauces (see figure 13.6 for a six-meal plan). Eat all you want of fruits, low-fat cereals, whole-grain breads (try olive oil instead of butter), vegetables, and water. Consider several servings of low-fat dairy products each day. Some think that milk and calcium contribute to fat and weight loss.

Avoid eating at establishments that promise all you can eat or offer supersized meals. If you're like us, you'll want to get your money's worth and will eat far more calories than you need.

Substitutions

The final step in this simple plan is to make substitutions. Substitute low-calorie snacks for high-calorie foods (e.g., pretzels for potato chips or peanuts). Substitute low-fat foods (nonfat milk, lean meats, nonfat salad dressing, low-fat cheese) for high-fat foods. When you begin to read labels, you will be on your way to a low-fat diet. Try to stay below 50 grams of

Meal	Menu
Breakfast	Egg or cheese Fruit Slice of whole-grain bread Coffee or tea
Midmorning	Fresh or dried fruit Milk (low-fat)
Lunch	Meat, fish, or peanut butter sandwich Milk, fruit, or vegetable juice
Midafternoon	Soup, fruit, and salad
Dinner	Meat, fish, poultry, or cheese Potato, rice, beans, corn, or whole grain Cereal product Fresh fruit Vegetables, including leafy greens Coffee or tea
Bedtime	Fruit and low-fat yogurt

FIGURE 13.6 Low-calorie six-meal plan.

fat daily. (If labels don't tell how much fat is in the food, the list of ingredients will help. Ingredients are listed in order of concentration, from highest to lowest. When fat comes early in the list, you are looking at a high-fat food.) Remember to avoid cottonseed, palm, and coconut oils, which are found in many snack foods, processed products, and coffee creamers. Watch out for hydrogenated oils found in all sorts of packaged foods. Oils that were otherwise safe, when hydrogenated, form a more solid fat (trans-fatty acids), which increases the risk of heart disease.

In food preparation, use olive oil and canola oil; both are high in monounsaturated fat, which is preferable to oil that is saturated or hydrogenated. Using this approach, you easily can achieve a daily caloric deficit of 500 calories. Because you are eating at least three meals a day, you won't feel weak and hungry. And when you combine the benefits of diet with those of exercise and fitness, you will be delighted with the results.

Finally, don't be tempted by low-fat snacks. Although they contain one-third less fat than the regular versions, they often have just as many calories, using sugar to make up the difference in taste.

Nutrition Facts

Serving Size 1/2 cup (114g)
Servings Per Container 4

Amount Per Serving

Calories 260   Calories from Fat 120

	% Daily Value*
Total Fat 13g	20%
Saturated Fat 5g	25%
Cholesterol 30mg	10%
Sodium 660mg	28%
Total Carbohydrate 31g	11%
Dietary Fiber 0g	0%
Sugars 5g	
Protein 5g	

Vitamin A 4%	Vitamin C 2%
Calcium 15%	Iron 4%

*Percent Daily Values are based on a 2000 calorie diet. Your daily values may be higher or lower depending on your calorie needs.

	Calories:	2000	2500
Total Fat	Less than	65g	80g
Sat. Fat	Less than	20g	25g
Cholesterol	Less than	300mg	300mg
Sodium	Less than	2400mg	2400mg
Total Carbohydrate		300g	375g
Dietary Fiber		25g	30g

Calories per gram:
Fat 9 • Carbohydrate 4 • Protein 4

FIGURE 13.7 To improve your diet, start by reading nutrition labels.

Label Reading

To lower the total amount of fat in your diet to 25 percent and to reduce saturated fat to one-third of total fat, begin by reading the labels on everything that you buy (see figure 13.7). Of course, ice cream and potato chips can be loaded with fat, but so are peanuts and many other snacks. If your goal is 25 percent of calories from fat and your daily intake is 2,000 calories, you can eat 500 calories of fat, or about 54 grams (500 ÷ 9.3 cal/g = 54). If you want to snack, choose pretzels with less than 1 gram of fat per serving instead of chips with 11 grams, or choose low-fat yogurt or ice cream with 0 grams of fat per serving versus 16 grams in the rich, creamy variety. In time, you will grow to prefer the low-fat version.

Reduced-Fat Diet

Reducing fat in the diet makes sense, up to a point. Fat is high in calories. In excess, it is related to heart disease, stroke, diabetes, and some cancers. Many good reasons exist for reducing the percentage of fat in your diet. Some fat is required for good nutrition, however, especially during early childhood. Essential fatty acids must be part of the diet. Moreover, fat-soluble vitamins are not absorbed unless fat is present. Fats improve the flavor of food and make it more filling. We would never suggest complete removal of fat from the diet, but we do suggest that you begin now to lower your percentage of calories obtained from fat from the 40 percent figure common in the United States to 25 or 30 percent, as recommended in the performance diet. We also urge you to reduce your intake of saturated fats to no more than one-third of total fat intake. Do this by substituting a cholesterol-lowering margarine for butter, replacing whole milk with nonfat milk and fatty meat with lean (including fish and fowl), and using more monounsaturated olive or canola oils. How far should you go to reduce the fat content of your diet?

Low-Fat, High-Carbohydrate Diet

The program recommended by Nathan Pritikin (1979) calls for the following daily energy intake (percentage of calories):

- 80 percent from carbohydrate (mostly complex)
- 10 percent from fat
- 10 percent from protein

Researchers at the California-based Longevity Research Institute have reported dramatic results among patients with heart and circulatory disorders and diabetes. The diet is a surefire way to reduce triglycerides and cholesterol. When accompanied by an exercise program, as it is at the institute, the diet may slow or even arrest the progress of atherosclerosis (Leonard, Hofer, and Pritikin 1974). Dr. Dean Ornish supports the low-fat diet (10% of cal from fat) for those with elevated risk of heart disease, with claims that the low-fat diet may reverse atherosclerosis (1993).

The low-fat diet has several advantages besides its effect on blood lipids and heart disease. Complex carbohydrate is high in fiber, and low-fiber diets are related to cancer of the colon. The high-carbohydrate diet is an excellent energy diet. When combined with a sensible exercise program, it will not lead to accumulation of fat. In fact, because carbohydrate has only 4 calories per gram, you can eat quite a bit without gaining weight. Finally, because fat seems to inhibit the action of insulin and because this diet reduces the level of fat in the blood, the low-fat diet could reduce the severity of adult-onset diabetes or reliance on insulin.

But the high-carbohydrate diet may not include enough protein for vigorous living. Let's assume that your weight is 70 kilograms (154 lb) and that your daily caloric intake averages 2,000 calories. If 10 percent of that energy comes from protein, you will take in 200 calories from protein. Protein averages 4.3 calories per gram, so 200 calories divided by 4.3 equals 47 grams of protein. That amount falls below the daily allowance for protein recommended by the National Research Council (.8 g of protein per kg of body weight × 70 kg = 56 g). For this reason, we do not recommend this level of protein intake. Instead, we recommend a diet that provides 15 percent of calories from high-quality protein, including lean meat, low-fat dairy, and plant sources.

How much fat does the very-low-fat diet allow? If daily intake is 2,000 calories, 10 percent fat allows 200 calories. Divide 200 by 9.3 calories per gram of fat, and you get 22 grams of fat, a very small amount. In our culture, this is a difficult diet. The author of the plan found it necessary to retrain the palates of his subjects because the drastic reductions of fat made food seem bland (Pritikin 1979). When one attempts to apply the diet in a restaurant, every page of the menu produces frustration.

> **B**e suspicious of any diet plan that promises rapid results of more than 2 pounds (.9 kilogram) of weight loss per week.

Diets to Avoid

Almost every popular magazine includes an article on dieting. Many offer a revolutionary new diet plan with such promises such as "Eat all you want," "Calories don't count," "Quick weight loss," and "Super energy." You've heard of the water diet, the drinking man's diet, the high-protein

Fasting

Fasting, the ultimate form of caloric restriction, is guaranteed to bring about a dramatic weight loss, as much as a pound (.45 kg) a day—for a while. An occasional day of fasting will do no harm unless you are under stress or in training for competition. But the risks of fasting are many, especially if you continue it for an extended period. If you are grossly overweight and are eager to fast, check into a clinic and proceed. Otherwise, avoid extended periods of fasting.

The Minnesota Semi-Starvation Study

While we are talking about diets to avoid, you should know about a famous study (probably unethical today) that was done during World War II from 1944 to 1945 at the University of Minnesota (Keys et al. 1950). This study would be classified as a very low-calorie, high-energy-expenditure study, where the average weight loss was about 25 percent of total body weight, including fat, muscle, bone, and water.

The purpose of the study was to understand how severe famine affects humans and to understand how to provide assistance to famine victims in Europe and Asia at the end of World War II. Thirty-six men participated. For the first 12 weeks, physiological and psychological baselines were established under normal food intake. Subjects then spent 24 weeks in a starvation phase, during which the caloric intake of each subject was drastically reduced. At the same time, subjects were required to do substantial moderate intensity exercise every day, causing them to lose an average of 25 percent of their body weight. In a final phase, various rehabilitative diets were attempted to renourish the volunteers. The results were used extensively by aid workers in Europe and Asia in the months following the cessation of hostilities. One author of this book treasures one of the few original copies of Key's two-volume treatise on this seminal research. It is fascinating reading and well worth the time for serious students of weight loss.

diet, the liquid-protein diet, the low-carbohydrate diet, and others. Unfortunately, these plans reach a far wider audience than do controlled studies, editorials, and warnings in medical journals.

Be suspicious of any diet plan that promises rapid results, more than 2 pounds (.9 kg) of weight loss per week. Certainly, you can lose more weight by fasting or by dehydration. Water is heavy, about 2 pounds per quart (about .5 kg/L). We could try to fool you into losing weight by sweating. You could easily lose 2 pounds in an hour; athletes lose 6 pounds (2.7 kg) or more in a hard workout. What is so bad about that? Your body needs the water and replaces it as soon as it can. Question any plan that calls for low intake of carbohydrate or protein, encourages high intake of protein or fat, or recommends dehydration as a means of weight loss.

Low-Carbohydrate Diet

One popular diet advocates near exclusion of carbohydrate. The creator of the diet states that the average overweight man should lose about 7 pounds (3.2 kg) in the first week of the diet! Remember, carbohydrate is stored with water. The diet allows a liberal intake of fat and all the protein you want, which should give you reason enough to question the plan. Low-carbohydrate diets are questionable for another reason: When blood-sugar levels are low, the fatty acid molecules from adipose tissue are shipped to the liver, where they are converted to ketone bodies to provide energy for the manufacture of glucose. Excess ketone bodies spill over into the blood and are carried to the tissues, where they are oxidized. During starvation or a low-carbohydrate diet, the production of ketone bodies can exceed the ability of the body to remove them metabolically. When this happens, the excess appears in the urine and in exhaled air. The condition is called ketosis, and the main danger is lowering of the blood **pH** (acidosis).

You should avoid simple sugars, but complex carbohydrates (whole-grain products, corn, brown rice, and beans) provide energy and nutrition. They are excellent sources of vitamins and minerals. Many are high in fiber as well. In those areas of the world where the diet consists largely of energy derived from complex carbohydrates, obesity is rare and atherosclerosis and heart disease are virtually nonexistent.

> *T*o think carbs make you fat is wrong.
> You're fat because you're not exercising.
>
> Chris Carmichael

High-Protein Diet

Advocates of the high-protein (low-carbohydrate) diet argue that carbohydrate stimulates insulin secretion and storage of fat and that a sustained high level of carbohydrate intake may lead to insulin resistance. Although this may be true for some sedentary people who eat excess simple carbohydrate, it is not a problem for the active person. In fact, regular exercise increases insulin sensitivity and reduces the risk of diabetes. Unless you are engaged in aerobic or muscular fitness training, you don't need more protein than the recommended dietary allowance (RDA). Excess protein is stored as fat or excreted in the urine. Because dietary protein often is associated with fat, as in meat or dairy products, you risk taking in more fat. Moreover, higher levels of meat and seafood consumption are associated with increased risk of gout (Choi et al. 2004).

- RDA for protein: .8 grams of protein per kilogram of body weight (2 oz for a 155 lb person, or 56 g for a 70 kg person)
- For aerobic training: 1.2 to 1.4 grams per kilogram of body weight (3 oz for a 155 lb person, or about 90 g for 70 kg person)
- For strength training: 1.4 to 1.8 grams per kilogram of body weight (4 oz for 155 lb person, or about 110 g for 70 kg person)

Some high-protein diets achieve temporary success because they are also low in calories and because significant water loss is associated with low carbohydrate intake. Unfortunately, they fail to provide the energy and some nutrients that you need to live a vigorous life. These diets appeal to those who intend to remain sedentary. They may be successful for short-term dietary needs.

Conversely, very low protein diets should be avoided. Any diet that restricts protein below the recommended dietary allowance makes no sense. During adolescence, such a plan could stunt normal development. Restricting protein intake is certain to cause muscle loss at any age. Muscle loss reduces resting metabolism and makes future caloric expenditure more difficult, leading to increased fat and body weight. And you cannot achieve the benefits of aerobic or muscular fitness training without adequate protein.

High-Fat Diet

Is there ever a reason to eat a high-fat diet? Probably not for the average American, even those participating in regular physical activity. However, endurance athletes tend to select a high-fat diet (50 percent of calories from fat) during periods of prolonged hard training. We've observed cross-country athletes from the U.S. ski team eating 50 percent of calories from fat during fall training camps, when they ski 50 kilometers (31 mi) or more daily. Wildland firefighters expend as many as 6,000 calories a day when they are working, and during those periods, they eat more fat (Ruby, Schoeller, and Sharkey 2001). Athletes who cross-country skied the entire length of the Iditarod dogsled race in Alaska (1,100 mi or 1,770 km), pulling a sled with food, tent, and sleeping bag, did so with the aid of high-fat snacks (e.g., balls of butter with bacon bits) to fuel their estimated energy expenditure of 10,000 calories per day! During periods of extreme endurance training, when energy requirements are high, increasing the percentage of fat in the diet to approximately 50 percent of total energy does not result in adverse changes in blood lipids (Brown and Cox 1998). However, a high-fat diet may interfere with the function of the immune system (Pedersen et al. 2000). For health reasons, one should return to a lower fat intake as soon as possible.

Diet Studies

Finally, after years of undocumented claims about various low-carb and other diets, we have some controlled studies to review. One study of obese men and women compared a low-carb diet to a conventional low-fat diet. Subjects on the low-carb diet lost more weight at 6 months (7.0% versus 3.2% body weight), but the differences were not significant at 12 months. No differences were found between the groups in total or low-density cholesterol, but increases in HDL cholesterol and decreases in triglycerides were greater on the low-carb diet. Both diets decreased blood pressure and the insulin response to oral glucose. The low-carb diet was associated with more improvements in CAD risk factors. Adherence was poor and attrition was high in both groups (Foster et al. 2003).

In a comparison of several popular diets, including the Atkins (low carb), Ornish (low fat), Weight Watchers (fewer calories), and Zone (fewer carbs), the authors studied adherence rates and the effectiveness of the diets on weight loss and reduction of cardiac risk factors (Dansinger et al. 2005). Each diet group began with 40 overweight or obese participants (22 to 72 years old), and the study lasted 18 months. Although differences among diets were not significant, weight loss ranged from 7.3 pounds (3.3 kg) on the Ornish diet to 4.8 pounds (2.1 kg) on the Atkins diet. Each diet reduced the ratio of LDL to HDL cholesterol about 10 percent. Cardiac risk reduction was somewhat better in the low-carb diets, but all diets reduced C-reactive protein approximately 20 percent. Benefits were limited to those who remained on the diets, but half of the Ornish and Atkins participants dropped out, and 35 percent of the Weight Watchers and Zone participants dropped out after a year. Weight loss predicted improvements in risk reduction. Each diet modestly reduced body weight. Increased adherence was associated with greater weight loss and risk-factor reductions for each diet group.

In a review of low-carb diet studies, the authors concluded that evidence is insufficient to make recommendations for or against use of low-carb diets, particularly among participants older than age 50, for use longer than 90 days, or for diets where 20 grams or less of carbohydrate are consumed per day. Among the published studies, weight loss on a low-carb diet was associated more with decreased caloric intake and increased diet duration than with reduced carbohydrate content (Bravata et al. 2003).

While we await future studies on the effectiveness of diets, consider this 12-week study on subjects with impaired glucose tolerance who had unlimited access to a low-fat, high-carb diet. Those on the low-fat (high-carb) diet lost 7 pounds (3.2 kg), whereas the group that ate a low-fat diet and exercised lost 10.6 pounds (4.8 kg), without caloric restriction. In addition, thigh fat area decreased in both groups, and no decrease occurred in resting metabolic rate or fat oxidation (Hays et al. 2004).

In a 2011 review of weight-loss programs to reduce metabolic syndrome, Church reported "for the purpose of weight loss, the combination of exercise training and reduced energy intake has been found to be more effective than either alone." The papers he reviewed suggest that modest diet restrictions combined with meeting physical activity health guidelines were the minimum for effective weight loss. These guidelines include obtaining at least 150 minutes per week of moderate-intensity physical activity, 75 minutes per week of vigorous-intensity physical activity, or a combination of the two, combined with at least 2 days per week of resistance training.

In our opinion, the low-carbohydrate (high-protein) diet may be a reasonable, short-term approach for people who intend to remain sedentary. But for those who are active or who intend to be, we recommend the performance diet (55 to 60 percent of calories from carbohydrate, 15 percent from protein, 25 to 30 percent from fat). The weight-loss results are similar to other diets. The carbohydrate provides energy for the active life and the activity reinforces long-term maintenance of the weight-control plan.

Health Clubs and Diet Centers

Do health clubs and diet centers figure in your weight-control program? Although both have experienced considerable growth, you should be a careful consumer of their services. You may be surprised to learn that state or local laws do not govern clubs or centers. No professional competence or qualifications are required. Hairdressers need a state license, but in most states, anyone can open and operate a health club or diet center. Here are some suggestions to help you become a discriminating consumer.

- *Health clubs*. To help you differentiate a good club from a bad one—an effective program and qualified staff from a fly-by-night organization—you should visit the club for a tour and free introductory session. Is the facility clean and well equipped? Does the equipment meet your needs? Are patrons satisfied? Do they encourage you to join? Ask about the staff's qualifications and credentials. Do they have degrees in the field from reputable institutions? Do they have experience? Are they certified? Are they all trained in emergency response? The American College of Sports Medicine (ACSM) certifies health and fitness instructors and program directors who meet educational and experience standards and who successfully complete a rigorous test. ACSM publishes standards for health clubs and a brochure to help you evaluate a health club. Write to ACSM at P.O. Box 1440, Indianapolis, IN 46206-1440 or visit their website (www.acsm.org) to request the brochure or other services.

Talk to club members before you join. When you decide to join a club, avoid long-term contracts. Be wary of discounts and other high-pressure come-ons, which may be signs of a failing business or high member turnover. Sign up for a few months or until you are certain that the club meets your needs. Then become active in a member advisory group that works with management to maintain and upgrade staff qualifications, facilities, and equipment.

- *Diet centers*. If you are considering the services of a diet center, follow the advice that we provided regarding health clubs. Visit, ask questions, and ask about qualifications. Is a registered dietitian on the staff? Is a reputable local physician associated with the center? Most important, ask about the long-term success rate of the program. Then ask to contact some of the diet center's clients. Ask yourself if the center provides any service that you cannot provide for yourself. The existence of so many centers suggests that the simple facts of energy balance and weight control have not reached enough people, or that people lack the information, opportunity, or will to take control of their eating and activity behaviors.

WEIGHT-CONTROL FALLACIES

Let's review some of the fallacies associated with weight loss. We'll consider false claims (lose girth, not weight), useless devices, drugs, and even smoking. Then we will examine the surgeries that extremely obese people sometimes consider.

Lose Girth, Not Weight

The idea that people can lose inches (cm), not pounds (kg), is the come-on of the figure salon. Such facilities try to appeal to people who don't want to work hard enough to achieve real fat and weight loss. Of course, you may be able to improve your appearance with exercises that merely tone muscles and improve posture. The fallacy is that while you are shaping the body, you are ignoring the engine, worn hoses, and other parts (i.e., the heart and blood vessels) and missing the health benefits associated with exercise and loss of body weight and fat. Typically, people do not lose girth at all; a slightly tighter pull on the measuring tape gives the impression of progress. Fitness and health, like beauty, are more than skin deep.

Spot Reduction

Evidence that fat can be removed from specific areas (spots) by localized exercises is extremely limited. One study showed a mere 1 millimeter of spot reduction after 6 weeks of exercise. Avid tennis players have approximately the same skinfold on both arms, even though the racket arm is more muscular.

Exercise Devices

You've seen the advertisements for passive exercise—electrical stimulation, vibrating machines, sauna shorts, and body wraps—devices that promise weight or fat loss without effort on your part. Sorry, they just don't work. Passive devices don't burn enough calories, electrical stimulation is not equivalent to voluntary exercise, vibrating devices do not break up fat and wash it away in the circulation, and tight pants or wraps do not remove fat with heat and massage. By spending the same amount of time in moderate exercise, you will get results, including the health benefits that you miss with passive exercise.

The advertising usually claims that with a few minutes of almost effortless activity, you will get a firm, healthy, athletic body. The promoters use attractive models, celebrities, or professional athletes to tout the product, and they usually offer a big discount if you act immediately. If you are uncertain, ask your physician or a certified health club

Dunlop's Disease

My friend Ted once tried sit-ups to get rid of what he called Dunlop's disease, in which his belly "done lopped" over his belt. He worked up to 400 sit-ups daily with no success. We showed him a study conducted by Dr. Frank Katch and colleagues at the University of Massachusetts. They collected fat biopsies from several sites before and after a 4-week training program consisting entirely of sit-ups. Posttraining analysis of fat cells revealed that the fat loss came from all the fat storage areas measured, not just abdominal fat (McArdle, Katch, and Katch 1994). What about Ted? He became an ultramarathoner, training for and running 100-mile (161 km) races, and his tummy ceased to be a problem. The moral of this story is that burning off sufficient calories will take care of the spots and inches (cm).

professional for advice. Our advice is to ask to see the results of research studies and to try the product before you buy. Don't sign a long-term contract for any type of exercise program or device. Remember, a brisk walk burns more calories than most passive devices do, and walking is a lot more fun.

Drugs

Laxatives and diuretics remove only water (dehydration). Amphetamines are sometimes prescribed to suppress the appetite, a dangerous approach to lifelong weight control. Reputable physicians prescribe anorectic agents (appetite suppressants) as part of a total program with diet, exercise, and behavior therapy. But they need to avoid increasing doses and the risk of dependency. One weight-control drug combination was associated with development of heart valve problems. Weight-control drugs, when they work, have to be taken forever to achieve lifelong weight control. Research on the genetic component of obesity may lead to future therapies, but such treatment will never remove the need to balance caloric intake and expenditure.

Smoking

Seeing people smoking cigarettes is sad, but it is tragic to hear that they continue the habit to avoid weight gain. Although it is true that smokers gain some weight when they quit, the amount is not so excessive that they can't eliminate it with diet and exercise. Moreover, the health consequences of smoking far outweigh the effect of any weight gain. Those who smoke should develop an addiction to exercise to replace the addiction to nicotine.

■ The best way to lose weight is through sensible dieting and exercise.

SENSIBLE WEIGHT GAIN

This section is intended to help underweight people achieve sensible nonfat weight gain. The plan is not meant to help you bulk up for sports like football. When normal-weight people bulk up, they assume considerable health risk. Coaches who encourage such procedures should be held responsible for conducting weight-loss programs when the athlete's season or career is over. As with weight loss, the weight-gain program includes exercise, diet, and behavior therapy.

• *Exercise.* This includes a strength-training program to build lean body weight and a reduction in calorie-burning activities (aerobic exercise, sports) to allow a positive caloric balance.

- *Diet.* This includes an overall increase in calories, with 750 extra calories on strength-training days and 250 extra on nontraining days. The extra calories should be largely from low-fat, protein-rich foods (lean meats, eggs, low-fat dairy products, or soy protein). A low-fat protein supplement can be used to provide an extra 20 grams (86 cal) of protein daily.

- *Behavior therapy.* If needed, develop a reinforcement schedule to reward gains in lean body weight. Determine a desirable weight and make steady progress toward that goal.

This program should lead to a gain of about 1 pound (.45 kg) of weight each week. If you attempt to gain weight too fast, much of the gain will be fat. So determine current eating behavior and plan needed modifications (e.g., more meals, nutritious snacks). Start strength training and watch the scale go up. Remember to return to aerobic exercise and weight control when you achieve the desired body weight.

SUMMARY

In the words of a leading obesity researcher, "Exercise is clearly beneficial as a means of losing weight and keeping it off. Given studies showing the association of exercise with weight maintenance, it would be difficult to argue that any factor is more important than exercise" (Brownell 1995, 124).

Activity is the positive way to achieve weight control without losing lean tissue. Dieting alone is a negative approach that uses deprivation to achieve results. Dieting by itself is seldom successful in the long run. Most weight-loss diets without physical activity end in failure, with more weight and fat than before the dieting began. Activities such as walking, jogging, or cycling may seem like slow ways to lose weight, but they work. If your activity burns 250 extra calories each day, you'll burn more than 1,500 calories a week. Even if your metabolic rate changes somewhat, you will begin to lose weight. Calories do count, and you should learn how to count them.

This chapter attempts to provide a lifelong approach to rational weight control.

- If you are slightly overweight, simply increase daily activity to achieve your goal.
- Twenty minutes of brisk walking each day (at 6 cal/min) will use enough calories to burn 1 pound (.45 kg) of fat each month.
- If your problem is moderate, use activity and food choices to gain control.
- Eliminate empty calories, substitute low-fat foods for high-fat foods, and eat moderate portions. This approach alone should help you lose an additional pound each month.
- Activity and diet can help you lose 4 pounds (1.8 kg) per month or more, but you should never attempt to lose more than 2 pounds (.9 kg) per week or 8 pounds (3.6 kg) per month.
- Finally, if your problem is significant and long-standing, you should add a behavioral approach to your program.

Proper use of any one of the three—activity, food choices, and eating behavior—will help you lose weight, but if you are interested in long-term weight loss, if your weight-control problem is significant, or if you want to gain complete and lasting control, consider combining the benefits of all three.

We have presented information on how to use activity, dieting, and behavioral therapy in your lifelong effort to achieve energy balance and weight control. In years past, young folks were more active and had more metabolically active tissue, so weight control wasn't a big problem. With inactivity and poor food choices, overweight and obesity are epidemic. As adults, we face new responsibilities, less time for activity, and a further decline in metabolically active tissue, including muscle. Eventually, winter weight gains fail to melt off in spring, and energy balance becomes a major issue. We've reached the stage of life where we must exercise more or eat less if we want to maintain body weight, waist size, blood lipids, and self-respect. Because some of us already engage in a considerable amount of exercise and have reduced the fat in our diets, we are faced with the unhappy prospect of life with fewer calories. But don't feel sorry for us. We've come this far enjoying an enormous appetite and a great love of food. It is time that we learn some self-control. For more information on behavior therapy, review chapter 5.

Performance

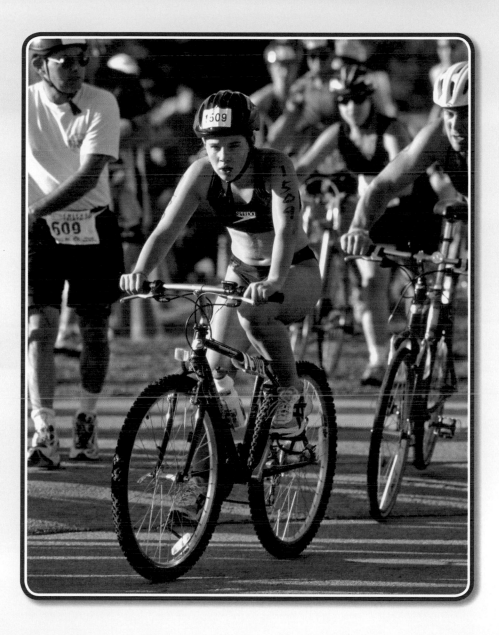

In a typical day, most of us spend about 8 hours asleep and 8 hours at work. The rest of the day is largely dedicated to preparation for one or the other, or to leisure-time pursuits, including activity and sport. If you improve fitness to enhance sport performance, sleep will take care of itself.

You may want to go beyond health, even beyond fitness, to perform at a high level and achieve your potential. To do this, you must set goals and then design and carry out a systematic plan to achieve them. The final step is to achieve what you trained for, sometimes in a public performance or event. We usually think of performing in sports, races, or other competitions; but some people train for cross-country bicycle trips, mountain climbs, or other personal goals.

This section will help you improve your performance. We'll show you how to use simple psychological skills so that you can play your best game more often. Furthermore, we'll discuss how to prepare for and perform in a variety of terrestrial environments, including heat, cold, and altitude.

chapter 14

Improving Performance

Work and Sport

> ❝Don't play sports to get in shape;
> get in shape to play sports!❞
>
> *Anonymous*

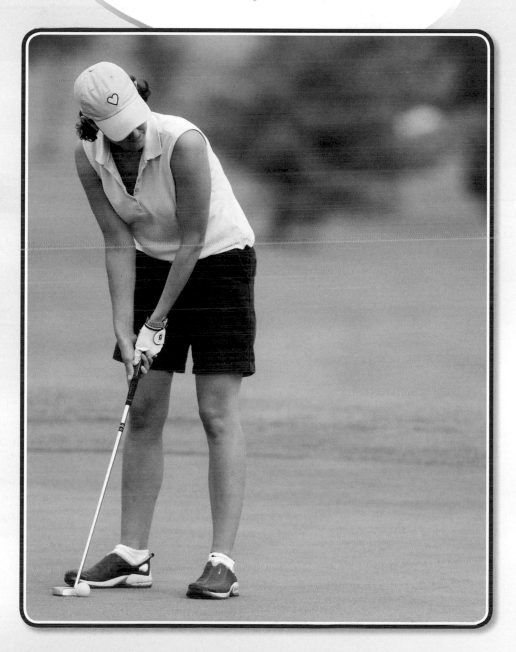

This chapter tells you how to prepare for athletic competition safely and effectively so that you can enjoy the intense pleasure and excitement of sport without the risk of fatigue, overtraining, injury, or illness. In athletic competitions, adults participate according to age group. Athletes often stay active into their 60s, 70s, and even 80s. A few continue to participate in races beyond their 100th birthdays, as did the late Larry Lewis, an indefatigable runner. If you like to train and you enjoy the thrill of competition and getting high on your own hormones, or if you have personal performance goals such as climbing Mt. Rainier, working as a wildland firefighter, or preparing for a more strenuous vacation, this section is for you. Please note that one chapter cannot begin to teach you all that you need to know about training for performance. This chapter aims to help you focus on the main principles and adapt a training program to fit your needs. See our companion book, *Sport Physiology for Coaches* (Sharkey and Gaskill 2006), for more on this and other principles. But remember, you must train before you compete.

This chapter will help you do the following:

- Use the principles of training
- Improve performance in your favorite sport
- Use diet to enhance performance
- Develop psychological skills to help you play your best game more often

TRAINING PRINCIPLES

This section introduces 15 important principles for making steady progress in your training and avoiding illness and injury. The principles are based on research studies and the insights of successful coaches. Coaches and athletes who plan and train in accordance with the following rules generally have positive results. By the end of this section, you should be ready to improve your performance or help others do the same. We focus on the adaptations and individual response to training.

• *Principle 1: Readiness.* The value of training depends on individual physiological and psychological readiness. Reasonable goals should be clearly defined, reasonable, and age appropriate. Take an inventory of available training equipment and of access to the necessary facilities and equipment. In order to benefit from training, you must prioritize time to do it, practice adequate nutrition, and get adequate rest.

• *Principle 2: Health.* Athletes need to be healthy when they train. A rational progression with appropriate periodization, rest, and recovery is critical. Additional factors include nutrition, sleep, and good hygiene. Pay attention to what your body is telling you and adjust training appropriately in order to stay healthy.

• *Principle 3: Individual response.* People respond differently to the same training for some of the following reasons: heredity, maturity, nutrition, rest, sleep, level of fitness, environmental factors, illness or injury, and motivation.

- *Principle 4: Overload.* Training must place a demand on the body system if desired adaptations are to take place. To begin, training must exceed the typical daily demand. As you adapt to increased loading, you should add more load. Three factors affect the training load: frequency, intensity, and time, or *FIT*. Remember, "If you always do what you always did, you will always get what you always got." In general, the training overload is generally increased in rotation steps by first increasing frequency, then duration, and, finally, intensity.

- *Principle 5: Adaptation.* Training induces subtle changes as the body adapts to the added demands. Dr. Ned Fredrick, a friend and a noted sport scientist, calls training for sport a gentle pastime in which we coax subtle changes from the body. The day-to-day changes are so small as to be immeasurable; weeks and even months of patient progress are required to achieve measurable adaptations. If you try to rush the process, you risk illness, injury, or both. See chapters 7, 8, and 9 to review adaptations to training. The principle of adaptation tells us that we can't rush training. We must follow a sensible program in alignment with these principles and learn to be satisfied with the results. Trying to do it all in one season is likely to do more harm than good.

- *Principle 6: Progression.* To achieve adaptations using the overload principle, training must follow the principle of progression. When you increase the training load too quickly, the body cannot adapt. Instead, it breaks down. You must observe progression in terms of FIT, or increases in frequency (sessions per day, week, month, or year), intensity (training load per day, week, month, or year), and time (duration of training in hours per day, week, month, or year).

- *Principle 7: Periodization.* Although the training load generally increases (progression), it must do so rationally to achieve optimal performance. Periodization describes the process of planning systematic variation into training. This variation occurs at several levels: daily, weekly, seasonal, and career. The next section discusses how to design a training plan with these levels of periodization.

- *Principle 8: Long-term training.* Changes resulting from the gradual overload of body systems lead to impressive improvements in performance, but it takes years of effort to approach high-level performance capability. Long-term training allows for growth and development, gradual progress, acquisition of skills, learning of strategies, and fuller understanding of the sport. Don't rush the process; too much training too soon may lead to mental and physical burnout and early retirement from the sport. Excellence comes to those who persist with an enjoyable, well-planned, long-term training program.

- *Principle 9: Specificity.* Exercise is specific. When you train, adaptations will take place in the muscle fibers used during the exercise. The adaptations to endurance training are different from adaptations to strength training. This concept means that the type of training you undertake must relate to the desired results. Specific training brings specific results. Of course, you can take any rule or principle to the extreme. Specificity does not mean that you should avoid training opposite or adjacent muscles. In fact, you should train other muscles to avoid muscle imbalances that could predispose the body to injury. You can train adjacent muscles to help you adapt to changes in conditions and to provide a backup when the primary muscle fibers become fatigued.

- *Principle 10: Rest and recovery.* Every athlete needs to recover following hard days or blocks of training. Build periodization and variation into your program to ensure that easier training follows harder periods. A training plan is an educated guess at what you will need. The essence of this principle is that you need to listen to your body and adjust the duration and intensity of each workout to what you are feeling. Remember, you need to stay healthy. Recovery is when adaptations occur.

• *Principle 11: Variation.* Vary your training program to maintain your interest and to avoid boredom, staleness, and poor performance. Successive sessions of hard work, if not followed by adequate time for rest and recovery, are certain to hinder progress in training. When workouts become dull, do something different. Run or bike a different route. Use cross-training to diminish monotony and lighten the physical and psychological burdens of heavy training.

• *Principle 12: Warm-up and cool-down.* A warm-up should always precede strenuous activity to increase body temperature, respiration, and heart rate, and to guard against muscle, tendon, and ligament strains. It should consist of calisthenics, gradual increases in exercise intensity, and stretching. Stretching is more effective after the warm-up.

The cool-down is just as important as the warm-up. Abrupt cessation of vigorous activity leads to pooling of the blood, sluggish circulation, and slow removal of waste products. It may also contribute to cramping, soreness, or more serious problems. High levels of the hormone norepinephrine are present immediately after vigorous exercise, making the heart more subject to irregular beats. Cooling down removes excess norepinephrine and reduces body temperature. Light activity and stretching continue the pumping action of muscles on veins, helping remove metabolic wastes through circulation.

• *Principle 13: Maintenance.* After reaching a performance goal, some athletes wish to stay at that level of training for a period of time. Maintenance of fitness requires less training than achieving the initial goal. Generally, you can decrease frequency and duration, but you must maintain intensity of training. The higher the level of fitness to be maintained, the greater the required training load. Furthermore, lower fitness levels can be maintained for longer than higher fitness levels can. Thus, when athletes peak, they are able to maintain that fitness level for only a few days or weeks.

• *Principle 14: Reversibility.* Most of the adaptations achieved from months of hard training are reversible. In general, it takes longer to gain endurance than it does to lose it. With complete bed rest, fitness can decline at a rate of almost 10 percent per week! Strength declines more slowly, but lack of use eventually causes atrophy of even the best-trained muscles. To avoid this problem, maintain a year-round program, with periods of hard work followed by periods of relative rest and variety.

• *Principle 15: Moderation.* The principle of moderation applies to all aspects of life. Too much of anything can be bad for your health. Temper dedication with judgment and moderation. If you train too hard, too long, or too fast, your body will begin to deteriorate. Practice moderation in all things. Remember, even elite athletes vary their training, taking easy days between hard training sessions.

TRAINING FALLACIES

Other so-called principles of training are fallacies or misconceptions. The following often-quoted statements are not true, and they have no basis in medical or scientific research.

• *Fallacy 1: No pain, no gain.* Although often difficult and sometimes unpleasant, serious training shouldn't hurt. Well-prepared athletes can perform difficult events in a state of euphoria, free of pain and oblivious to discomfort. Marathon winners sometimes seem to finish full of vitality, whereas others appear near collapse. Pain is not a natural consequence of exercise or training; it is a sign of a problem that you shouldn't ignore. During exercise, the body produces natural opiates, called endorphins, which can mask discomfort of the effort. If you experience real pain during training, you should back off. If the pain persists, have the problem evaluated.

Discomfort, on the other hand, can accompany difficult aspects of training such as heavy lifting, intense interval training, or long-distance effort. Discomfort is a natural consequence of the lactic acid that accompanies the anaerobic effort of lifting or intervals, or of the muscle fatigue, microscopic muscle damage (microtrauma), and soreness that come with long-distance training. We would accept this statement: No discomfort, no excellence. Overload sometimes requires working at the upper limit of strength, intensity, or endurance. That state can be temporarily uncomfortable. If exercise results in pain, it is probably excessive. The next two fallacies are also associated with this first misconception.

• *Fallacy 2: You must break down muscle to improve.* Microtrauma sometimes occurs in muscle during vigorous training and competition, but it isn't a necessary or even a desirable outcome of training. Runners have shown significant microtrauma at the end of a marathon with long downhill stretches that require eccentric muscular contractions (contractions of a lengthening muscle). Eccentric contractions are a major cause of muscle soreness, which is associated with muscle trauma, reduced force output, and a prolonged (4- to 6-week) period of recovery. Excessive trauma doesn't help training; it stops it.

Weightlifters can traumatize muscle with excess weight or repetitions, but that result is not a necessary stage in the development of strength. Neither pain nor injury is a normal consequence of training, and you should avoid both.

• *Fallacy 3: Go for the burn.* This popular maxim is often heard among bodybuilders who do numerous repetitions and sets to build, shape, and define muscles. The burn they describe is probably due to the increased acidity associated with elevated levels of lactic acid in the muscle. Although this sensation isn't dangerous, it isn't a necessary part of a strength program designed to improve performance.

• *Fallacy 4: Lactic acid causes muscle soreness.* This fallacy has been around for years, without any basis in fact. Although contractions that lead to soreness may produce lactic acid, it isn't the cause of the soreness. Lactic acid is cleared from muscle and blood within an hour of the exercise. Soreness comes 24 hours or more after unfamiliar exertion or a long layoff, long after the lactic acid has been removed or metabolized. It is probably associated with microtrauma to muscle and connective tissue and the swelling that results. After recovery, additional exposure to the activity will yield less soreness.

• *Fallacy 5: Muscle turns to fat (or vice versa).* Another common misconception is that when an athlete stops training, muscle can turn to fat. Muscle will no more turn to fat than fat will

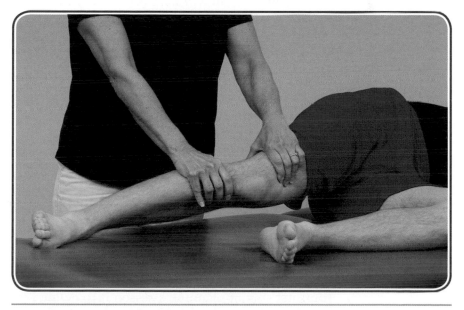

■ Normal training should not cause pain or injury.

Senior Success

Dr. Thomas K. Cureton was a pioneer in exercise physiology and the study of fitness at the University of Illinois during the 1950s and 1960s. During the week, this vigorous teacher and researcher taught classes, conducted research studies, and wrote books and articles about exercise and fitness. On weekends, he took to the road to preach the gospel of fitness and health to the lay public. His YMCA workshops were legendary for the enormous energy he exhibited. He was so busy that he had little time for himself.

Sometime after his retirement, he returned to the pool, the site of his youthful success in competitive swimming. Before long, he was setting national and then world records in his age group. We'll never forget his contributions or his delight at finding athletic success in his eighth decade. It's never too late to start, or to start over.

turn to muscle. Both are highly specialized tissues with specific functions. Muscles are composed of long, spaghetti-like fibers with contractile proteins designed to exert force. Fat cells are round receptacles designed to store fat. Training increases the size of muscle fibers (hypertrophy), and detraining reduces their size (atrophy). Excess caloric consumption causes fat cells to grow in size as they store more fat. The cells shrink when you burn more calories than you eat. But long, thin muscle fibers do not change into spherical blobs of fat, or vice versa.

• *Fallacy 6: I ran out of wind.* Athletes often have the sensation of running out of wind when they run too fast for their level of training. The sensation comes from the lungs and reflects another discomfort of exertion. But this circumstance is more likely to be due to an excess of carbon dioxide than it is to lack of oxygen or air. Carbon dioxide is produced during the oxidative metabolism of carbohydrate, and it is the primary stimulus for respiration. So when carbon dioxide levels are high, as they are during vigorous effort, they cause distress signals in the lungs. The respiratory system thinks that ridding the body of excess carbon dioxide is more important than bringing in more oxygen. Excess carbon dioxide is a sign that you have exceeded your lactate threshold and that you are working above your level of training. Become familiar with the sensation and what it is telling you; if you ignore it, you will soon become exhausted.

DESIGNING YOUR TRAINING PROGRAM

Putting together a training program can be a daunting task. We recommend a systematic approach to design both individualized and group programs. You can use this four-step plan to develop a successful training program:

1. Set goals.
2. Analyze your needs.
3. Periodize the training plan.
4. Monitor your progress and health (or that of your athletes).

We have discussed steps 1, 2, and 4 elsewhere in this book and will only briefly review before showing you how to divide the training plan into periods.

1. *Goal setting.* Goals provide a destination. They give direction, drive, and motivation. Your first step in planning a season is to define your goals. A training plan may need to include specific goals for muscular and **energy fitness**, technique, tactics, and psychological

skills. See chapter 4 for more information, or consult a book on psychological skills that includes a good section on goal setting, such as *Coaching Young Athletes* by Rainer Martens.

2. *Needs analysis.* In planning a trip, you need to know where you are, where you want to go, and how you can get there. When planning training, athlete assessment defines where you are. Goal setting determines where you want to go, and an analysis of the muscular- and energy-fitness needs will guide your route to your destination. Once you have completed the assessment and goals, develop the training plan.

3. *Plan and periodize the program.* It is generally best to look at the long-term picture (principle 8) first and then determine how to periodize your year, each week within a period, and the days within each week. Figure 14.1 is a schematic of this long-term, yearly, weekly, and daily training. It shows how a general program of planned progression and variation with rest and recovery (periodization) might proceed. The principle of individual response (principle 3) implies that you will need to vary the basic plan to fit your particular

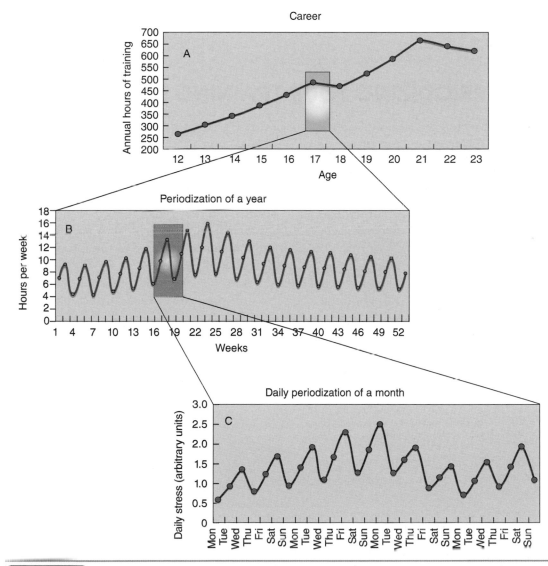

FIGURE 14.1 Periodization of training: *(a)* yearly training hours for a young athlete, *(b)* weekly hours in one year, and *(c)* daily periodization for one month.

needs. Graph A shows a hypothetical increase in training hours per year for a developing athlete. The dips in the progression indicate years during which training volume was decreased to reduce stress and increase performance. Typical years for reducing volume might include senior years in high school and college and Olympic years. Graph B shows weekly hours for a single training year. Note the overall progression, with total volume peaking around week 25, and then a gradual reduction of volume as more high-intensity training is done to prepare for competitions. Note also the 3-week cycle of medium-, high-, and low-volume weeks to allow for stress and recovery. Graph C shows the **daily periodization** of a month of training. Note the 3-day cycle of medium, hard, and easy days within the larger weekly cycles.

4. *Monitoring health and training.* As we hinted throughout the periodization sections, the most important concern of training is to maintain health and to recover adequately. You can best maintain health and optimal performance with a properly periodized program that varies stress, intensity, duration, and activities. Pay attention when you are feeling more tired than you anticipated. The **fatigue index** (see page 375) is an excellent method to monitor recovery and health. Figure 14.6 lists a number of methods used by successful athletes and coaches to monitor overtraining, which is discussed later in this chapter on page 373.

PERIODIZING YOUR TRAINING PROGRAM

Each of the following sections on how to periodize training first discuss the **energy training**, followed by muscular training. To tailor a training program suited to your needs, you first must know the energy sources required in the activity. Figure 14.2 illustrates the relative contribution of anaerobic and aerobic energy sources in relation to the distance or duration of running events (use the time scale to estimate energy sources for other activities).

Next, it helps to know something about your individual capabilities, both anaerobic and aerobic. If you are eager to prepare for a marathon, you should be as strong as possible in aerobic fitness. If your event is primarily anaerobic, like a 100-meter swim, you will need anaerobic capability, along with the aerobic capacity to support training and enhance recovery. When you know the energy sources used in the activity and your own capabilities, you can begin to design your training program. Decide where your sport falls in the continuum of 100 percent anaerobic to 100 percent aerobic. A sport such as soccer may be 70 percent aerobic for a midfielder but 80 percent anaerobic for a goalie,

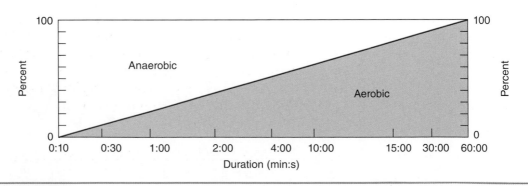

FIGURE 14.2 Anaerobic and aerobic energy sources in relation to distance and duration of events. Shorter events are primarily anaerobic. For distances greater than 1,500 meters (longer than 4 min), training should concentrate on aerobic fitness.

while baseball is probably 90 percent anaerobic. The following sections discuss training intensity and interval training.

Training Intensity Levels

In order to keep training simple, we can divide it into three intensity levels: **easy aerobic training**, race pace–plus intervals, and maximal effort intervals. With this division, you will quickly see that you can adapt a general program to nearly any need.

Easy Aerobic Training

This intensity should feel easy for most athletes. Elite endurance athletes may spend 80 to 90 percent of their total training time at this level. They obviously spend long hours running, biking, or swimming. While the easy aerobic training is not the largest portion of a sprinter or anaerobic athlete's program, it remains an important component to improve recovery and the ability to complete multiple intervals.

Race Pace–Plus Intervals

This intensity is unique to each athlete. The concept is that race pace–plus intervals are always adjusted to your current performance speed. Thus, for long aerobic events, the intervals are generally aerobic. For high-intensity sports, they may be done at maximal effort with an assistive device, such as a bungee cord, or while sprinting slightly downhill. By doing intervals slightly faster than current race speed, you will both train the appropriate energy system and gain the neuromuscular coordination to move slightly faster. After a few weeks of training, you should do a time trial or a competition, or test your actual performance. You should be slightly faster. From there, you can reset your interval times slightly. Over a training season, we have seen dramatic improvements in race times for athletes who have used this system.

The rest period between race pace–plus intervals is generally up to each athlete, but it needs to be long enough for recovery so that the target time can be achieved. In general, rest periods start out long during the basic training period, and gradually get shorter through the precompetition and early competition periods.

For endurance sports, the duration may be around 20 minutes, but it is seldom longer than one-fourth of the race distance. For sprint sports, these intervals include maximal efforts, with some sort of assistance to allow a higher velocity. The distance may be just a portion of the event or the entire race length. These differ from **maximal intervals** in that they are assisted. In general, race pace–plus intervals become longer (with shorter rest) as the season progresses. This is especially true for endurance sports.

The number of intervals varies with the sport, stress, and athlete. A general rule is that athletes should do as many intervals as possible (time permitting) within a workout as long as they are able to maintain their target pace. In general, the number of intervals within a workout will decrease slightly as the training year progresses due to the increasing intensity and decreasing rest period. However, the number of interval sessions typically increases during the training year, with a peak during the early competition period.

Maximal Intervals

These intervals involve maximal effort for short periods of time. Their purpose is to train high-energy systems.

For endurance athletes, these intervals typically last 30 to 60 seconds, with long rest periods. For runners, cyclists, and cross-country skiers, these are often done uphill to increase the resistance. The intervals are not used until late in the early competition period

Definitions for Race Pace and Race Pace–Plus Intervals

Race pace: This is the current speed that an athlete can maintain for a designated race length.

Race pace–plus intervals: Intervals that are done at a speed slightly (1%–5%) faster than current race pace, but are generally done for a distance shorter than the race length. Examples: (1) A 5-minute miler might do .25-mile (.4 km) intervals in 72 seconds, which is slightly (4%) faster than his current pace of 75 seconds per .25 mile. (2) A 13.5-second 100-meter sprinter practices bungee assisted starts or finishes. The bungee allows the sprinter to run slightly faster than her current race speed for a portion or all of the distance. (3) A marathon runner who can sustain 8-minute miles during a marathon (3:29:36 marathon) might do 2-mile intervals in 15:30, or about 3 percent faster.

to begin a peaking program for the most important competitions. The number of intervals completed depends on each athlete's sport. Some evidence exists that short rest periods during these intervals can also be successful.

For anaerobic athletes, these intervals are shorter, lasting from 10 to 30 seconds. They may be resisted. They are similar to the race pace–plus intervals, but they do not use assistive devices to increase speed. Resistance devices include bungee cords, weights, parachutes, or a slight uphill grade.

Heart Rate Monitors

Athletes often use heart rate monitors to make sure that they are training at the correct intensity. The best monitors are those that use the electrical signal from the heart (ECG). One popular version transmits the signal from the chest to a wrist monitor that displays the rate and stores heart rates for later analysis.

If you decide to use a monitor, you will still need to listen to your body to become familiar with respiratory problems and other signs of distress. Use the monitor to estimate your lactate threshold, and then become aware of your breathing at that level of exertion. You'll need to be able to sense your effort when you race.

Coaches and physiologists will tell you that no race was ever won or judged by heart rate. Speed is the only criteria. Heart rate monitors are good for helping athletes go slowly, but to go fast, you need to monitor speed.

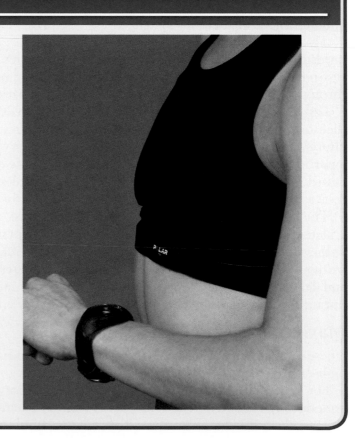

Multiyear Periodization

Figure 14.1 presents a hypothetical long-term energy plan for an athlete. For multiyear planning, the most important years have reduced volume and increased intensity. Within each year, there are seasonal and weekly variations in training load, with a gradual increase through the precompetition periods, then a reduction or tapering of training as the competition period approaches. Variation also comes with easy, moderate, and hard training days. The shape of the curves is fairly typical for all sports, but people need to individualize the hours to their sport, what they can personally handle, and what their available time and environment allow.

Ages 6 to 12

Countries with the highest per capita Olympic and World Championship medals have programs that generally encourage participation in many sports and activities without specialization. Youth are encouraged to be active, but they have little structured training. A mix of skill, speed, and endurance activities is considered optimal, since it allows youths to find out where they excel.

Resistance training for this age group is generally not encouraged. If resistance training is done, the focus should be on technique, low resistance, and high repetitions.

Ages 12 to 18

Note that the total energy-training hours increase each year up through age 17 in accordance with the principles of progression and overload. It is generally agreed that by age 14, young athletes may start specializing in sports of their choice. The principle of individual response will help them find those activities at which they excel if they are allowed to explore many options up to age 14 or 15. During this period of time, the hours of higher intensity training are probably also increasing slightly. Up to age 16, data support that longer duration with low- to moderate-intensity training and limited interval training is most effective for long-term development. Obviously, athletes in sports that are more anaerobic will do less long-distance training and more speed and muscular training than aerobic athletes do. In this model, the total hours drop slightly at age 18 (high school senior) to allow for improved performance by increasing rest and recovery, while also slightly increasing interval and speed training to enhance peak performance. Resistance training during this age period may start to increase to heavy weights postpuberty, with care for growth plates. Focus on maintaining good technique and increasing muscle mass. During the later years, athletes may begin to do more power training.

Ages 18 to 30

These are generally the years of peak performance. During these years, energy training volume (total annual hours) may increase gradually. However, athletes will find a unique training load that their physiology can sustain without injury or illness. Many athletes find that level by overtraining for 1 year or more, resulting in increased injury, illness, and loss of performance. Athletes who listen carefully to their bodies and monitor fatigue and recovery are more likely to find their personal **training plateau** without loss of performance. During this life period, it is common to gradually increase the hours of higher intensity training while maintaining or slightly decreasing lower intensity hours, as shown in figure 14.1a, for ages 22 and 23. Each sport requires a different mix of training modes and intensities, and much is written about individual sports elsewhere. Keep the general principles in mind. When participating in team sports, remember that everyone responds differently to training. We all need to adjust our training for optimal performance.

Training Plateau?

If your training has reached a plateau and you aren't making satisfactory progress, try adding additional high-intensity training. Cross-country skiers who had not responded well to high-volume, low-intensity training switched to a program with twice the volume of high-intensity training. They demonstrated improvement in $\dot{V}O_2$max, **anaerobic threshold**, and competitive results (Gaskill et al. 1999). Add intensity with race pace intervals, **fartlek** (speed play), time trials, and races, but be sure to cut back on overall volume to avoid fatigue and overtraining. This study was done with mature athletes; it does not apply to athletes less than 24 years old.

Muscular training focuses on specific training for each sport. In general, volume of both strength and power training increases. Endurance athletes increase strength and power, as well as power endurance.

Age 30 and Above

Great performances continue to occur, and the same training principles apply. As we get older, we also need to train smarter and apply the principles of specificity and individual response, as well as pay close attention to rest and recovery. There is no denying that after the peak younger years, there is a gradual decline in both our energy systems and our muscular system. Smart training can greatly attenuate those declines, while training and competing smarter often result in improved performances well past age 30.

Muscular training remains vital for mature athletes. It is common for muscle mass to decrease with aging. Resistance training can attenuate the loss of muscle protein. Focus should be on sport-specific needs as well as muscular balance to reduce injury risk.

Annual Periodization

Seasonal periodization is the planning of your training year into periods with specific goals. Although you can make significant improvements in both aerobic and anaerobic energy sources in as little as 2 months, a year-round program is both safer and more effective (see figures 14.3 and 14.4). The concept of moving from general training to specific training within each yearly cycle is important. For energy training, all programs begin with an aerobic buildup, a period of slow distance work that builds stamina and neuromuscular efficiency.

Figure 14.3 shows relative volumes for each energy training type during each season of training. Part *a* covers aerobic sports. The volume of easy aerobic, race pace–plus intervals, and maximal intervals for each period is relative to the largest volume that you might do during the year. Thus, if your maximum weekly load was 10 hours (line M) you would be doing about 8 hours of easy aerobic training, 1.6 hours (including rest) of race pace–plus intervals, and 25 minutes (including rest) of maximal intervals training during a week. During the off-season (line O), you would be training for about 4 hours, with 3 hours and 45 minutes of easy aerobic training and 15 minutes of race pace–plus intervals during the week.

Figure 14.3*b* covers anaerobic sports, such as running, cycling, cross-country skiing, and soccer. The volume of easy aerobic, race pace–plus intervals, and maximal intervals for each period is relative to the largest volume that you might do during the year. Thus, if your weekly load was 10 hours at the line marked M, you would be doing about 4.5 hours of easy aerobic training, 3 hours (including rest) of race pace–plus intervals, and 1 hour and 30 minutes (including rest) of maximal intervals during a week. During the off-season

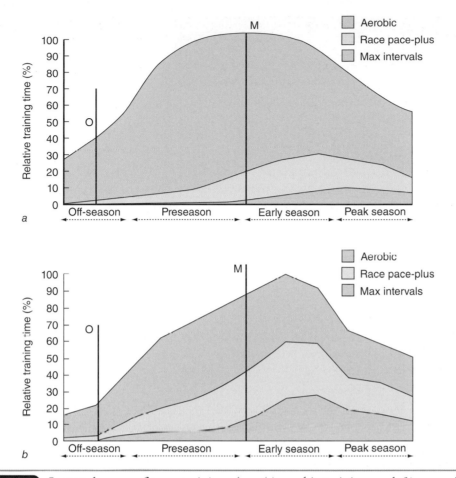

FIGURE 14.3 Seasonal energy fitness training plan: (*a*) aerobic training, and (*b*) anaerobic training.

(line O), you would be training for about 1 hour and 45 minutes of easy aerobic training and doing 20 minutes of race pace–plus intervals during a week.

These graphs are general plans that you can adjust based on goals, sport, and individual capabilities.

Figure 14.4 is a schematic of relative volumes of muscular training across a training season for aerobic and anaerobic sports. You will need to adjust the plan to where your sport falls on the continuum between the two ends of the spectrum. Part *a* covers aerobic sports. The volume of light preparatory, strength, power, and muscular endurance training for each period is relative to the largest volume that you might do during the year. Thus, if your maximum weekly load was 2.5 hours of muscular fitness training (line M), you would be doing about 45 minutes of strength training (2 to 6RM), 1 hour and 15 minutes of power training (8 to 15RM), and 30 minutes of muscular endurance training (15 to 25RM) during a week. During the off-season (line O) you would gradually increase lifting of light weights to about 30 minutes a week, slowly increasing the weights to a point where you are ready to begin strength training.

Figure 14.4*b* covers anaerobic sports, such as sprints or football. The volume of light preparatory, strength, and power for each period is relative to the largest volume that you might do during the year. Thus, if your maximum weekly load was 10 hours of muscular fitness training (line M), you would be doing about 7 hours of strength training (2 to

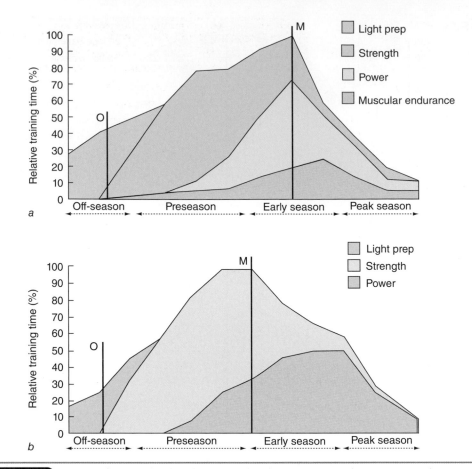

FIGURE 14.4 Seasonal training plan for muscular fitness: *(a)* aerobic sports, and *(b)* anaerobic sports.

6RM) and 3 hours of power training during a week. During the off-season (line O), you would gradually increase lifting of light weights to about 2 hours and 20 minutes per week, slowly increasing the weights to a point where you are ready to begin strength training.

These graphs are general plans that you can adjust based on goals, sport, and individual needs.

To help with the annual planning process, we generally divide the year into four training periods. The general plan starts with an off-season (postcompetition) period of easy, nonspecific training, followed by a period of basic training (often called the preseason) to develop the aerobic base and foundation for strength. After laying the foundation, athletes increase anaerobic capacity, power, and speed during the period leading into and including the early competitions (early competition period). Finally, the peak performance period is a time of reduced total training volume, increased speed and power work, and, most important, increased rest and recovery to allow optimal performance.

It is common for many sports to have two or three major competition periods within a year. In those cases, it is possible to use the models in figure 14.3 and 14.4 as 4- or 6-month programs. Another alternative is to develop an annual program focusing on the most important competitions. Make minor adjustments to the program for the 2 to 4 weeks prior to less important competitions. The timing of the seasonal training periods will depend on your sport, your season, and the needs of each individual athlete.

Off Season

This is a time of recovery from the previous competitive season. It includes nonspecific, nonstructured activities done at a low intensity. The duration depends on the motivation of each athlete. Many athletes do physical activities that they enjoy, but which may be unrelated to their competitive sports. Vedar Ulvang, one of the great Norwegian cross-country skiers, was well known for his sea kayaking and mountaineering exploits during the recovery period. This postcompetitive period generally ranges from a few weeks to a few months in length. Sport-specific conditioning declines during this period, and little muscular training is done. Research has shown that without this period of recovery, athletes do not perform as well the following year.

Official Seasons

In many academic and professional sports, the year may include an **official training season**, when coaches run practices with the athletes, and an unofficial season, when the athletes are expected to train on their own. For academic programs, the official season generally corresponds with the precompetition, early competition, and peak performance seasons, which means that athletes need to complete off-season and basic training periods on their own. Most coaches understand that it takes time to develop strength and endurance, so they encourage their athletes to participate in running and strength training during the basic training period prior to their official season. Doing this allows appropriate time to systematically develop the physiological systems necessary to achieve individual and team goals. This additional training requires self-motivation on the part of the athlete and an effort by coaches to encourage participation.

Basic Training

This period marks the beginning of planned training. The focus of this time is to build a foundation of strength and energy fitness to support the higher intensity work that will be done as the competition season approaches. For both anaerobic and aerobic energy sports, high-intensity training is minimal during this period.

For endurance sports, most training will be done as easy distance or recovery training, with only minimal volumes of higher intensity intervals or sustained training. Speed and power, which are critical for all sports, can be maintained with a few short duration, moderate- to high-intensity intervals done once or twice a week. Most sports require various degrees of aerobic energy. This is true across the continuum from long-distance endurance sports to sprinting and explosive events. It is clear that endurance athletes require more aerobic fitness than sprint or power athletes do. Improved aerobic function enhances recovery and allows sprinters and power athletes to do more repetitions and improve their performance. Changes in aerobic fitness often require extended periods of training. Thus, training of the aerobic energy system begins in this cycle.

Muscular training during this period of time focuses on strength training. After a short period of using lighter weights to adapt the body back to resistance training, you can gradually increase the weight until using heavy weights with low repetitions results in increased strength. Power and sprint athletes continue strength training for up to 16 weeks until a plateau is reached and muscle hypertrophy has occurred. Endurance athletes also do strength training, but will stop after 6 to 12 weeks, before significant hypertrophy occurs.

Skill development may also be a priority, using imagery, drills, and easy practice. Sport psychologists have shown that changing technique requires patience, feedback, and visualization. The recovery and basic training periods are a great time to work on technique, allowing athletes time to master new skills before competitions begin.

The basic training period lasts a minimum of 8 weeks and as long as 5 months in order to optimize muscle recruitment for strength and lay an adequate foundation for aerobic energy. For sports with limited training periods, such as high-school and college programs, the training during this period is generally done individually, not as a part of the structured season. For academic programs, this period needs to be at least 8 weeks and as long as 12. For year-round sports, the basic training period may last 4 or 5 months. During the period, there will be a gradual increase in total training hours and intensity of training as the precompetition period approaches.

Precompetition

This period is the transition from basic training to competition. It lasts 6 to 8 weeks for school sports, and 12 to 14 weeks for year-round programs, extending up through the first competition. Energy-fitness training will include more interval and high-intensity training. The speed and intensity of the intervals depends on the energy system needed, but it is common practice to use race pace–plus intervals for all events. This means learning to move slightly faster during intervals, but for a shorter distance than athletes can currently perform for their event (see the following sections for more on interval training). Moderate competition simulations begin with an emphasis on speed, skill, and tactics.

Muscular training during this period transitions to power training, with slightly lighter weights and high speeds of movement with sport specificity. Strength may be maintained with a few sets of heavy weights each week. Both endurance and sprint athletes do power training specific to their sport.

This period is often the start of the training season for many school-based programs. If no systematic training has been done before the official-season, athletes will begin without adequate strength and endurance. They need to understand that it is their responsibility to prepare before the official academic season. Without basic training, it is more likely that athletes will become injured and that their performances will suffer. Those who have not adequately prepared should not do high-intensity training until they are ready.

Athletes who compete in multiple sports may finish one competitive cycle in the fall and head into a new sport during the winter. In these cases, athletes need 1 or 2 weeks for rest and recovery before beginning the new season.

Early Competition

The early competition period generally lasts 4 or 5 weeks for school sports, and as long as 10 weeks for yearlong programs. This period may include scrimmages and early competitions to prepare for important league and championship contests. Many athletes include all but their most important event in this period. Generally, overall training volume decreases from the precompetition period, while sport-specific speed and power endurance increase. Competitive success can be high, but the emphasis remains on power endurance, speed, and race pace–plus interval training, along with maintaining an endurance base in line with the needs of the sport. Speed training is generally increased, while resistance training is reduced to maintenance status. More time will be spent on technique and tactics. Athletes need to recover more between training sessions in order to be able to do high-quality, competition-specific training. Toward the end of the early competition period, training volume will begin to decline (taper) in preparation for major competitions. The early competition period ends about 2 to 4 weeks before peak performances.

Muscular training for sprint and power athletes during the early competition period continues, with a somewhat reduced volume of power training and strength maintenance. Endurance athletes transition to a specific power-endurance program, with low-resistance, high-repetition training.

Peak Performance

Depending on the sport, training during the peak performance period will continue with high-intensity work, but the total volume of training will be reduced so that athletes can rest for important competitions. The main training emphasis is on speed, skill, and tactics, while maintaining sport-specific power, power endurance, and aerobic fitness.

In the 1 or 2 weeks leading to the most important event, athletes may taper their training in an effort to peak for an important event. Effective tapers gradually reduce training volume and stress by 40 to 60 percent. This allows athletes time for complete recovery between high-quality workouts and competitions. In addition to the taper, coaches may wish to focus on slight adaptations to the race pace–plus intervals. For aerobic, mid-distance, and intermittent events, we recommend intervals at about 5 percent above current race speed. During the early and peak competition periods, it is effective to gradually lengthen the intervals while gradually decreasing the recovery period. Reduce the number of intervals and stop before speed deteriorates. This slight increase in intensity and reduction in rest will help athletes peak. Combining a taper with assisted race pace–plus intervals at maximal intensity, while maintaining long rest periods, will help sprint athletes improve their performance. Peaking can improve performance by 2 to 4 percent.

Annual Periodization and Specificity of Muscular Training

In a study of junior cross-country skiers, a periodized sport-specific muscular fitness training (arm work on an inclined ramp duplicating the poling motion in cross-country skiing) was found superior to lifting weights or even roller skiing to improve arm power and performance. The athletes first developed strength on a steeply inclined ramp (with low repetitions) during the basic training period. They then focused on power, using explosive contractions, on a lesser incline during the precompetition period. During the later parts of the precompetition period and into the early competitions, they trained for muscular endurance with high repetitions and low resistance. The cross-country skiers in the periodized program improved race performance 15 percent more than traditional weight-training and roller-ski programs for cross-country skiers (Nesser et al. 2004).

Muscular training decreases during the peak performance period, and it may be minimal for endurance athletes. However, muscular power activities remain an important component for sprint and power sports, but with a much reduced lifting schedule and adequate rest prior to competitions.

Weekly Periodization

Within the four structured training periods, systematic variation in stress of physical training needs to be planned. We recommend using a 3-week cycle of medium, hard, and recovery weeks (see figures 14.1c and 14.5). When you plan an average training week appropriate for the time of the year, use figure 14.3 to estimate the total training volume and proportions of easy aerobic training, race pace–plus intervals, and maximal intervals. The same procedure can be used to plan appropriate training volumes of strength, power, and power endurance from figure 14.4. During an average week, athletes should feel tired after hard workouts, but they should easily recover by the following morning. Once an average week is determined, the following week should be a hard week, which requires 20 to 50 percent more effort, generally by making each workout 20 to 50 percent longer

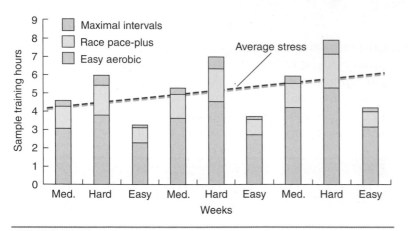

FIGURE 14.5 This periodization graph represents a theoretical model of weekly energy fitness progression for an aerobic sport during the basic endurance and strength period, using a 3-week periodization. The dotted line shows the average progression of training stress. During moderate weeks, race pace–plus training is about 10 percent of energy fitness training. Muscular fitness training is scheduled 3 days per week, with 3 sets of strength (3–6RM). During hard weeks, race pace–plus training is increased to 15 percent, and muscular fitness includes 3 days of 2 sets for strength and 1 set for power training. For easy weeks, race pace–plus training is reduced to 7 percent, and muscular fitness is reduced to 2 days with 2 sets of strength and 1 set for muscular endurance with higher repetitions.

Intensity and Specificity

High intensity requires more rest: The closer you are to competition, the greater the need for high-intensity training. This added stress requires added rest. Don't try to quickly get into shape coming into the major competitions. That work needs to be done much earlier. In the few weeks leading up to competitions, focus on sport-specific tasks and fine-tuning. Your high-intensity training now should build on the foundations established in the previous months. Athletes who have not laid an appropriate foundation are not ready for higher intensity training. They may become overtrained or get injured. Lower fit athletes should be encouraged to continue basic fitness training through the competitions to prepare for future years. The use of the fatigue index (page 375) is a great tool to ensure that your athletes are getting adequate rest.

Start with general training and move toward sport-specific training. During periods of transition, overlap types of training within each week. When moving from strength to power training, it is appropriate to include both types in practice, just as it is common in aerobic fitness to require days of long-duration training mixed with days of speed work.

or by increasing intensity. The athletes may not recover well after each workout. By the end of the week, athletes should feel tired. The third week in the cycle can then be an easy week, about 20 to 50 percent less strenuous than the average week. Here, the focus is lower duration and intensity and on recovery. More is not always better. Adding easy weeks to training may seem counterintuitive, especially with short official seasons, but their value has been shown repeatedly. Coaches who fail to allow time for recovery pay for it with poor performance, illness, and injuries. Figure 14.5 shows a typical planned progression using a 3-week cycle.

One difficulty for athletes and coaches is to determine the optimal training load or stress for a training program. In order to adjust the stress of easy, moderate, and hard weeks, we recommend that athletes use the fatigue index, described in figure 14.7 on page 374 and form 14.1 on page 375. The fatigue index is a simple morning evaluation in which the sum of resting, exercise, and recovery heart rates is used to monitor fatigue.

The peak performance period requires a more structured **weekly periodization** to ensure that major competitions follow easier weeks of training. If you know the dates of competitions in both the early competition and peak performance periods, mark them on your calendar. Classify the weeks before important competitions as easy weeks, and allow 2 weeks for peaking before the most important competition. Note: Not all competitions can be considered important, especially during the early competition period. Some less important competitions may follow medium- or even high-stress training weeks.

Daily Periodization

By now, you should have a picture of training as a gradual increase in specificity and intensity, with decreasing hours during the competition period. You should also visualize the undulating weekly change with medium, hard, and easy weeks. This concept of layers of planned variation should continue down to the weekly level.

Within each training week, be sure to vary the physical stress of the training days. Just like the periodization of weeks, vary the days within each week in a regular cycle of medium, hard, and easy days. It is fine to vary this to best accommodate training. It is no problem to do 2 or 3 days of hard training in a row, but be sure to have a few easier days afterward. This daily periodization helps athletes recover for high-intensity training days and stay healthy. The training stress needs to be appropriate for each athlete's maturity. The best gauge will be how you respond to your plan. At the end of hard weeks, you should be tired, but you should recover easily during the following easy week. Vary the overall stress of the training days so that you seldom have more than 2 or 3 high-stress days in a row without allowing an easier day for recovery. During the precompetition and competition periods, it is better to follow every hard day with an easier day.

Concurrent Strength and Endurance Training

Many athletes conduct concurrent strength and aerobic endurance training in the same muscle group. Early research suggested that endurance training interfered with full development of strength (Hickson 1980). A study of 45 male and female subjects supports the contention that combined strength and endurance training can suppress some of the adaptations to strength training. Gains in strength were greater with strength-only training. With female subjects, the combined training raised the level of the stress hormone cortisol. Surprisingly, the combined training augmented the number of capillaries per muscle fiber, a measure important to endurance (Bell et al. 2000). A review confirmed that endurance athletes benefit greatly from concurrent combined training (Aagaard and Andersen 2010), but if you need high levels of strength, focus on strength training with modest endurance training. Experienced athletes seem to thrive in concurrent strength and endurance training. Because concurrent training requires synthesis of strength and endurance proteins, consuming up to 1.8 grams of good-quality protein per kilogram of body weight each day is important.

Stress comes in many forms for athletes. For example, during exam periods in college or high school, athletes find that the mental stress and lack of sleep may require them to reduce their training load. They also need to be aware that endurance days, even if the pace is slow, may be stressful if the duration is long. Pay attention to how you are feeling. If you are more tired than you had anticipated, adjust your practice for the day.

Easy days do not mean that athletes don't do a full practice or that they need to spend less time working. It simply means that they need to use activities that will allow full recovery. These are great days to do technique and skill work, watch game films, practice psychological skills, work on tactics, or even do game simulations. Allow plenty of recovery time.

PSYCHOLOGY OF PERFORMANCE

Psychologist Nathaniel Ehrlich (1971) draws a distinction between competitors and performers in athletic competition. Competitors evaluate their performances strictly on a win–loss basis, with little regard given to the absolute level of performance. Performers attach secondary importance to winning. They evaluate their performances against an absolute scale, an ideal.

The competitor subscribes to the Vince Lombardi dictum "Winning isn't everything; it's the only thing." The performer, on the other hand, would give the nod to "It isn't whether you win or lose; it's how (and how well) you play the game." Ehrlich draws an analogy between Maslow's self-esteem and self-actualization levels of motivation (see chapter 4). Competitors seek recognition and fear competition as a threat to their self-esteem; performers seek to realize their potential. We would hope to find a mature, self-actualizing approach to competition among adult athletes. Each would be seeking his or her potential, and competition would serve as a means to that end.

If you value your mental health and you don't want to be frustrated by defeat and lose your self-esteem, become a performer. Performers never fail. If their performance is flawed, they know that time and practice will bring them closer to their goal. Focus on the quality of the experience, not the outcome. Don't get angry when you lose; you need good competition to improve. Analyze, but don't judge your performance. Approach weaknesses positively (I need to get my racket back earlier), not negatively (My forehand stinks). Set goals in terms of performance instead of wins, medals, or trophies. You may find that those come as your performance improves. If not, you can still find satisfaction in the game, and you won't feel regret when it's over.

Play Your Best Game

Have you noticed that you do well on some days and poorly on others? Have you ever wished that you could play your best game more often? Sport psychologists Tutko and Tosi (1976) offered suggestions to help you do just that and to improve your ability to deal with the emotional side of your game.

Relax. Contract and then relax your muscles, and think *Let go* as you learn muscle relaxation, as in Jacobson's progressive relaxation (1938). Concentrate on your breathing and think *Easy* with each exhale, as in Benson's **relaxation response** (1975). Eventually, you can use the relaxation techniques in competition to help relieve tension.

• *Concentrate.* Focus your attention on an object in the game (e.g., tennis ball) to free the mind of fears and negative judgments and to allow your best performance. When your opponent tosses the ball for the serve, think *Ball*, concentrate on the ball, and let your body do what it has learned to do.

• *Mentally rehearse.* Do this before and during practice and before competition to help focus on key elements of the game. Imagine yourself performing well.

• *Physically rehearse.* Practice to hone your skills in days preceding competition and as skill rehearsal in the warm-up just before the event.

You will notice that these sport psychologists neglected to include advice on how to psych yourself up for the game or how to psych out your opponent. Did they forget? Probably not. Most of us fail because we are overaroused. We are so psyched up and concerned that we are literally tied in knots, unable to execute the skills that we worked so hard to perfect. If we think too much and try too hard, we are bound to fail. So Tutko and Tosi provide advice aimed at helping you free your mind, relax, and reach the state called flow. Then and only then can you produce your best performance. You'll find yourself saying, "I played over my head," "I was out of my mind," "I couldn't miss; everything I hit went in." Don't get us wrong; we're not suggesting that you enter an event and then forget why you're there. On the contrary, you're there to play well and have fun. You should savor every moment.

The theory behind this approach is based on the different roles played by the right and left brains. The left brain is absorbed with details. It is analytical and judgmental, whereas the right brain is concerned with movements, patterns, and the overall picture. After we learn skills, we should perform them without the critical review of the left brain. Relaxation and concentration allow us to play our best game more often.

Successful distance runners tend to associate during a race. They tune in to their bodies so that they will know how fast they dare run. They are consciously aware of pace, position, key opponents, and features along the course. Less successful runners tend to disassociate, to lose track of time and place. Form becomes less efficient, and their pace slows.

By learning to handle your emotions, you'll enjoy the game more. Eliminate the

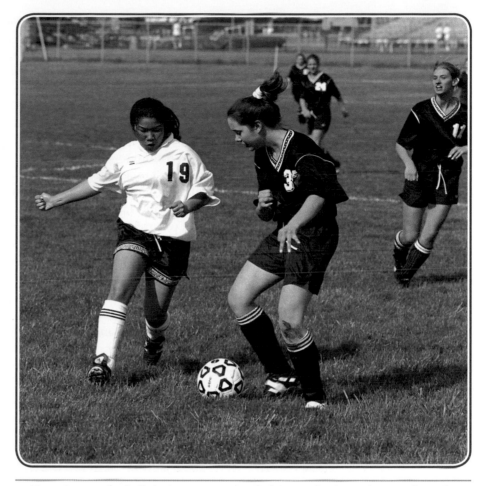

■ Focusing on the ball during a game can help you eliminate fears and reach your potential.

tensions, fears, and frustrations, and you may win more often. If you can do all these things and devote sufficient time to practice and training, you will be well on your way to achieving your potential. More important, the enjoyment and success that you experience will keep you involved in a lifelong pursuit of excellence.

Performance Potential

Researchers published a fascinating account of the restraints on performance in running (Ryder, Carr, and Herget 1976). Using running records from the previous 50 years, they plotted the rate of improvement and made some surprising conclusions. On average, the rate of improvement in distances ranging from 100 meters to 30 kilometers has been a steady but slow .75 meter per minute per year. Because record breakers seldom participate in further assaults on the record, the investigators concluded that good runners just don't work as hard after they have set a record. The researchers contend that running records are still well below human physiological limits, that the restraints on performance are largely psychological and pathological. The major obstacle is not the race but the amount of time devoted to daily training. In recent years, athletes have had to train many hours a day to achieve record-breaking status. After achieving the record, the athlete is likely to turn attention to other, more mundane matters, such as starting a career, earning a living, getting married, and having a family.

Thus, time is the obstacle, time and the injuries associated with overuse and overtraining. If you feel stymied in your training, if you are stuck on a plateau, invest more time to resume your progress. Barring injury, you should be able to improve. Following this line of reasoning, progress in world records will begin to slow when men and women have invested as much training time as is humanly possible. Thereafter, progress will depend on improved equipment and new techniques. Today, nearly 40 years after this analysis, training has become a full-time job for world-class athletes, and world records continue to decline. Of course, specialists in sports medicine are actively engaged in repairing the bodies battered by relentless training.

Most of us are unable to invest excessive time in training, so we must define our potential as the level that we attain following the maximum possible time and effort. Given the limitations imposed by job and family, as well as by heredity, physique, sex, and age, you can still make dramatic progress toward your potential. Consider the case of petite Michiko Suwa from Japan. She came to the United States at the age of 28 and changed her first name to Miki. Five years later, she began jogging. In 1973 at age 38, she ran her first marathon. Later that year, she astounded the running world with a woman's world record. Neither physique nor age predicted her potential. Look at Priscilla Welch, a two-pack-a-day smoker who quit smoking, started running, and went on to become a world-class competitor in the marathon. Or consider Sister Marion, a nun who started running in 1979. Within 5 years, she qualified for the 1984 Olympic marathon trials, at the age of 54! As we wrote this book, Janet Evans, who won three swimming gold medals at the Seoul Olympics in 1988 and continued winning in 1992 and 1996, was working to come back and swim in the 2012 London games even after having two children. Although she did not make the U.S. Olympic team, her accomplishments at age 40 are inspiring.

OVERTRAINING

Training, when overdone, can be a stressor that reduces the ability of the immune system to resist infection. Yet athletes at all levels seem prone to overtrain. We grew up believing the old fallacy "No pain, no gain." Yet the risks of overtraining are many, including illness, injury, and lost time. Athletes should expect to be tired after a hard workout, but they should recover by the following morning. This tiredness is simply the application of the overload principle, which requires that you do more than you have previously been doing to get a training response. Thus, athletes can expect to be tired at the end of a long or high-intensity workout. Another term for this tiredness is **overreaching**. This suggests that we have put an excess load on our bodies, but one from which we can recover. Some athletes will even link several days of hard training together until they recognize that they are pushing past the symptoms of overreaching and beginning to move toward overtraining. Athletes in tune with their bodies will back off and take a few easy training days at this point to recover.

Symptoms of overtraining include lethargy, fatigue, poor performance, sleep loss, loss of appetite, and illness. Because the symptoms arise slowly, overtraining is difficult to diagnose. Causes of overtraining include boredom, overwork relative to rest, immune suppression because of exhaustion and stress, hormonal imbalance, poor nutrition, rapid weight loss, and inadequate hydration. Scientists have used measures such as the wake-up heart rate and temperature, cortisol to testosterone ratio, and mood scales to try to help people avoid overtraining.

Increases in the ratio of cortisol to testosterone have been correlated with overtraining. Blood levels of cortisol, a hormone from the adrenal gland, increase when the body is under physical or psychological stress (Neary et al. 1994). Testosterone is an anabolic (growth-stimulating) hormone that decreases with overtraining. The ratio is a sensitive but expensive indicator of overtraining. If you undertake serious training, you should become familiar with some simple ways to detect overtraining and use them regularly (see figure 14.6). The fatigue index is an excellent way to monitor fatigue and avoid overtraining.

The fatigue index is a simple way to detect the early stages of overtraining in athletes. It is an inexpensive but accurate way to judge when an athlete is accumulating fatigue on a collision course with overtraining. The results correlate closely with immune function: When the fatigue index goes up, immune function declines, and vice versa. All you need to conduct the test is a sturdy 8-inch (20 cm) bench (or bottom stair) and a stopwatch. A heart rate monitor is recommended, but not required. Form 14.1 details the procedure for the fatigue index. After a baseline is established, subsequent tests can be used to gauge the extent of fatigue. Large increases in the fatigue index suggest the need for additional rest, or a break from hard training.

Athletes who use the fatigue index daily will find it very helpful to have a visual image of their stress and recovery, as shown in figure 14.7. Using a graph, it is easy to establish baselines and to evaluate when thresholds of overtraining (form 14.1) have been exceeded.

The treatment for overtraining is relative rest. Serious cases demand time off or bed rest, but most people respond to reduced training, more time for recovery, attention to nutrition, and a change of pace. Remember that you should approach training as a gentle pastime. If you make haste slowly, you will eventually reach your goals. If you overtrain, you'll lower your resistance to infection. For more about training and overtraining, see *Sport Physiology for Coaches* (Sharkey and Gaskill 2006).

CROSS-TRAINING

As the triathlon attracted multisport athletes, the concept of cross-training gained attention. Cross-training can be viewed as systematic variety that prevents overuse injuries. It allows addicted athletes to train hard every day with little risk of overuse or repetitive

Index	How to use
Pulse index	Take your pulse rate daily (for 60 sec), in the morning before rising. Average the daily rates. When the morning pulse is 5 or more beats above normal, you should suspect illness or overtraining. Take an easy day to get back to normal.
Weight index	Check your weight daily, in the morning (after using the toilet but before eating breakfast). Average daily weights. A rapid or persistent weight loss could indicate impending problems because of poor eating habits, failure to replace fluids, nervousness, or excessive fatigue.
Temperature	Take your morning temperature daily for a week to establish your normal reading. Then use it to determine whether the morning temperature is elevated. A fever usually indicates infection. Take a day off.
Step test	After rising in the morning, but before breakfast and coffee, do this procedure. Step up and down on the bottom step of stairs (8 in., or 20 cm). Use 2 steps per second, moving both feet up on the 1st second and both down on 2nd second. Continue for 1 min, then immediately take your pulse for 15 sec (multiply by 4 to obtain the rate per min). Average the daily rates for a week to get a baseline. When the posttest pulse is 10 or more beats above the normal baseline, you should suspect illness or overtraining. Take a day or two of easy training until your step test pulse is back to normal. For a more sensitive variation, use the fatigue index listed in form 14.1.

FIGURE 14.6 Overtraining indexes.

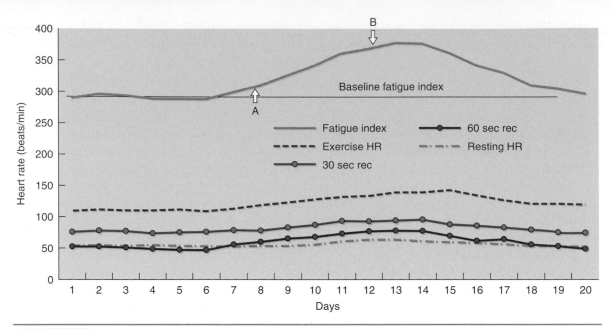

FIGURE 14.7 Data from an athlete during a 3-week competition period. The athlete chose to ignore the signs of fatigue appearing at day 8 (*a*). By day 12 (*b*), this person had developed a serious cold and sore throat and could not compete for the next 2 weeks. See form 14.1 for this procedure.

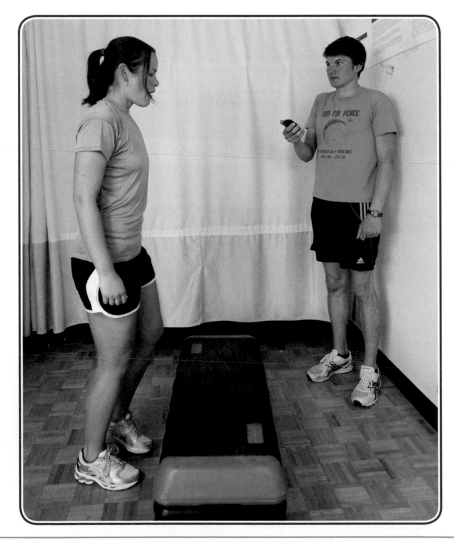

■ Monitoring your training using the fatigue index will help you optimize your training load and reduce the risk of overtraining.

Form 14.1   The Fatigue Index

Procedure

After rising in the morning, but before eating breakfast or consuming stimulants (tea or coffee):

- Sit quietly for 3 to 5 minutes until your heart rate is stable. You can read the paper during this time.
- Take the resting heart rate at the wrist for 10 seconds, and then multiply the number of beats by 6 to get the rate per minute.
- Start the stopwatch and begin stepping up and down stairs (up with one foot then the other, then down with the first foot and then the other). The entire sequence of stepping up and down should take 2 seconds. Repeat this 30 times in 1 minute.
- Stop after 1 minute of stepping. While standing, take the postexercise heart rate (10 sec x 6 = bpm), then sit down immediately.
- Sit quietly and relax. At 30 seconds after exercise, take your heart rate (10 sec x 6 = bpm).
- At 60 seconds after exercise, take the final heart rate (10 sec x 6 = bpm).

Resting heart rate   = _____

Postexercise heart rate   = _____

30-second postexercise heart rate   = _____

60-second postexercise heart rate   = _____

Fatigue index (sum)   = _____

To calculate the fitness index, sum all heart rates (resting, postexercise, and 30 sec and 60 sec recovery). The total is the fatigue index. The index is unique for each person, and should be compared to the athlete's average index for several days during a rested period.

Criteria for Evaluating the Fatigue Index

The higher the index is above baseline values, the greater the likelihood that the athlete has not recovered from prior training. When the fatigue index is more than 20 above the normal baseline, the athlete is at increased risk for depressed immune function and upper respiratory infections.

Increase in fatigue index	Risk of overtraining
0 to 20 above baseline	Not generally a concern unless sustained higher intensity training is planned
20 to 30 above baseline	Slightly increased (Suggest no race pace or high intensity training)
30 to 45 above baseline	Increased risk (Suggest only short, easy training)
More than 45 above baseline	High risk (Suggest no training)

From B.J. Sharkey and S.E. Gaskill, 2013, *Fitness and health, seventh edition* (Champaign, IL: Human Kinetics).

Mood States

The profile of mood states (POMS) has been used to study the effects of overtraining. The POMS test uses the responses to 65 words, such as *tense, hopeless, bitter, lively, worn out,* and *bewildered,* to yield mood scores. Subjects are asked to indicate the answer that best describes to what degree they have experienced those particular moods during the past week, including the day of the test. Response options are 0—not at all, 1—a little, 2—moderately, 3—quite a bit, and 4—extremely. Responses are categorized into six mood scores: tension–anxiety, depression–dejection, anger–hostility, vigor–activity, fatigue–inertia, and confusion–bewilderment. The classic iceberg profile depicts an athlete low in all scores except vigor. Overtraining lowers vigor while it raises all the other scales (Morgan et al. 1988).

Neck Check

What should you do with an upper respiratory tract infection? Dr. Randy Eichner recommends the neck check. If symptoms are above the neck, such as a stuffy nose, sneezing, or a scratchy throat, try a test drive at half speed. If you feel better after 10 minutes, you can increase the pace and finish the workout. If symptoms are below the neck, with aching muscles or coughing, or if you have a fever, nausea, or diarrhea, take the day off (Eichner 1995). You can return to training when the fever is gone for at least 24 hours without the aid of aspirin or other antifever medications.

trauma injuries. Some people extol the virtue of training a variety of muscle groups, as in swimming, cycling, and running. Triathletes train for all three disciplines, and they do sport-specific weight training to enhance performance. Cross-training allows athletes and fitness enthusiasts the option to train more than they could in a single sport and to achieve balance in their training.

Does cross-training provide special performance benefits? Probably not. Specificity is still the best rule to follow if you want to improve in a sport. Swimming will not improve performance in running or cycling, and vice versa. Activities that use similar muscles may contribute some to performance, but not to the same degree as increases in specific training (Foster et al. 1995). Of course, cross-training is a necessity if you are preparing for a multiple-discipline event, and it is a great way to remain active and fit as you grow older.

FITNESS AND WORK

Workers in construction, agriculture, forestry, firefighting, law enforcement, and the military are often required to engage in strenuous effort. Without proper conditioning, the stress of arduous work can be unpleasant or worse, so concern for employee health and safety has prompted screening procedures to make sure that the worker is capable of meeting job demands. Some companies have instituted employee fitness programs to help workers meet and maintain required levels of work capacity. Work capacity is defined as the ability to accomplish production goals without undue fatigue and without becoming a hazard to oneself or coworkers. Work capacity can also be viewed as sustainable capacity, the level of effort that one can sustain throughout the work shift. Obviously, both energy and muscular fitness are necessary for different physical jobs and training programs greatly enhance job performance. For more information on this topic, we recommend the book *Hard Work* (Sharkey and Davis 2008).

SUMMARY

This chapter presents a simple approach to the development of a year-round training program that provides for the systematic development of aerobic and anaerobic energy sources and for muscular strength, endurance, and power. If you are ready for some serious training, consider the program recommended by Rob Sleamaker (1989). The SERIOUS training program includes the following:

Speed

Endurance

Race or pace

Intervals

Overdistance

Up or vertical (e.g., hills) if applicable

Strength

For more detailed information on training and programming consult *Sport Physiology for Coaches* (Sharkey and Gaskill 2006).

If you are not that serious, forget speed and pace, but don't ignore variety in your training. Alternate hard with easy, short with long, speed with distance—and don't forget to include rest days for recovery. Outline a program and get started. Keep simple records, and change the program as your goals change. As your interest grows, look for books or magazines that focus on your activity. In time, you will become an expert on training and your body's response. Knowledge, coupled with adequate training, will improve your performance.

Environment

Acclimate, Then Perform

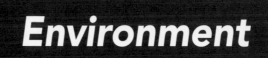

> " No athlete is crowned
> but in the sweat of his brow. "
>
> *St. Jerome*

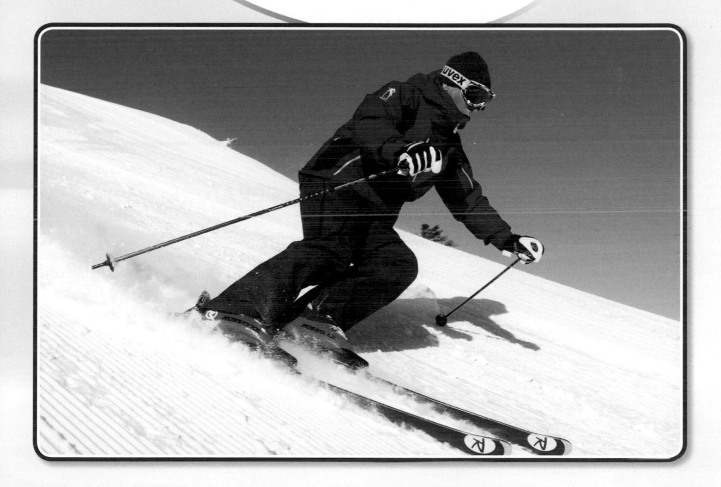

When you move to Montana, you expect to face a cold and sometimes hostile environment, and you know that you will have the opportunity to spend time at higher elevations. But would you expect high temperatures in the summer or air pollution in a state with less than one million residents spread out over 150,000 square miles (388,500 km²) of open space? Over the years, we've learned some tricks for coping with and even enjoying environmental extremes.

Environmental factors such as heat and cold, humidity, altitude, and air pollution can profoundly affect health and performance. Failure to consider these effects can lead to serious problems, even death. On the other hand, you can adjust or acclimate to the environment, enabling you to perform well and comfortably under a wide range of conditions. Let's consider the problems caused by extremes of temperature, humidity, altitude, and air pollution to see how fitness and proper planning can minimize their effects.

This chapter will help you do the following:

- Anticipate the effects of the environment on performance
- Take appropriate steps to minimize environmental effects
- Understand how fitness enhances your ability to acclimatize and perform in difficult environments

---

REGULATING TEMPERATURE

The body's temperature-regulating mechanism consists of four parts:

1. A regulating center located in the hypothalamus, an area at the base of the brain that serves as a thermostat to maintain body temperature at or near 37 degrees Celsius (98.6 °F)
2. Heat and cold receptors located in the skin to sense changes in environmental temperature conditions
3. Regulators such as muscles that increase body heat with shivering or exercise
4. Vasomotor (nervous system) controls that constrict or dilate arterioles to conserve or lose body heat

The temperature-regulating center responds to the temperature of the blood flowing by the hypothalamus. If the blood cools, the thermostat sends information for the body to conserve heat by constricting blood vessels in the skin and the extremities. Shivering also can generate some heat.

If the blood temperature rises above the desired level (sometimes called a *set point*), the regulating center can cause dilation of cutaneous (skin) blood vessels and stimulate the production of sweat. Consequently, blood moves from the warmer core of the body to the surface, allowing heat loss by conduction, convection, and radiation, as well as by evaporation of sweat from the surface of the skin. Complete evaporation of 1 liter of sweat leads to a heat loss of 580 calories. When the sweat does not evaporate and drips off the body, little heat is lost.

Heat and cold receptors in the skin also help maintain body temperature. The cold of the ski slopes will cause constriction of blood vessels, especially in the hands and feet. The extremities will stay cold until you raise body temperature, warm the blood, and reopen the blood vessels. The best way to do this is by vigorous exercise. Of course, you can put on more clothing or seek relief in the lodge.

The stifling heat of the tennis court will cause dilation of blood vessels, which diverts a significant amount of blood from the muscles to the skin. The heart rate increases in an effort to maintain blood flow to the working muscles and the skin. Sweating will eventually reduce blood volume, and unless you replace the water, your performance will suffer. If you persist in the activity and fail to replace the water loss, you may end up with heat exhaustion or heatstroke. So you are wise to listen to your body's call for rest, shade, and fluid replacement.

Individual differences in body fat, number of sweat glands, fitness level, and possibly sex may influence your response to heat.

• *Body fat*. Body fat serves as a layer of insulation beneath the surface of the skin. People with more subcutaneous fat may have better insulation from the cold, but they are not significantly less prone to lose excess heat to the environment because the body learns to route blood around the fat for cooling purposes. Excess fat is a handicap because the body needs extra energy just to carry it around.

• *Sweat glands*. Each of us inherits a certain number and pattern of sweat glands. Because evaporative heat loss is the most important protection against heat stress, a good supply of active sweat glands is important. Like almost everything else, sweat glands respond to use. If you use them a lot, they become more efficient.

• *Physical fitness*. Fitness seems to enhance the ability to regulate body temperature during work in the heat. It does so by lowering the temperature (set point) at which sweating begins. Thus, fit people can work or play with lower heart rates and core temperatures than those of their unfit counterparts. In our lab, a highly fit subject had a heart rate of 118, whereas less-fit people had rates of 170 beats per minute while doing the same work in the heat on the treadmill (Cordes and Sharkey 1995). Acclimatization further lowers the point at which sweating begins. Therefore, the physically fit and heat-acclimated person is even better prepared for work in the heat (Nadel 1977). Evidence indicates that fitness hastens the process of acclimatization.

• *Sex*. Men produce more sweat than women do for a given increase in body temperature, perhaps too much. Women are efficient sweaters. Their sweat production is more suited to the heat load, so they don't waste water. When men and women are compared on the same task, men seem better able to work in the heat, but the difference may be due to fitness, not sex. When the fitness level is the same or when the workload is equal in terms of a given percentage of maximal oxygen intake, women are quite able to work in the heat. In several recent marathons, women seemed to tolerate the heat as well as or better than many men did, probably because they sweat more efficiently.

Other factors that can influence your response to heat are illness, medications, drugs, and alcohol. If you have been ill, your thermoregulatory system will take several days to recover. Many prescription and over-the-counter medications, as well as all recreational drugs and alcohol, can influence the body's response in a hot environment. If you are in doubt about medications or drugs, check with a physician or pharmacist before you risk exposure in a hot environment.

Fitness seems to enhance the ability to regulate body temperature during work in the heat.

EXERCISING IN THE HEAT

When exercise begins, the temperature-regulating center increases the usual set point of the body, allowing body temperature to increase. The rise in temperature depends on the intensity of exercise. In a moderate environment, the temperature will increase about 1 degree Celsius (1.8 °F) at 50 percent of maximal oxygen intake and will rise to about 39 degrees (102 °F), a rise of 2 degrees Celsius (3.6 °F), at the maximal level. This resetting of the core temperature during exercise can be viewed as an adjustment favorable to the enzyme activity within the muscles. The higher set point also serves to reduce the problem of heat dissipation. Under moderate environmental conditions, the body does not employ methods of heat dissipation until the elevated set point has been reached.

In hot environments, we are able to maintain temporary thermal balance during exercise by virtue of circulatory adjustments and evaporation of sweat. The body gains heat when the air temperature exceeds the temperature of the skin. When humidity is low, the evaporation of sweat maintains thermal equilibrium. But when humidity is high and evaporation cannot take place, heat is stored and body temperature rises, severely impairing performance. Blood is diverted from muscles to the skin, blood volume is reduced through sweating, and water and electrolytes are lost in the sweat. Stroke volume declines, heart rate increases, and lactic acid may accumulate. Blood may even begin to pool in the large veins, further reducing venous return and cardiac output. The result, an alarming rise in body temperature called **hyperthermia**, sets the stage for heat stress disorders, heat exhaustion, or even heatstroke, the potentially fatal collapse of the temperature-regulating mechanism (see section on heat stress in this chapter, page 384).

Fluid Replacement

In a normal day, we lose and must replace about 2.5 liters of water (1 L = 1.057 qt; 1 qt = .946 L). Of this water loss, about .7 liter comes from the lungs and skin (insensible water loss), 1.5 liters from the urine, .2 liter from the feces, and about .1 liter through perspiration. During heavy exercise in the heat, the water lost through sweating can exceed 2 liters per hour. Sweat production may amount to as much as 12 liters per day. Because work capacity becomes impaired as water loss progresses, the fluid must be replaced. Dehydration in excess of 5 percent of body weight leads to a marked decline in strength, endurance, and work capacity. Estimate 1 quart for each 2-pound (.9 kg) weight loss; therefore, if you weigh 150 pounds (68 kg) and lose 8 pounds (3.6 kg), or more than 5 percent, you will be about 4 quarts (3.78 L) low on fluid!

The thirst mechanism always underestimates fluid loss during work in the heat and after work ends. Therefore, you should take frequent drinks throughout the work period. If you drink 250 milliliters (about 1 cup) every 15 minutes, you can replace 1 liter per hour. If the sweat rate is higher, you will find it extremely difficult to keep up with fluid needs. Marathon runners are wise to drink as much as possible (up to 500 ml) before the event to offset the tremendous water loss and difficulty of replacement. If, during prolonged periods of work in the heat, weight loss exceeds 2 percent (e.g., 3 lb for a 150 lb person, or 1.4 kg for a 68 kg person), the person should rehydrate before returning to work or exercise.

You can assess your level of dehydration by observing the color of your urine. When the urine is clear or wheat colored, you are hydrated. When it is dark, you are dehydrated; you should begin replacing fluids immediately (Armstrong 2000). Sweating rates and evaporative cooling depend on adequate hydration. Moderate **hyperhydration**, or excess fluid

> *B*ecause work capacity becomes impaired as water loss progresses, the fluid must be replaced.

intake, allows you to sweat more and work with a lower rectal temperature and heart rate, enabling increased work performance in hot work or sporting environments.

Electrolytes

Water replacement will not compensate for the loss of electrolytes (sodium, chloride, and potassium) in the sweat. For each liter of sweat lost, approximately 1.5 grams of salt are lost as well. Because the average meal includes 3 to 4 grams of salt, three meals per day will satisfy most salt needs. For long periods (8 hr or more) of work in the heat, when considerable loss of water and salt will occur, workers and athletes

> ## Hyponatremia
>
> Is it possible to drink too much water during prolonged exertion? Yes, it is: Excess water intake during prolonged exertion can disturb the body's electrolyte balance and can lead to abnormally low levels of plasma sodium (less than 135 mmol/L) and a condition called **hyponatremia**. Symptoms range from weakness, disorientation, seizures, severe headache, and coma; even death is possible if plasma sodium falls below 120 mmol/L. Unfortunately, the early symptoms sometimes lead to even greater water intake. When excess water intake is combined with a loss of sodium in sweat, the risk of hyponatremia grows. Problems occur when athletes consume 3 or more liters of water per hour in a long event such as a marathon, or in military training. For example, nine U.S. Marines experienced hyponatremia after drinking 10 to 22 quarts of water over a few hours of exertion. All survived after emergency treatment (Gardner 2002). You can avoid hyponatremia by drinking up to 1 liter of fluid per hour, using a mix of electrolyte drinks (sport drinks) and water.

should salt food liberally (8 hr at 1.5 g/L of salt = 12 g salt loss). We do not recommend salt tablets for several reasons. They are slow to dissolve and leave the stomach, so they will not provide aid for several hours. While they are dissolving, they take needed water from the bloodstream through osmosis. In addition, excessive salt intake can cause stomach cramps, weakness, high blood pressure, and other problems. Recently developed electrolyte supplements help athletes maintain electrolyte balance during daylong competitions.

You have several choices for replacement of water and salt. You can buy solutions containing the necessary electrolytes as well as some glucose (carbohydrate–electrolyte beverages), but remember that you may have to replace several quarts (L) of fluid. Replacing water and salt in this way could become expensive. You can save money by using the saltshaker at mealtime, drinking citrus fruit drinks for potassium, and obtaining the balance of fluid needs with water. Alternatively, you can prepare your own solution by adding a bit of salt to a quart of half-strength frozen lemonade. Another approach is to replace some of your fluid needs with tomato juice and the rest with water. When long periods of work in the heat make it necessary to replace electrolytes, use commercially available carbohydrate–electrolyte beverages or add a quarter teaspoon of salt to each quart (L) of water. Be sure to replace potassium during mealtime with citrus fruits or drinks, bananas, or other potassium-rich foods.

Carbohydrate–electrolyte sports drinks may offer several advantages. Their palatability ensures greater fluid intake, they help maintain blood glucose levels and performance during prolonged exertion, and the electrolytes reduce fluid loss through the urine. In addition, the carbohydrate helps maintain immune function (Ruby et al. 2003), and the elevated blood sugar serves to maintain cognitive function (Puchkoff et al. 1998).

Avoid very high glucose levels (more than 8%) in fluid-replacement solutions while running in the heat; the glucose could retard emptying of the stomach and reduce delivery of essential fluid. In a marathon or other long-duration race, runners should drink cool (40 °F, or 4 °C) electrolyte solutions that are relatively low in carbohydrate (40–80 g/L, or

4%–8%). Cyclists and cross-country skiers can tolerate higher carbohydrate concentrations during exercise, especially in cool temperatures.

To maintain proper hydration, you should drink water and low-carbohydrate electrolyte solutions before, during, and after vigorous activity.

- Before: Drink 2 to 3 cups (about 500–750 ml) before the event.
- During: Drink a cup (about 250 ml) or more of fluid every 15 to 20 minutes, or 1 quart (1 L) per hour.
- After: Replace fluid and carbohydrate after the event.

> **T**o maintain hydration, you should drink before, during, and after vigorous activity.

Of course, when it is not hot, or if you are not sweating a lot, you will not need to drink as much. Overdrinking without replacing sodium can lead to hyponatremia (see earlier box).

After exercise, drink plenty of fluids and begin to replace carbohydrate to replace muscle glycogen. The best postexercise strategy is to eat high-glycemic foods (e.g., sweets, breads, potatoes) in the first 2 hours after exercise, a critical period for glycogen replacement. A 4:1 carbohydrate-to-protein ratio may help speed muscle recovery.

Heat Stress

When the body is at rest, metabolic heat production amounts to about 1.2 calories per minute, or 72 calories per hour. Moderate exercise can elevate heat production to 600 calories or more per hour. You can see that exercise by itself can create considerable heat. Normally, heat is lost by convection, radiation, or evaporation of sweat. But when exercise is performed in a hot environment or when the humidity is high, metabolic heat cannot be dissipated. Both the body temperature and the risk of heat disorders rise.

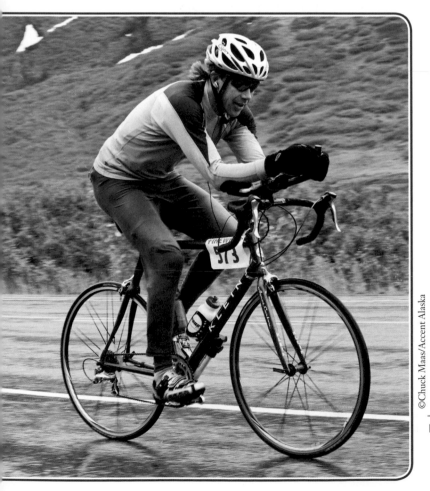

©Chuck Maas/Accent Alaska

- **Heat cramps** occur when electrolytes are lost in the sweat. Take a sport drink and use stretching and massage to relieve the cramp.
- **Heat exhaustion** occurs when the heat stress exceeds the capacity of the temperature-regulating mechanism. A person with cold, pale skin, body temperature of 39 to 41 degrees Celsius (102–106 °F), a weak pulse, and dizziness should be given fluids and allowed to rest in a cool environment.

■ Replacing fluids and electrolytes is essential after vigorous exercise in the heat, but moderate exercise in mild or cold weather requires less fluid intake.

- **Heatstroke** means that the temperature-regulating mechanism has failed. The skin is flushed, hot, and dry. Sweating stops, and the body temperature may rise above 41 degrees Celsius (106 °F). Heatstroke can lead to permanent damage of the temperature-regulating center of the brain, or even to death. This is a medical emergency! Cool the victim rapidly and administer fluids, if possible, while awaiting transport.

As you may have guessed, we cannot predict heat stress based on air temperature alone. Relative humidity is an important factor in determining how effective sweating will be. If sweat cannot evaporate, if it merely drips from the body, little heat is lost, and the water loss only adds to a circulatory problem. Air movement and radiant heat also are important factors to consider in evaluating the effect of a given environment on human comfort and performance. Even the type and color of clothing affect heat loss. Finally, we must consider metabolic heat production resulting from physical activity, which is the major heat source.

One way to assess the risk of heat stress is to use the heat stress index (figure 15.1). This chart is based on the shaded air temperature, moderate radiant heat from the sun, a light breeze, and a moderate work rate. Unfit or nonacclimated people will suffer at lower levels of heat, humidity, or work.

In sport or the workplace, the **wet bulb globe temperature (WBGT)** provides a simple and accurate indication of the effect of environmental factors on active people. The index uses dry bulb and wet bulb thermometers to assess air temperature and relative humidity (see form 15.1). The black copper globe thermometer indicates radiant heat as well as air movement. The several temperatures are weighted to indicate their relative contribution to the total heat stress. As you can see in the figure, the wet bulb temperature, or relative humidity, is the greatest contributor to heat stress (70% of the total).

Heat Stress Chart

When heat and hard work combine to drive the body temperature up, the temperature-regulating mechanism begins to fail and the worker faces serious heat stress disorders. This dangerous- often deadly–combination of circumstances can be avoided by monitoring the environment with simple measurements of temperature and humidity. This chart can help alert individuals to dangerous heat stress conditions.

Extreme heat stress conditions. Only heat-acclimated individuals can work safely for extended periods. Take frequent breaks and replace fluids.

Watch for changing conditions. Heat-sensitive and nonacclimated individuals may suffer. Increase rest periods and be sure to replace fluids.

Little danger of heat stress for acclimated individuals. Lack of air movement, high radiant heat, and hard effort can raise danger.

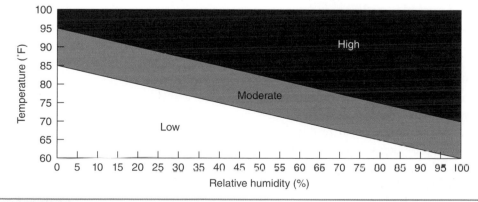

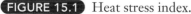

FIGURE 15.1 Heat stress index.

Reprinted from B.J. Sharkey, 1997, *Fitness and work capacity*, 2nd ed. (Missoula, MT: USDA Forest Service).

Form 15.1　WBGT Heat Stress Index

Sum the wet bulb, dry bulb, and black globe contributions to get the heat stress index.

							Example			
Wet bulb	=	_____	°F	×	.7	=	_____	80	× .7 =	56
Dry bulb	=	_____	°F	×	.1	=	_____	90	× .1 =	9
Black globe	=	_____	°F	×	.2	=	_____	120	× .2 =	24
				WBGT	=	_____°F		WBGT	=	89 °F

The wet bulb indicates humidity, the dry bulb measures the ambient temperature, and the black copper globe measures radiant heat and air movement.

Standards for work or exercise:

Above 80 °F—Use discretion.

Above 85 °F—Avoid strenuous activity.

Above 88 °F—Cease physical activity.*

*Trained people who have been acclimated to the heat can continue limited activity.

From B.J. Sharkey and S.E. Gaskill, 2013, *Fitness and health, seventh edition* (Champaign, IL: Human Kinetics). Reprinted from B.J. Sharkey, 1974, *Physiological fitness and weight control* (Missoula, MT: Mountain Press), 92. By permission of B.J. Sharkey.

The U.S. Marine Corps uses the WBGT to determine when to reduce or cancel physical training activities, and many high school and college athletic trainers and coaches use it to determine when to schedule practice sessions or distance runs. Bear in mind that the WBGT does not allow an estimate of the effect of clothing or energy expenditure. Dark or nonporous clothing can increase radiant heating or reduce evaporation. High levels of energy expenditure can create internal heat problems in moderate environments. No simple index tells you everything about heat stress, but for moderate energy expenditures (up to 425 cal/hr), while you are wearing light clothing (in color and weight), the WBGT is an excellent indicator of heat stress.

Heat Acclimatization

On the first day of vigorous exercise in a hot environment, you may experience a near-maximal heart rate, elevated skin and core temperatures, and severe fatigue. But after just a few days of exposure to work in the heat, you can accomplish the same task with a lower heart rate, made possible by improved blood distribution and increased blood volume. Skin and core temperatures are lower, because sweating begins at a lower temperature (Wenger 1988). The loss of water in the urine diminishes, and the salt concentration of the sweat gradually declines. This increase in circulatory and cooling efficiency is called **heat acclimatization**, and most of the process occurs after 5 to 10 days of work in a hot environment (increases in sweat rate may take longer).

Highly fit people become acclimatized in 4 or 5 days, whereas sedentary subjects take twice as long. The best way to acclimatize is to work in the actual conditions (temperature and humidity) that you'll have to endure. If you live in a cool climate and don't have a heat chamber in which to achieve acclimatization, high-intensity training can get you halfway there, probably because of the heat generated during vigorous effort. Using a nonrubberized sweat suit will increase the temperature close to the skin. Fit people start to sweat at a lower body temperature, and they increase sweat production at a faster rate. Acclimatization helps move the set point for sweating even lower.

Less-fit people should acclimatize using periods of light to moderate activity in a hot environment, alternated with rest periods during which they replace fluid. Electrolytes can be replaced with commercial drinks or the saltshaker at meals, plus potassium-rich citrus fruits or bananas. The vitamin C in the citrus drinks may hasten the acclimatization process.

In summary, the prescription for exercise in a hot, humid environment includes the following advice:

- Wear porous, light-colored, loose-fitting clothing.
- Acclimatize to the expected environment and workload (i.e., do 50% the first day, 60% the second, and add 10% each day until you do 100% on the sixth day).
- Take 250 to 500 milligrams a day of vitamin C while acclimatizing.
- Always replace water and electrolytes.
- Find a cool place for rest periods.
- Always work or train with a partner.
- Don't be too proud to quit when you feel the symptoms of heat stress (dizziness, confusion, cramps, nausea, or clammy skin).
- Keep a record of body weight during prolonged periods of work or training in the heat. Weigh in before and after exercise to gauge fluid loss. To check for day-to-day rehydration, weigh yourself in the morning, after using the toilet but before eating breakfast.
- Maintain aerobic fitness. The enhanced circulatory system and blood volume will help you work better in the heat, acclimate faster, and hold your acclimatization longer.

If you follow these suggestions, you can join the "mad dogs and Englishmen" out in the midday sun.

> **H**ighly fit people become acclimatized in 4 or 5 days, whereas sedentary subjects take twice as long.

Rhabdomyolysis

A final word about another heat-related risk of exertion, exertional **rhabdomyolysis**. In this condition, damaged skeletal muscle tissue releases the products of breakdown into the bloodstream. The muscle damage may be caused by physical factors, including strenuous exercise (especially in the heat and when dehydrated), medications, drug abuse, and infections. Some people have a hereditary muscle condition that increases the risk of rhabdomyolysis. This dangerous condition has been reported in military personnel and in law enforcement and firefighting trainees during hot, humid conditions. It has occurred when unprepared people engage in multiple sets of heavy lifting. Damage occurs to muscle membranes, allowing cellular components (such as creatine kinase, myoglobin, and potassium) to leak out. Rhabdomyolysis can lead to renal failure, irregular heartbeats, and even death (Parekh, Care, and Tainter 2012). Risk factors include a sedentary lifestyle, high ambient temperatures, and intense or extreme exercise. Military and fire department records indicate that the risk goes down as fitness improves. People taking cholesterol-lowering statin drugs may be at higher risk, as are those with sickle cell anemia, some viral infections, and dehydration, and those susceptible to hyperthermia (Clarkson and Sayers 2008). Some people appear to be more genetically susceptible to rhabdomyolysis (Clarkson et al. 2005).

EXERCISING IN THE COLD

Because of the metabolic heat generated during exercise, cold temperatures do not pose a threat similar to that posed by hot, humid conditions. But severe exposure to low temperatures and high winds can lead to frostbite, freezing, **hypothermia**, and even death. Constriction of blood vessels (vasoconstriction) increases the insulating capacity of the skin, but it also results in a marked reduction in the temperature of the extremities. The body almost seems willing to lose a few fingers or toes to save the more important parts. Protective vasoconstriction often leads to severe discomfort in the fingers and toes. To relieve the pain, warm the affected area or raise the core temperature to allow reflexive return of blood to the extremities. Although shivering may cause some increase in temperature, gross muscular activity is far more effective in restoring heat to the troubled area. Because large-muscle activity takes considerable energy, the cold-weather enthusiast must maintain a reserve of energy for use in emergencies. Excessive fatigue is the first step toward hypothermia and possible death.

Windchill

Windchill describes the effect of wind speed on heat loss (see figure 15.2). When the wind speed is 20 miles (32.2 km) per hour, a reading of 10 degrees Fahrenheit (minus 12 °C) is equivalent to minus 9 degrees Fahrenheit (minus 23 °C). Runners, skiers, and skaters can create their own windchill. Skiing at 20 miles per hour on a 10-degree-Fahrenheit day is equivalent to minus 9 degrees Fahrenheit. If the skier is moving into a wind, the effect is even worse. When possible, run, ski, or skate away from the wind. If you must face into the wind on a cold day, be sure to cover exposed flesh, including earlobes and the nose, and be on the lookout for frostbite.

Windchill chart

									Temperature (°F)									
Calm	40	35	30	25	20	15	10	5	0	-5	-10	-15	-20	-25	-30	-35	-40	-45
5	36	31	25	19	13	7	1	-5	-11	-16	-22	-28	-34	-40	-46	-52	-57	-63
10	34	27	21	15	9	3	-4	-10	-16	-22	-28	-35	-41	-47	-53	-59	-66	-72
15	32	25	19	13	6	0	-7	-13	-19	-26	-32	-39	-45	-51	-58	-64	-71	-77
20	30	24	17	11	4	-2	-9	-15	-22	-29	-35	-42	-48	-55	-61	-68	-74	-81
25	29	23	16	9	3	-4	-11	-17	-24	-31	-37	-44	-51	-58	-64	-71	-78	-84
30	28	22	15	8	1	-5	-12	-19	-26	-33	-39	-46	-53	-60	-67	-73	-80	-87
35	28	21	14	7	0	-7	-14	-21	-27	-34	-41	-48	-55	-62	-69	-76	-02	-89
40	27	20	13	6	-1	-8	-15	-22	-29	-36	-43	-50	-57	-64	-71	-78	-84	-91
45	26	19	12	5	-2	-9	-16	-23	-30	-37	-44	-51	-58	-65	-72	-79	-86	-93
50	26	19	12	4	-3	-10	-17	-24	-31	-38	-45	-52	-60	-67	-74	-81	-88	-95
55	25	18	11	4	-3	-11	-18	-25	-32	-39	-46	-54	-61	-68	-75	-82	-89	-97
60	25	17	10	3	-4	-11	-19	-26	-33	-40	-48	-55	-62	-69	-76	-84	-91	-98

Wind (mph)

Frostbite times   ■ 30 minutes   ■ 10 minutes   ■ 5 minutes

FIGURE 15.2 Windchill index.

Courtesy of the National Oceanic and Atmospheric Administration. www.noaa.gov.

Frostbite

Frostbite is damage to the skin resulting from exposure to extreme cold or windchill. As you can see on the windchill index, the danger of frostbite is minimal at temperatures above 20 degrees Fahrenheit (minus 7 °C). A temperature or windchill of minus 20 degrees Fahrenheit (minus 29 °C) seems necessary to produce the condition.

At first, frostbite appears as a patch of pale or white skin, because of the constriction of blood vessels in the area. After mild frostbite, the skin appears red and swollen when the blood returns. In severe frostbite, the skin may appear purple or black after it is warmed. Immersion in warm (not hot) water will hasten the return of blood to the area. Do not massage the affected part. Protect the groin and other sensitive areas to avoid the excruciating pain that occurs when circulation returns. If your feet become frostbitten on a winter outing, do not remove your boots to warm your feet. Your feet could swell and prevent you from being able to put your boots back on. Walk or ski out before removing your boots and warming your feet.

If you're worried about freezing the delicate tissues of the lungs during cold-weather exercise, don't. Cold air may make your breathing uncomfortable because it is so dry, but the danger of damage to the tissue is small. The respiratory system has a remarkable ability to warm and humidify air. Humans tolerate air temperatures well below minus 20 degrees Fahrenheit (minus 29 °C) without damage. The cold air is warmed to above 32 degrees Fahrenheit (0 °C) before it reaches the **bronchi**. When the temperature goes below minus 20 degrees Fahrenheit, however, you should modify or curtail your exercise plans. The danger to earlobes, nose, fingers, and toes is great, and at much lower temperatures, respiratory tract damage is possible, though unlikely. Very cold air constricts airways and makes vigorous effort difficult. Use a scarf or mask to cover the mouth and nose if effort in very cold temperatures is necessary.

Hypothermia

When your body begins to lose heat faster than it can produce it, you are undergoing exposure. Prolonged exertion leads to progressive muscular fatigue. Shivering and vasoconstriction are attempts to preserve body heat and the temperature of vital organs. Exhaustion of energy stores and neuromuscular impairment lead to the virtual termination of activity. As exposure continues and your body loses additional heat, the cold reaches the brain. You then lose judgment and the ability to reason. Your speech becomes slow and slurred, you lose control of your hands, walking becomes clumsy, and you want to lie down and rest. Don't do it! You are hypothermic. Your core temperature is dropping. Without treatment, you will lose consciousness and die.

You may be surprised to learn that most hypothermia cases occur in air temperatures above 30 degrees Fahrenheit (minus 1 °C). Cold water, windchill, and fatigue combine to set the stage for hypothermia. Avoid the problem by staying dry. If you become wet, dry off as soon as possible. Be aware of the windchill and how wind refrigerates wet clothing. During a cold-weather hike or ski tour, take off layers of clothing before you perspire and put them back on as you begin to cool. Eat and rest often to maintain your energy level. Stop or make camp when you still have energy. Don't wait until the situation is critical.

If someone exhibits the symptoms of hypothermia, transport the victim to a medical facility as quickly as possible. The heart may begin to fibrillate during rewarming, and emergency equipment will be needed. If immediate transport isn't possible, or if the case isn't severe, do the following:

- Get the victim out of the wind and rain.
- Remove all wet clothing.
- Provide dry clothing, warm drinks, and a warm, dry sleeping bag for a mildly impaired victim.
- If the victim is only semiconscious, try to keep the person awake and put him or her, unclothed, into a sleeping bag with another person.
- Build a fire.

Cold-Weather Clothing

Physiologists rate the insulating value of clothing in **Clo units**, with 1 Clo unit being equivalent to the clothing that will maintain comfort at a room temperature of 70 degrees Fahrenheit, or 21 degrees Celsius (roughly equivalent to a cotton shirt and slacks). Figure 15.3 illustrates how the insulating requirements change during vigorous activity, such as cross-country skiing or hiking (heavy work), light work, and rest. That variation is precisely why it is necessary to dress in layers in cold weather. At 0 degrees Fahrenheit (minus 18 °C), a light shirt will be adequate during vigorous effort, whereas you may need 2 inches (5 cm) of insulation to maintain comfort at rest, and more for a good night's sleep.

Because perspiration is a major problem during exercise in the cold, you would be smart to buy a set of synthetic undergarments. These fabrics wick perspiration away from the skin so that evaporative cooling won't strip heat from the body. Next, you should put on a wool or fleece layer for warmth. Layers of clothing provide an insulating barrier of air, and you can peel off layers as your temperature rises and put them back on as it falls.

A windproof and rainproof garment should be all the additional clothing that you need during exercise. Invest in breathable clothing if you can afford it, but don't expect any garment to handle the tremendous moisture load created during vigorous skiing or running. You can carry a down or pile coat in your pack for use at lunch or in camp. Modern, light, synthetic fabrics have several advantages over goose down. They are less expensive, easier to care for, and don't mat and lose insulating qualities when wet.

Of course, you'll also need a hat and gloves. If you get very hot during exercise, try a polypropylene ear band that allows heat loss from the top of the head. When you stop, put on a pile or wool hat to retain body heat. The same goes with gloves. Wear lighter ones during vigorous exercise, but be ready to put on warm mitts for extended breaks. With the right clothing, you can enjoy outdoor activity in all but the most severe conditions.

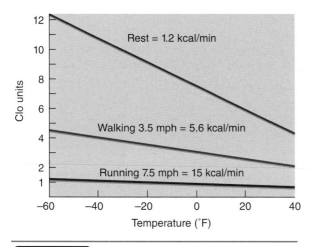

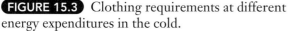

FIGURE 15.3 Clothing requirements at different energy expenditures in the cold.

With the right clothing, you can enjoy outdoor activity in all but the most severe conditions.

Cold Acclimatization

Can we adjust to the cold in the same way that we acclimatize to hot environments? If so, what are the physiological mechanisms involved? Specific examples of cold acclimatization appear in the research literature (Folk 1974). One mechanism is a metabolic adjustment, wherein metabolism increases as much as 35 percent. The female divers (known as Ama) of the Korean Peninsula evidence this adjustment, as well as improved tissue insulation during the winter months when the water temperature falls to 50 degrees Fahrenheit (10 °C). Australian Aborigines are able to sleep in cold conditions through a hypothermic response, a lowering of the core temperature from 98.6 degrees Fahrenheit (37 °C) to a more easily maintained 95 degrees Fahrenheit (35 °C). Of course, natural selection and heredity play important roles in adaptation to cold environments. Large body mass, short extremities, high levels of body fat, and deep routing of venous circulation also help.

Repeated exposure to cold seems to lead to physiological and psychological adjustments that allow one to tolerate and enjoy physical activity in cold environments (Young 1988). We may perceive near-freezing temperatures as bitter in November but balmy in February. The extra calories that we consume in fall and winter lead to extra weight and an increase in the insulating layer of subcutaneous fat. The extra fat may be why we can cross-country ski barehanded at 25 degrees Fahrenheit (minus 4 °C) in February!

Finally, remember the need for hydration during exercise in the cold. Your body perspires and loses water vapor as you exhale. Plan to carry and use a water bottle or hydration system, and consider a carbohydrate drink and energy snacks to help maintain energy levels.

EXERCISING AT ALTITUDE

More than 40 million people live at altitudes above 10,000 feet (3,000 m), and some live above 17,000 feet (5,200 m). No permanent habitations are found above 18,000 feet (5,500 m), however, indicating that such an elevation may be incompatible with adaptation and long-term survival. Indeed, the upper reaches of 29,000-foot-high (8,840 m) Mount Everest have been called the death zone. Although **arterial oxygen desaturation** begins as we move upward from sea level, elevations below 5,000 feet (1,500 m) have little noticeable effect on otherwise healthy people. But as you ascend to higher elevations to ski, hike, climb, or even to live, barometric pressure declines along with available levels of atmospheric and alveolar oxygen. When this occurs, the arterial blood is unable to become highly saturated, less oxygen is transported, and the tissues are forced to operate with a reduced supply (see table 15.1). Thus, in spite of the heroic efforts of the oxygen

Table 15.1 Altitude and Oxygen

Altitude (ft)	Barometric pressure (mmHg)	PO$_2$ in air (mmHg)	PaO$_2$ alveoli* (mmHg)	Resting arterial O$_2$ saturation (%)	Aerobic fitness (% of sea level max)
0	760	159	105	97	100
3,200 (980 m)	680	142	94	96	
6,500 (1,980 m)	600	125	78	94	90
10,000 (3,050 m)	523	111	62	90	
14,100 (4,300 m)	450	94	51	86	75
18,400 (5,600 m)	380	75	42	80	
23,000 (7,000 m)	305	64	31	63	50
29,141 (8,800 m)	230	48	19	30	

*Partial pressure of oxygen in lungs.

intake and transport systems, altitude always leads to a reduction in aerobic fitness and associated endurance performance.

In this age of easy travel, you can quickly ascend to a national park or ski resort located above 5,000 feet (1,500 m). When you arrive, you'll have to adjust cardiac output for a given workload. The heart rate is higher, but the stroke volume may be lower because of diminished oxygen supply to the heart muscle. You bring more air into the lungs each minute. This hyperventilation leads to increased carbon dioxide exhalation and the acid–base disturbances associated with mountain sickness. The symptoms—headache, shortness of breath, rapid heartbeat, loss of appetite—appear at 8,000 feet (2,400 m) or above. Work capacity declines at altitude, as does the motivation to perform hard work.

Does a high level of physical fitness provide some advantage to the newcomer? On arrival, conditioned people maintain their sea-level advantage over unfit people, but no more. Trained people are able to do less than they could at sea level, and are just as likely as others are to suffer mountain sickness. At very high elevations, some highly trained endurance athletes have been found to be nonresponders, whose respiration fails to adjust adequately to the added demands of the altitude (Jackson and Sharkey 1988).

Altitude Acclimatization

Profound changes occur soon after one ascends to a higher elevation, through a process called **altitude acclimatization**. Pulmonary ventilation increases, so more air can be moved into the lungs. This increase doesn't take more energy, because the air is less dense at higher elevations. Oxygen transport gradually improves through increases in red blood cells, hemoglobin, and blood volume. Above 15,000 feet (4,600 m) the red blood cells increase from 5 million per cubic millimeter to 6.6 million, and hemoglobin rises from 15 grams per 100 milliliters to above 20. These changes make the blood more viscous, but that isn't a problem because the hypoxia (lower oxygen tension) of altitude vasodilates, or relaxes, the arterioles. Altitude exposure may cause an increase in lung and muscle capillaries. Myoglobin, the molecule that serves to store oxygen in muscles, also is increased at higher elevations (Smith and Sharkey 1984).

A good adjustment to higher elevation occurs in about 3 weeks, or about 1 week for each 1,000 feet (300 m) above 5,000 feet (1,500 m). Once acclimated, your oxygen intake and transport systems will be better able to supply oxygen to the working muscles. These adjustments reduce but never eliminate the effect of altitude on aerobic fitness. Endurance performance will always decline at altitude, regardless of your state of acclimatization.

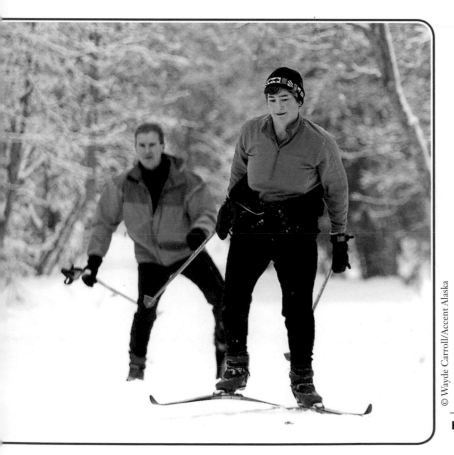

© Wayde Carroll/Accent Alaska

■ Exercise at a lower intensity for a shorter duration when training at altitude.

Unfortunately, these hard-earned changes (they occur only when you work at altitude) are reversible; they return to prealtitude values within weeks after you leave the mountains.

Altitude Training

Because of the reduced ability to take in oxygen at altitudes above 5,000 feet (1,500 m), your usual pace will be more anaerobic than usual. You have several options. You can do your usual distance but go more slowly, go at your usual pace but for shorter distances, or (our favorite) slow down and enjoy the view. Go sightseeing and forget about distance or pace. If you are training to compete at altitude, you should realize that the slower pace may cause your speed to slip a little. Occasional shorter but faster runs should help avoid that problem (athletes sometimes drop to lower elevations for speed work).

For years, coaches and athletes have sought the ultimate training stimulus at a moderate altitude of 5,000 to 10,000 feet (1,500-3,000 m). They believe that reduced availability of oxygen to muscles (hypoxia) is the stimulus that causes changes in aerobic fitness, and that exercise at moderate altitude ensures extreme tissue hypoxia. So they travel to a training site at 6,000 to 9,000 feet (1,800-2,700 m) to train for several weeks or months before returning to sea level for a major event such as the Olympic Games. Unfortunately, the effort may not be worth it for all athletes. One study showed that a small benefit resulted from altitude training on return to sea level, but the study did not use a control group. A replication of the study with a control group found that altitude training was no more effective than equally arduous sea-level training. The subjects were highly trained middle-distance runners, 17 to 23 years old, who trained for 3 weeks either at sea level or at 7,500 feet (2,300 m) (Adams et al. 1975). Arduous effort at sea level also leads to tissue hypoxia.

Live High, Train Low

The benefits of altitude training do not seem to help all athletes equally. A study helps explain why some respond and others do not. Male and female collegiate runners participated in a 28-day live-high, train-low investigation (2,500 m and 1,250 m, respectively, or 8,200 ft and 4,100 ft) of the effects of altitude. Those who improved in performance (in a 5,000 m run) were called responders; those who did not were labeled nonresponders. Responders displayed a significant increase in **erythropoietin (EPO)**, a compound that stimulates production of red blood cells in bone marrow. The authors concluded that the improvement in performance depended, in part, on (a) living high enough to increase EPO, red blood cell volume, and $\dot{V}O_2$max, and (b) training low enough to maintain interval-training velocity near sea-level values (Chapman, Stray-Gunderson and Levine 1998). Over the last decade, the use of altitude tents and rooms with reduced oxygen content to simulate sleeping at higher elevations has become popular with high level endurance athletes. Vogt and Hoppeler (2010) reviewed the literature on hypoxic training and suggest that little evidence supports improved sea-level performance following hypoxia or altitude chamber use. This debate continues.

Casual observers of sport may be quick to conclude that athletes' performances are due to their residence at high altitude. Outstanding African athletes have emerged to perpetuate the practice of altitude training. The athletes live above 7,000 feet (2,100 m), but many observers forget that the athletes were born there and lived there most of their lives. Their parents were born there, as were their grandparents. So the benefit that these observers identify as resulting from training at altitude is, in reality, a product of natural selection combined with long-term residence at a higher elevation, not just a few weeks of altitude training.

AVOIDING THE EFFECTS OF AIR POLLUTION

Long-term exposure to respirable particulate has been associated with heart and lung disease, ozone exposure has been associated with lung and heart problems, and carbon monoxide exposure has been associated with central nervous system and heart problems. Do we need to check the local air pollution index before going outside to exercise? In some cities, children's school recesses and sporting events are canceled when pollution rises. If you fly over any major city in the United States, you'll see the pall of pollution that daily diminishes the quality of our lives. Although some forms of pollution are most dangerous for old or weak people, young children, and those with respiratory and cardiac problems, other forms attack physically active people. Exercise increases the volume of air taken into the lungs each minute. Because pollution-related respiratory disorders often are related to the degree of exposure, avoiding or reducing exercise in polluted atmospheres seems wise.

We are beginning to recognize the many sources of air pollution as threats to the quality of life and to life itself. Efforts are under way to lower carbon monoxide, dust, and soot (respirable particulate), as well as sulfur dioxide and other pollutants. Some pollutants are relatively harmless by themselves, but in combination with others, they can exert potent biological effects.

The biological effects of air pollution include the following:

- Deadening of ciliary action
- Reduction of oxygen-transport capacity (because carbon monoxide competes for space on hemoglobin molecules)
- Suppression of the immune system
- Chronic obstructive pulmonary disease, including alveolar breakdown in emphysema, irritation of airways in chronic bronchitis, and loss of diffusing surfaces in pulmonary fibrosis
- Lung and other cancers
- Heart disease via exposure to fine (<2.5 um/m^3) particulate (Brook et al. 2004)

Although many forms of industrial, urban, and automotive pollution are troublesome, nauseating, or even fatal, no single source of pollution is as deadly as the cigarette, which causes most of the biological effects listed previously. Smoking can irritate the bronchial tubes, deaden ciliary action, reduce oxygen transport, cause lung cancer and heart disease, and make the smoker more susceptible to infection, chronic bronchitis, and emphysema.

Studies have shown that smoking contributes to depression and impotence, and it has been associated with musculoskeletal and lower back problems and with long-term disability.

In the United States, cigarette smoking is responsible for 400,000 deaths annually! Studies have shown that smoking contributes to depression and impotence. It has been associated with musculoskeletal and lower back problems and with long-term disability (Amoroso et al. 1996).

To gain a perspective on the risks of smoking versus industrial pollution and the extreme risk of combining the two, consider the risks of dying from lung cancer. Although an asbestos worker has a lung-cancer mortality rate 5 times that of the general population, a smoker's rate is 10 times greater, and the asbestos worker who smokes has a rate 87 times greater than that of the population (USDHEW 1979).

We must continue the fight for clean air so that we don't have to regulate our activities in accordance with the air pollution index or see our enjoyment of physical activity decline because of humankind's mistreatment of the environment. In the meantime, you should avoid exercise in obviously dangerous areas (along expressways, near industrial pollution) and when air pollution warnings are in effect. That recommendation doesn't mean that you shouldn't exercise; you just need to find a way to avoid the pollution. Be sure to add your voice to the growing fight against all forms of pollution, including the worst of all, the cigarette.

SUMMARY

In this chapter, we've outlined the problems encountered in different environments and provided practical advice on how to minimize the problems and maximize performance and enjoyment. Solutions range from improving fitness and acclimatization to dressing properly and maintaining hydration and energy. Fitness, although especially important in the heat, improves performance in all environments. Acclimatization is necessary for heat and altitude and useful in the cold. Fluid replacement is critical in the heat, but it is also extremely important in the cold and at altitude, where breathing causes the loss of considerable fluid. Maintaining energy levels is essential to prolonged performance in all environments. Finally, proper clothing is required to cope with the demands of the environment.

But what about air pollution? What can we do to minimize its effects? The answers are simple. Minimize exposure and maintain your immune system with regular exercise, rest, and good nutrition. Include immune-friendly foods in your diet (see chapter 12). If your diet is inadequate, consider antioxidant supplements to counter the free radicals found in pollutants. Minimize exposure by exercising where or when pollution levels are lowest. If you are particularly sensitive to pollutants or allergens, you may want to use a dust mask to filter particles or a mask impregnated with activated charcoal to absorb pollutants. Unfortunately, simple masks do not remove carbon monoxide, so avoid high-traffic areas during exercise.

Appendix

Section I: Coronary Heart Disease (CHD) Risk Factors					
Cholesterol	<160	160–200	200–240	240–280	>280
Chol/HDL ratio	<3	3–4	4–5	5–6	>6
Score:_____	+2	+1	–1	–2	–4
Blood pressure: Systolic	<110	110–120	120–150	150–170	>170
Blood pressure: Diastolic	<60	60–80	80–90	90–100	>100
Score:_____	+1	0	–1	–2	–4
Smoking	Never	Quit	Smoke cigar or pipe or close family member smokes	One pack of cigarettes daily	Two or more packs daily
Score:_____	+1	0	–1	–3	–5
Heredity	No family history of CHD	One close relative over 60 with CHD	Two close relatives over 60 with CHD	One close relative under 60 with CHD	Two or more close relatives under 60 with CHD
Score:_____	+2	0	–1	–2	–4
Body mass index (BMI, use chart on page 308)	<19	19–24	25–29	30–39*	>40*
Score:_____	+2	0	–1	–3	–5
Sex	Female under 55 years	Female over 55 years	Male	Stocky male	Bald, stocky male
Score:_____	0	–1	–1	–2	–3
Stress	Phlegmatic, unhurried, generally happy	Ambitious but generally relaxed	Sometimes hard-driving, time-conscious, competitive	Hard-driving, time-conscious, competitive (type A)	Type A with repressed hostility
Score:_____	+1	0	0	–1	–3
Physical activity	High intensity, 60 min most days	Moderate, 30 min most days	Moderate, 20–30 min, 3–5 times per week	Light, 10–20 min,1–2 times per week	Little or none
Score:_____	+3	+2	+1	–1	–3

*If waist is under 40 in. (102 cm) subtract one less (e.g., –2 or –4)

Total: CHD risk factors _____

(continued)

Section II: Health Habits (Related to Good Health and Longevity)					
Breakfast	Daily	Sometimes	None	Coffee	Coffee and doughnut
Score:_____	+1	0	−1	−2	−3
Regular meals	Three or more	Two daily	Not regular	Fad diets	Starve and stuff
Score:_____	+1	0	−1	−2	−3
Sleep	7–8 hr	6–7 hr	8–9 hr	9 hr	6 hr
Score:_____	+1	0	0	−1	−2
Alcohol	None	Women 3/wk	Men 1–2 daily	3–6 daily	>6 daily
Score:_____	+1	+1	+1	−2	−4

Total: Health habits _____

Section III: Medical Factors					
Medical exam and screening tests (blood pressure, diabetes, glaucoma)	Regular tests, see doctor when necessary	Periodic medical exam and selected tests	Periodic medical exam	Sometimes get tests	No tests or medical exams
Score:_____	+1	+1	0	0	−1
Heart	No history of problems, self or family	Some history	Rheumatic fever as child, no murmur now	Rheumatic fever as a child, have murmur	Have ECG abnormality or angina pectoris
Score:_____	+2	0	−1	−2	−3
Lung (including pneumonia and tuberculosis)	No problem	Some past problem	Mild asthma or bronchitis	Emphysema, severe asthma, or bronchitis	Severe lung problems
Score:_____	+1	0	−1	−1	−3
Digestive tract	No problem	Occasional diarrhea, loss of appetite	Frequent diarrhea or stomach upset	Ulcers, colitis, gallbladder, or liver problems	Severe gastrointestinal disorders
Score:_____	+1	0	−1	−2	−3
Diabetes	No problem or family history	Controlled hypoglycemia (low blood sugar)	Hypoglycemia and family history	Mild diabetes (diet and exercise)	Diabetes (insulin)
Score:_____	+1	0	−1	−2	−4
Drugs	Seldom take	Minimal but regular use of aspirin or other drugs	Heavy use of aspirin or other drugs	Regular use of mood-altering or psychogenic drugs	Heavy use of mood-altering or psychogenic drugs
Score:_____	+1	0	−1	−2	−3

Total: Medical factors _____

Section IV: Safety Factors

Driving in car	<7,000 mi (11,000 km) per year, mostly local	7,000–10,000 mi (11,000–16,000 km) per year, local and some highway	10,000–15,000 mi (16,000–24,000 km) per year, local and highway	>15,000 mi (24,000 km) per year, highway and some local	>15,000 mi (24,000 km) per year, mostly highway
Score:_____	+1	0	0	–1	–2
Using seat belts	Always	Most of time (>75%)	On highway only	Seldom (<25%)	Never
Score:_____	+1	0	–1	–2	–4
Risk-taking behavior (motorcycle, skydive, mountain climb, fly small plane, and so on)	Some with careful preparation	Never	Occasional	Often	Try anything for thrills
Score:_____	+1	0	–1	–1	–2

Total: Safety factors _____

Section V: Personal Factors

Diet	Low fat, low calories, fruits and vegetables	Balanced with complex carbohydrate	High protein, limited fat	Extra calories, low carbohydrate	Fad diets and fat
Score:_____	+2	+1	0	–1	–2
Longevity	Grandparents lived past 90, parents past 80	Grandparents lived past 80, parents past 70	Grandparents lived past 70, parents past 60	Few relatives lived past 60	Few relatives lived past 50
Score:_____	+2	+1	0	–1	–3
Love and marriage	Happily married	Married	Unmarried	Divorced	Extramarital relationship(s)
Score:_____	+2	+1	0	–1	–3
Education	Postgraduate or master craftsman	College graduate or skilled craftsman	Some college or trade school	High school graduate	Grade school graduate
Score:_____	+1	+1	0	–1	–2
Job satisfaction	Enjoy job, see results, room for advancement	Enjoy job, see some results, able to advance	Job OK, no results, nowhere to go	Dislike job	Hate job
Score:_____	+2	+1	0	–1	–3
Social	Have some close friends	Have some friends	Have no good friends	Stuck with people I don't enjoy	Have no friends at all
Score:_____	+1	0	–1	–2	–3

(continued)

Section V: Personal Factors *(continued)*					
Race	White or Asian	Black or Hispanic	American Indian		
Score:_____	0	–1	–2		

Total: Personal factors _____

Section VI: Psychological Factors					
Outlook	Feel good about present and future	Satisfied	Unsure about present or future	Unhappy in present, don't look forward to future	Miserable, rather not get out of bed
Score:_____	+2	+1	0	–1	–3
Depression	No family history of depression	Some family history, feel OK	Family history and mildly depressed	Sometimes feel life isn't worth living	Thoughts of suicide
Score:_____	+1	0	–1	–2	–3
Anxiety	Seldom anxious	Occasionally anxious	Often anxious	Always anxious	Panic attacks
Score:_____	+1	0	–1	–2	–3
Relaxation	Relax or meditate daily	Relax often	Seldom relax	Usually tense	Always tense
Score:_____	+1	0	–1	–2	–3

Total: Psychological factors _____

Section VII: For Women					
Health care	Regular breast and Pap tests	Occasional breast and Pap tests	Never have exams	Treated disorder	Untreated cancer
Score:_____	+1	0	–1	–2	–4
Birth control pill	Never used	Quit 5 years ago	Still use, under 30 years	Use pill and smoke	Use pill, smoke, over 35
Score:_____	+1	0	0	–2	–3

Total: For women only _____

Section VIII: Summary

You can now estimate your longevity. Add your total score from the previous sections to your normal life expectancy (from the chart below) to find your longevity estimate. If you would like to improve your longevity estimate, go back and decide on some lifestyle areas you would like to improve.

Category	Score (+ or – from previous sections)
I. CHD risk factors	
II. Health habits	
III. Medical factors	
IV. Safety factors	
V. Personal factors	
VI. Psychological factors	
VII. For women only	
Total	

_____ + _____ = _____

Totals from sections I-VII   Life expectancy for your age from table below   Your longevity estimate

Life expectancy*		
	Expectancy (all races)	
Nearest age	**Male**	**Female**
30	77.1	81.5
35	77.5	81.7
40	77.8	81.9
45	78.3	82.2
50	79.0	82.7
55	79.9	83.2
60	80.9	83.9
65	82.2	84.9
70	83.7	86.0
75	85.6	87.5
80	87.9	89.9

From B.J. Sharkey and S.E. Gaskill, 2013, *Fitness and health, seventh edition* (Champaign, IL: Human Kinetics). Centers for Disease Control and Prevention, 2011, *National vital statistics reports.* Available: www.cdc.gov.

Glossary

absolute intensity (of physical activity)—The rate of energy expenditure during exercise. This is usually expressed in metabolic equivalents, or METs, where 1 MET equals the resting metabolic rate of ≈ 3.5 ml $O_2 \cdot kg^{-1} \cdot min^{-1}$. It can also be expressed as L $O_2 \cdot mm^{-1} \cdot min^{-1}$ or cal/min.

acclimatization—The process of adjusting to an environmental change, such as altitude, temperature, or humidity, that allows a person to maintain performance in the new environment. Acclimatization may occur in a short period of time (days or weeks) or across an organism's lifetime. It may eventually, for populations who live in an extreme environment for many generations, result in genetic selection.

actin—One of the major proteins in a muscle that make up the crossbridges that allow muscle contraction.

action stage—Stage of behavior change where a person is fully engaged in a new behavior.

adenosine triphosphate (ATP)—The high-energy compound that fuels muscular contractions (and all metabolism) by releasing the energy stored in a phosphate bond to produce adenosine diphosphate (ADP) and a free phosphate ion (Pi). The metabolism of carbohydrates and fats (and a little protein) is used to produce ATP from ADP and Pi, which then fuels muscle contraction.

adipose tissue—Tissue in which fat is stored.

adoption stage—Stage of behavior change where activity is internalized as part of lifestyle.

aerobic—In the presence of oxygen; aerobic metabolism utilizes oxygen.

aerobic capacity—$\dot{V}O_2$max expressed in liters per minute. (i.e. total aerobic capacity, see maximal oxygen intake).

aerobic enzymes—Enzymes associated with aerobic metabolism.

aerobic exercise—Exercise intensity below the point at which blood–lactic acid levels rise.

In simple terms, aerobic exercise includes all large-muscle activities that can be comfortably sustained for 15 minutes or more.

aerobic fitness—How well someone can take oxygen from the atmosphere into the lungs and then into the blood, and then pump it through the heart and circulatory system to the working muscles, where it is used to oxidize carbohydrate and fat to produce energy.

aerobic power—$\dot{V}O_2$max expressed in oxygen use relative to body mass (ml $\cdot kg^{-1} \cdot min^{-1}$), see maximal oxygen intake.

aerobic training zone—The range of intensities over which aerobic fitness improves, generally thought to occur between the first and second lactate thresholds.

agility—The ability to change position and direction rapidly, with precision and without loss of balance.

altitude acclimatization—The physiological processes that lead to an improved ability to live and work in a high-elevation environment.

alveoli—Tiny air sacs in the lungs where exchange of oxygen and carbon dioxide takes place.

amino acids—The molecular units from which proteins are made. Different arrangements of the 22 amino acids form the various proteins (muscles, enzymes, hormones, and so on).

anaerobic—In the absence of oxygen, nonoxidation metabolism.

anaerobic exercise—Exercise that relies increasingly on nonoxidative energy production and increases the production of CO_2 and lactic acid to levels that begin to inhibit muscular contraction and cause breathing to become labored.

anaerobic threshold—More properly called the *lactate threshold*, or the point at which lactic acid produced in muscles begins to accumulate in the blood. It defines the upper limit that can be sustained aerobically.

angina—Properly termed *angina pectoris*, this is chest pain due to ischemia (a lack of blood, thus a lack of oxygen supply and waste removal) of the heart muscle, generally due to obstruction of the coronary arteries (the heart's blood vessels).

anorexia nervosa—An eating disorder characterized by excessive dieting and subsequent loss of appetite.

antidiuretic hormone (ADH)—A hormone that assists in the maintenance of fluids and electrolytes (sodium, potassium, calcium, and chloride).

anxiety—A diffuse apprehension of some vague threat, characterized by feelings of uncertainty and helplessness.

appestat—The control center for food intake in the brain. The appestat is located in the hypothalamus, an area of the brain that functions like a thermostat to turn on eating behavior and then turn it off when the desire or hunger has been satisfied.

arterial oxygen desaturation—A condition where arterial blood carries less oxygen than it is capable of. The desaturation is measured as a percent of maximal oxygen that can be carried (i.e., all oxygen binding sites on hemoglobin in red blood cells are bound to oxygen).

asymptomatic—Without symptoms.

atherogenic—Likely to clog arteries (i.e., cause atherosclerosis).

atherosclerosis—A condition in which an artery wall thickens as a result of the accumulation of fatty materials such as cholesterol. The process of clogging arteries.

atrophy—Loss of size of muscle.

balance—Ability to maintain equilibrium.

behavior change (behavior modification)—The methods that have been shown to effectively change or modify behavior.

behavior therapy—A system of record keeping and motivation that helps change a behavior (e.g., overeating).

bioelectric impedance—A technique that estimates percentage of body fat from body water content. The technique, based on the fixed amount of water in fat, requires strict adherence to hydration standards to achieve acceptable accuracy.

blood lipids—Lipids (fats) found in the blood. Blood lipids are mostly transported in a protein-fatty complex such as chylomicrons or lipoproteins. The concentration of blood lipids depends on intake and digestion from the intestine along with an uptake into cells and adipose tissue. Blood lipids are mainly fatty acids and cholesterol.

blood pressure—Force exerted against the walls of arteries.

body composition—The relative amounts of fat and lean tissue.

body mass index (BMI)—A common measure that relates weight to height. It can be calculated as weight in kilograms divided by the square of height in meters (kg/m^2) or in pounds and inches as ($lb/in.^2 \times 703$).

bonk—A term that cyclists and endurance athletes use to describe the utter fatigue, confusion, and lack of coordination that result when blood glucose falls below the level required by the nervous system.

bronchi—Smaller branches of the airway.

buffer—Substance in blood that soaks up hydrogen ions to minimize changes in acid–base balance (pH).

bypass surgery—Properly called *coronary artery bypass graft (CABG) surgery.* Open-heart surgery in which harvested veins from the leg or abdominal wall are surgically grafted on the outside of the heart to bypass an area that has been blocked or that has serious plaque (atherosclerotic) buildup.

calisthenics—A form of exercise, generally using body weight or a partner as the resistance, consisting of a variety of simple, often rhythmical, movements.

calorie—Amount of heat required to raise 1 kilogram of water 1 degree Celsius; same as kilocalorie.

calorimeter—Tool used to measure the caloric value of foods. A small amount of food is placed in a chamber and burned in the presence of oxygen. The heat liberated in the process indicates the energy content of the food (1 cal is the heat required to raise 1 kg of water 1 °C).

capillaries—Smallest blood vessels (between arterioles and venules) where oxygen, food, and hormones are delivered to tissues and carbon dioxide and wastes are picked up.

carbohydrate—Simple (e.g., sugar) and complex (e.g., potatoes, rice, beans, corn, and grains) foodstuff that we use for energy; stored in liver and muscle as glycogen, while excess can be stored as fat. Simple sugars include glucose, sucrose, and fructose, while complex carbohydrates include starches and other long chains of carbohydrates.

carbohydrate loading—A strategy used by endurance athletes, such as marathon runners, to maximize the storage of muscle glycogen to enhance duration of performance, generally during events of 90 to 120 minutes or longer.

cardiac—Pertaining to the heart.

cardiac catheterization—The insertion of a catheter into a chamber or vessel of the heart. This is done for both investigational and interventional purposes.

cardiac contractility—How well the heart contracts with each beat.

cardiac output (Q)—The amount of blood in liters (L) pumped by the heart each minute. Cardiac output is the result of heart rate × stroke volume (HR × SV). Resting cardiac output is typically about 5 L/min.

cardiorespiratory fitness—Synonymous with aerobic fitness or maximal oxygen intake. Our ability to take in, transport, and utilize oxygen. Cardiorespiratory fitness can be measured in absolute terms (L O_2/min) or in relative terms adjusted for body weight (ml $O_2 \cdot kg^{-1} \cdot min^{-1}$).

cardiovascular—Related to heart and blood vessels.

central nervous system (CNS)—The brain and spinal cord.

cholesterol—Fatty substance found in nerves and other tissues; excessive amounts in blood have been associated with increased risk of heart disease.

chylomicrons—Digested fat clumps in the lymphatic system. These are the first form of digested fat. Chylomicrons are carried by the lymphatic system to the circulation for transport to cells for energy or to adipose tissue for storage.

circuit weight training (CWT)—Training where one set of each exercise is completed in order before beginning on the second set of all exercises. Resistance is generally low, with short rest periods to promote muscular endurance, although strength benefits are fewer.

Clo units—A unit of clothing insulation. One Clo unit is equivalent to the clothing that will maintain comfort at a room temperature of 70 °F, or 21 °C (roughly equivalent to a cotton shirt and slacks).

concentric contraction—A muscular contraction in which a muscle shortens, such as the bicep during the lifting potion of a bicep curl exercise. Concentric contractions are generally flexion movements. They occur while lifting an object or during the power phase of an activity, such as the push-off during running.

contemplative stage—Stage of behavior change where a person is thinking about it.

contraction—Development of tension by muscle: Concentric muscle shortens and eccentric muscle lengthens under tension; static contractions are contractions without change in length.

contract/relax stretch—A variation of the static stretch. Do a static stretch, relax, and then contract the muscle for a few seconds. Then repeat the static stretch. When performed on muscles like those in the calf, the technique seems to help the muscle relax so that the tendon can be better stretched. This technique is also often termed *proprioceptive neuromuscular facilitation stretching* (PNF stretching).

cool-down—Postperformance exercise used to dissipate heat, maintain blood flow, and aid recovery of muscles.

coordination—A harmonious relationship of muscle action with a smooth union or flow of movements in execution of a task. Coordination is synonymous with *skill*.

core muscles—Different muscles that stabilize the spine and pelvis. Many run the entire length of the torso. When contracted, these muscles stabilize the spine, pelvis, and shoulder girdle to create a solid base of support.

core training—Training that focuses on core muscles that anchor and stabilize the arms and legs involved in work, sport, and recreational activities. The core muscles stabilize the spine, pelvis, and shoulder girdle to create a solid base of support. Core exercises recruit one or more large muscle areas (abdominal, back, trunk, chest, shoulders, and hip) and involve two or more primary joints (multi-joint). They are a high priority in terms of health and performance.

coronary angioplasty—Properly known as *percutaneous coronary intervention* (PCI), angioplasty is a procedure used to treat the narrowed coronary arteries of the heart that result from coronary heart disease. PCI involves inserting a catheter into the coronary arteries, which is generally fed up from the femoral artery. The catheter expands the narrowed coronary artery by using a balloon. Generally, a meshlike stent is also expanded by the balloon and left in place to keep the artery open.

coronary arteries—Blood vessels that originate from the aorta and branch out to supply oxygen and fuels to the heart muscle.

coronary artery disease (CAD)—Buildup of plaque in the coronary (heart) arteries that supply blood to the heart muscle (myocardium). This is also called coronary heart disease (CHD). CAD is the leading cause of death worldwide.

C-reactive protein—A protein marker associated with higher risk of heart disease.

creatine phosphate (CP)—Energy-rich compound that backs up ATP in providing energy for muscles.

cross-sectional research—A research method that involves observation of a population or a representative subset at a specific point in time.

daily periodization—Varying the daily stress to allow for periods of both overload and rest.

dehydration—Loss of essential body fluids.

delayed-onset muscle soreness (DOMS)—Muscle soreness that occurs about 24 hours after exercise as a result of muscle damage. DOMS occurs mainly as a result of eccentric contractions and unfamiliar exercise.

deoxyribonucleic acid (DNA)—The source of the genetic code housed in the nucleus of the cell.

depression—An illness characterized by sadness, low self-esteem, pessimism, hopelessness, and despair.

detraining—Cessation of training, used to observe the decline of important measures (e.g., blood volume) associated with performance.

diabetes (diabetes mellitus)—A disease characterized by problems associated with the hormone insulin, which is needed to get blood sugar into cells, including fat cells. There are two main types of diabetes: (1) insulin-dependent diabetes mellitus (IDDM or type 1 diabetes), where the patient does not produce insulin and requires exogenous (external) insulin to survive, and (2) non-insulin-dependent diabetes mellitus (NIDDM or type 2 diabetes), where the patient produces insulin, but his insulin receptors are insulin resistant.

diastole—The period of time during which the heart is filling (not beating).

diastolic blood pressure—Lowest blood pressure in an artery during the resting phase of the heartbeat.

dieting—Eating according to a prescribed plan.

direction of behavior—Where and how one behaves when aroused.

dose—In physical activity, the total amount of energy expended.

duration—Distance or length of time (or calories burned, in the case of the exercise prescription).

dynamic balance—The ability to maintain equilibrium while in motion.

dynamic strength—The ability to use muscular power during movement. The maximal weight that a person can lift one time.

dynamic stretching—This method requires going through the range of motion with control, working at either end to increase the range. It mimics sport movements such as the golf swing. Dynamic stretches help loosen your swing before a round of golf. Use care to remain gentle in your motions.

easy aerobic training—This is an intensity below the first lactate threshold that should feel easy for most athletes and that can be sustained for long periods of time.

eccentric contractions—A muscular contraction in which the muscle lengthens, such as the bicep muscle resisting the load and lengthening during the lowering potion of a bicep curl exercise. Eccentric contractions are generally resistive movements. They occur while lowering an object or during the deceleration or landing phase of an activity, such as the heel strike during running.

electrocardiogram (ECG or EKG)—A method of viewing the electrical activity of the heart and evaluating the rate, rhythm, and electrical or conduction abnormalities of the heart.

electrolyte—Any substance made electrically conductive by the presence of free ions. In the human body, the primary electrolytes are sodium (Na^+), potassium (K^+), calcium (Ca^{2+}), magnesium (Mg^{2+}), and chloride (Cl^-). Sodium is the main electrolyte found in extracellular fluid, and it is involved in fluid balance and blood pressure control.

endocrine system—The system of many glands and their associated secretions (hormones) that are distributed by the circulatory system.

endurance—The ability to persist or to resist fatigue.

energy balance—A comparison between the calories consumed in the diet and the calories burned in the course of all daily activities. Thus, [energy balance = energy intake – energy expenditure].

energy expenditure—All of the energy that a person metabolizes to live, including energy required for basal metabolism, digestion of food, and physical activity.

energy fitness—How we produce the energy needed for muscular movement. This includes both aerobic (with oxygen) and anaerobic (without oxygen) means.

energy intake—The energy (calories) that one consumes in food in the form of carbohydrate, fat, and protein.

energy training—Refers to how we train our energy systems, including both the anaerobic and aerobic systems.

enzymes—Proteins that catalyze (increase the rates of) chemical reactions. In the human body, nearly all metabolism requires enzymes at every step.

epidemiology—The study of the distribution and patterns of disease and illness and their causes in specific populations.

epinephrine—A hormone released from the adrenal medulla and nerve endings of the sympathetic nervous system during times of stress. It is also a neurotransmitter. It increases heart rate, constricts blood vessels, dilates air passages, helps mobilize energy, and participates in the fight-or-flight response of the sympathetic nervous system.

ergometer—A device, such as a bicycle, used to measure work capacity.

erythropoietin (EPO)—A hormone compound that stimulates production of red blood cells in bone marrow.

essential amino acids—Amino acids that cannot be synthesized in the human body and that must be obtained through diet.

evaporation—Elimination of body heat when sweat vaporizes on the surface of the skin; evaporation of 1 L of sweat yields a heat loss of 580 cal.

excess post-exercise oxygen consumption (EPOC)—The amount of oxygen used that exceeds the resting level after exercise. As oxygen is consumed, calories are also utilized at the rate of about 5 cal/L of oxygen consumed.

exercise—A subset of physical activity that is planned and structured. It is repetitive, and purposeful in the sense that improvement or maintenance of physical fitness is the objective.

exercise duration—The length of time that an exercise session lasts. Duration can also be measured in terms of distance covered or calories burned.

exercise frequency—Number of times a week that a person completes physical activity or exercise sessions.

exercise intensity—A measure of how much work is done during exercise. The intensity has an effect on which fuel the body uses. Many ways exist to measure intensity, including heart rate, utilization of oxygen, rating of perceived exertion, and speed of movement. For resistance training, intensity refers to the resistance, the speed of movement, the rest period, and the total load lifted.

Exercise is Medicine campaign—An initiative launched by the American College of Sports Medicine (ACSM) and the American Medical Association (AMA). The initiative calls for physical activity and exercise to be standard parts of disease prevention and medical treatment, urging health care providers to assess and review patients' physical activity programs at every visit and to include exercise clearance and prescriptions or referrals to a qualified health or fitness professional in standard office visits.

exercise mode—The specific type of exercise being done.

exercise stress test—A graded exercise test (starts at a low intensity and gradually increases intensity until the test is stopped or volitional exhaustion is reached) during which symptoms of heart disease (ECG, heart rate, and blood pressure, and symptoms such as balance and ischemia) are evaluated.

external locus of control—Belief that chance or others control the lives of individual people.

extrinsic motivation—Motivation that is external, such as awarding trophies for a competition.

false negative—When a diagnosis incorrectly identifies the absence of a disease (i.e., the patient does have the disease).

false positive—When a diagnosis incorrectly identifies the presence of a disease (i.e., the patient does not have the disease).

fartlek—Swedish term meaning speed play; a form of training in which participants vary speed according to mood as they run through the countryside.

fast-twitch muscle fibers—Muscle fibers with high force output, low aerobic capacity, and high anaerobic capacity. They fatigue quickly. These are generally grouped into fast, oxidative-glycolytic (FOG) and fast, glycolytic (FG) fibers.

fatigue—Diminished work capacity, usually short of true physiological limits; real limits in short, intense exercise are factors within muscle (muscle pH, calcium); in long-duration effort, limits are glycogen depletion or central nervous system fatigue, due in part to low blood sugar.

fatigue index—A morning test of recovery from training using resting, submaximal, and recovery heart rates.

fat—Important energy source; it is stored for future use when excess calories are ingested.

fibrin—A protein involved in the clotting of blood.

first lactate threshold—The early rise in blood lactic acid that is associated with long-term endurance or sustainable fitness.

fitness—A combination of aerobic capacity and muscular strength and endurance that enhances health, performance, and the quality of life.

flexibility—The range of motion through which the limbs are able to move.

free radicals—Highly reactive compounds with one or more unpaired electrons. Many that are produced during exercise and oxidation of foods can damage muscle tissue, especially in untrained people who have limited antioxidant capabilities.

frostbite—Damage to the skin resulting from exposure to extreme cold or windchill.

genotype—A person's genetic constitution.

glucose—Energy source transported in blood; essential energy source for brain and nervous tissue.

glycemic index—An index ranking foods on the rate of carbohydrate digestion and its effect on the rise of blood glucose.

glycogen—A molecule formed from branching chains of linked glucose molecules. This is the way that we store carbohydrates in our body, mainly in muscle and the liver.

group cohesion—A dynamic process reflected by the tendency of a group to stick together and remain united in the pursuit of its objectives and for the satisfaction of its members' needs.

half-life—In reference to enzyme activity, the time it takes to lose one-half of the benefit.

health—A state of complete physical, mental, and emotional well-being, not merely the absence of disease or infirmity.

heart attack—Death of heart muscle tissue that results when atherosclerosis blocks oxygen delivery to heart muscle; also called myocardial infarction (MI).

heart rate—Frequency of contraction, often inferred from pulse rate (expansion of artery caused by a heartbeat).

heart rate reserve—The difference between the resting and maximal heart rates, calculated as maximal heart rate (HRmax) – resting heart rate.

heat acclimatization—The physiological processes that improves one's ability to live and work in a hot environment.

heat cramps—Cramps occurring as a result of electrolyte loss (generally from sweating).

heat exhaustion—When the heat stress exceeds the capacity of the temperature-regulating mechanism. Symptoms include cold, pale skin, body temperature of 39 to 41 °C (102 to 106 °F), a weak pulse, and dizziness.

heat stress—Temperature-humidity combination that leads to heat disorders such as heat cramps, heat exhaustion, or heatstroke.

heatstroke—When the temperature-regulating mechanism of a person has failed. The skin is flushed, hot, and dry. Sweating stops and body temperature may rise above 41 °C (106 °F). Heatstroke can lead to permanent damage of the temperature-regulating center of the brain, or even to death. Heatstroke is a medical emergency! Cool the victim rapidly and administer fluids, if possible, while awaiting transport.

hemoglobin (Hb)—The molecule in red blood cells that carries oxygen from the lungs to tissues. Hb binds oxygen when oxygen pressures are high (lungs) and releases it when oxygen pressures are low (tissues).

hemoglobin saturation—The percentage of oxygen binding sites on hemoglobin that are bound to oxygen.

high-density lipoprotein (HDL) cholesterol—A carrier molecule that takes cholesterol from the tissue to the liver for removal. It is inversely related to heart disease risk. HDL cholesterol is thus called good cholesterol.

hydrostatic (underwater) weighing—A method to estimate percent body fat using Archimedes's principle that density = weight in air / (weight in air – weight in water). Density can then be converted into % fat using sex, age, and race-specific equations.

hyperhydration—Excess fluid intake.

hypertension—High blood pressure defined as systolic blood pressure greater than 130 mmHg (millimeters of mercury) or diastolic blood pressure greater than 85 mmHg.

hyperthermia—(1) Body temperature above that expected for the physical activity state or a person. (2) An alarming rise in body temperature that sets the stage for heat stress disorders.

hypertrophy—Increased muscle mass and cross-sectional area.

hypoglycemia—Low blood sugar, generally defined as blood glucose below 80 mg/dl.

hypokinetic—Meaning low movement, this term is used to describe poor range of movement (poor flexibility).

hyponatremia—Dangerously low concentration of sodium in body fluids, usually measured in blood. This can be a result of excess water intake during vigorous activity, leading to a loss of salt.

hypothalamus—An area at the base of the brain that serves, among other duties, as a thermostat to maintain body temperature at or near 37 °C (98.6 °F).

hypothermia—Low body temperature; life-threatening heat loss brought on by rapid cooling, energy depletion, and exhaustion.

indirect calorimetry—Indirectly quantifying caloric use by measuring oxygen consumption and converting it to energy expenditure (with the knowledge of how much oxygen is required for each calorie produced for each fuel source). An average value is 5.0 calories per liter of oxygen consumed, but this can vary: 4.43 cal/L for protein, 4.7 cal/L for fat, and 5.06 cal/L for carbohydrate.

inhibition—Opposite of excitation in the nervous system.

insulin—A hormone secreted by the pancreas in response to rises in blood sugars. Insulin acts to stimulate the uptake of blood glucose into muscle cells and the liver, as well as promoting the uptake of triglycerides and excess glucose into adipose tissue for storage.

insulin resistance—A condition in which insulin is produced, but where insulin receptors become less sensitive to insulin. It is often associated with overweight, hypertension, low HDL cholesterol, and elevated triglycerides and blood glucose.

intensity (of physical activity)—The rate of energy expenditure during physical activity that can be defined in either absolute or relative terms. It is also defined as the relative rate, speed, or level of exertion.

internal locus of control—Belief that people can control outcomes in their lives.

interval training—Training method that alternates short bouts of intense effort with periods of active rest.

intrinsic motivation—Motivation that comes from within, such as running for the personal enjoyment one receives.

ischemia—A lack of blood to an area of the body resulting in reduced oxygen supply and waste removal. Ischemic heart disease refers to reduced blood flow and oxygen supply to the heart muscle.

isokinetic strength—Maximal force that can be generated at any set speed.

isometric strength—Same as static strength, the maximal force exerted against an immovable object.

isotonic strength—Contraction against a constant resistance.

lactate thresholds—The first lactate threshold (LT1) occurs as muscles produce more lactic acid than can be cleared from the blood. This generally occurs at a moderate intensity and represents long-duration sustainable capacity. The second lactate threshold (LT2) occurs when blood lactate accumulates rapidly and breathing becomes labored. Exercise over LT2 cannot be sustained long. Above LT1 and especially above LT2, more blood lactate accumulates because FG fibers produce more lactic acid and because most muscle fibers are active and therefore unable to remove (take up) lactate.

lactic acid—A by-product of glycogen metabolism that also transports energy from muscle to muscle and from muscle to the liver; high levels in muscle poison the contractile apparatus and inhibit enzyme activity.

lean body weight—Body weight minus fat weight.

leptin—A hormone produced by fat cells that helps regulate body weight and metabolism.

lipase—An enzyme that facilitates the splitting of triglyceride molecules into glycerol and fatty acids, which are then able to enter the circulation system.

lipid—Fat.

lipoprotein—A fat–protein complex that serves as a carrier in the blood (e.g., high-density lipoprotein cholesterol).

lipoprotein lipase (LPL)—The enzyme responsible for the uptake of plasma triglyceride fatty acids (TGFA) from plasma chylomicrons and other sources in the blood.

low-density lipoprotein (LDL) cholesterol—Cholesterol that is transported in the blood on low-density lipoproteins (LDL), which move cholesterol from the liver throughout the circulatory system, delivering it as needed. When cholesterol levels are high, LDL cholesterol may be deposited in excess. This is a precursor to atherosclerosis (plaque buildup) in arteries. LDL cholesterol is thus called bad cholesterol, even though normal levels are necessary for cell health.

lymphatic system—A system of tiny vessels and nodes that transports and filters cellular drainage and also transports digested fat in the form of chylomicrons to the circulatory system.

macronutrients—The three energy sources of carbohydrate, fat, and protein.

maintenance stage—Stage of behavior change where a person has been active for months.

maximal aerobic fitness—Maximum ability to take in, transport, and utilize oxygen.

maximal fat oxidation—The intensity of exercise at which the absolute rate of fat oxidation is maximized.

maximal intervals—These intervals are maximal effort for short periods of time. Their purpose is to train high-intensity energy systems.

maximal oxygen intake ($\dot{V}O_2$max)—Our maximal capacity to take in, transport, and use oxygen. This is considered the definition of aerobic fitness.

maximal oxygen intake ($\dot{V}O_2$max) test—An exercise test that involves increasing intensity of exercise, starting at an easy rate and grade, with increases every minute or two. Oxygen intake is computed each minute as the test proceeds toward maximal effort. The test ends when oxygen intake levels off in spite of increased treadmill rate or grade, or when the person can no longer keep up with the treadmill. The highest level of oxygen used is called the maximal oxygen intake ($\dot{V}O_2$max), or peak aerobic fitness.

metabolic equivalent (MET)—The resting metabolic rate. This is generally about 3.5 ml $O_2 \cdot kg^{-1} \cdot min^{-1}$. Intensity of physical activity is often given in terms of METs, or how many times resting energy expenditure is being used for a given activity.

metabolic syndrome—A combination of medical disorders that, when occurring together, increase the risk of developing cardiovascular disease and diabetes. A number of different organizations have criteria for this syndrome. A common criterion is that used by the U.S. National Cholesterol Education Program Adult Treatment Panel III, which requires at least three of the following. Central obesity: waist circumference ≥102 cm or 40 in. (male), ≥88 cm or 35 in. (female). Dyslipidemia: tri-

glycerides (TG) ≥1.7 mmol/L (150 mg/dl); HDL cholesterol <40 mg/dl (male), <50 mg/dl (female). Blood pressure: ≥130/85 mmHg. Fasting plasma glucose: ≥6.1 mmol/L (110 mg/dl).

metabolism—Energy production and utilization processes, often mediated by enzymatic pathways.

micronutrients—Vitamins and minerals are called micronutrients because we need only small amounts on a daily basis.

mitochondria—Cellular organelles where oxidative metabolism, the enzymatic breakdown of carbohydrate and fat to produce energy for muscular contractions, takes place. Mitochondria are often called the powerhouses of cells.

mode—The specific type of exercise used such as walking, running, cycling, or swimming.

moderate-intensity activities—Those activities performed at a relative intensity of 40%–60% of $\dot{V}O_2$max or absolute intensity of 4 to 6 METs.

morbidity—Disease.

mortality—Death.

motivation—The arousal, direction, and persistence of behavior.

motor area—Portion of cerebral cortex that controls movement.

motor neuron—Nerve that transmits impulses to muscle fibers.

motor unit—The motor neuron (nerve) and the muscle fibers it controls.

muscle biopsy—A hollow needle is inserted though an incision in the skin and fascia into the muscle. By removing a small piece of muscle about the size of a popcorn kernel, it is possible to measure aerobic and anaerobic enzymes, muscle glycogen stores, and gene expression, as well as to study an ever-increasing list of muscle functions.

muscle fiber—Long muscle cells with multiple nuclei.

muscle-fiber types—Fast-twitch fibers are fast contracting but quick to fatigue; slow-twitch fibers contract somewhat more slowly but are fatigue resistant.

muscle tone—Muscle firmness in the absence of a voluntary contraction.

muscular endurance—The ability of a muscle to persist. In practical terms, it is the ability to complete repeated repetitions of submaximal contractions or submaximal holding time (static or isometric endurance).

muscular fitness—The ability of muscles to produce force and persist. Muscular fitness includes muscular strength, muscular endurance, flexibility, power, speed, agility, and balance. The strength, muscular endurance, and flexibility needed to carry out daily tasks and avoid injury.

muscular training—Often referred to as resistance training, this is how we train muscles to become stronger and more powerful and to persist longer.

myocardial—Pertaining to heart muscle.

myocardial infarction—A heart attack that results from the interruption of blood supply to a part of the heart, causing heart cells to die. The resulting ischemia (restriction in blood supply) and ensuing oxygen shortage, if left untreated for a sufficient period of time, can cause damage or death.

myogenic changes—Changes in muscle tissue.

myoglobin—The compound in muscle (and some tissue cells) to transport oxygen within the cell primarily from the cell membrane to the mitochondria.

myosin—One of the major proteins in a muscle that make up the crossbridges that allow for muscle contraction.

neurogenesis—The growth of new brain cells.

neurogenic—Training that influences the nervous system.

neuron—Nerve cell that conducts an impulse; basic unit of the nervous system.

norepinephrine—A stress hormone. Along with epinephrine, norepinephrine is a main hormone in the fight-or-flight response, directly increasing heart rate, triggering the release of glucose from energy stores, and increasing blood flow to skeletal muscle.

nutrition—Provision of adequate energy (calories), as well as needed amounts of fat, carbohydrate, protein, vitamins, minerals, and water.

nutritional calorie (calorie listed on a food package)—The amount of energy necessary to raise 1 liter of water (1.057 quarts) 1 degree Celsius (1.8 °F).

obesity—An excessive accumulation of fat beyond what is considered normal for one's age, sex, and body type. Obesity is defined as having more than 20% fat for men or more than 30% fat for women (or as being more than 20% above desirable weight, or having a BMI of 30 or greater).

official training season—Period in academic sports and some professional leagues when the coaches are allowed to work with athletes.

osteoporosis—Weakening of bones through the loss of bone minerals.

outcome-oriented goals—Goals that are the result or outcome of a performance or action.

overload—A greater training load than normally experienced; used to coax a training effect from the body.

overreaching—Tiredness as a result of hard training from which we can rapidly recover. In the overreached state, athletes have put an adequate overload on their body to stimulate training adaptations.

overtraining—Excess training that leads to staleness, illness, or injury, or tiredness and reduced performance as a result of too great an overload with too little recovery time. Overtraining results in a condition from which athletes will recover only slowly, often requiring multiple weeks or even months.

oxygen debt—Recovery oxygen intake in excess of resting needs. The debt, or excess postexercise oxygen consumption (EPOC), is used to repay the oxygen deficit, to replace ATP and phosphocreatine (PCr), to remove lactic acid, and to replace some of the energy used during the exercise.

oxygen deficit—Lack of oxygen in early moments of exercise.

oxygen intake—Oxygen used to provide energy through oxidative pathways.

perceived exertion—Subjective estimate of exercise difficulty.

performance diet—A recommended diet for active people, with 55%–60% of calories coming from carbohydrate (mostly complex), 25%–30% from fat (low in saturated fats), and 15% from protein.

periodization—The process of planning systematic variations and rest in the training program. Variation occurs at daily and weekly and even seasonal levels.

peripheral fatigue—Fatigue that occurs locally in a muscle as a result of fuel reductions or acid–base balance.

persistence—The ability to go on resolutely or stubbornly in spite of difficulties.

pH—Acidity or alkalinity of a solution; below 7 is acid, and above 7 is alkaline.

phenotype—The observable appearance of a person resulting from the interaction of the genotype and the environment.

physical activity—Any bodily movement produced by skeletal muscles that results in energy expenditure beyond resting expenditure.

physical fitness—(1) Cardiorespiratory fitness, muscle strength, body composition, and flexibility, comprising a set of attributes that people have or achieve that relate to the ability to perform physical activity. (2) The ability to perform the necessary tasks of daily living and to have energy for leisure activities at the end of the day.

physiology—The study of how organisms function.

physiology of fitness—The study of how muscular contractions move the body to participate in exercise, sport, and strenuous work. How do these muscles function? What makes them move, and what causes fatigue? What is the energy for muscular contractions, and how is oxygen central to movement and performance? And why is physical activity good for your health?

physiological age—Also called *functional age*, as contrasted to chronological age, this defines one's ability to perform physically. The best single measure of physiological age is probably the aerobic fitness score. That number tells you about the health and capacity of the respiratory, circulatory, and muscular systems.

plaque—A growth of cellular debris and low-density lipoprotein cholesterol that impedes blood flow in the coronary artery.

plyometrics—Explosive movements designed to improve power. A plyometric contraction involves first a rapid muscle-lengthening (eccentric stretch) movement, then an explosive muscle-shortening (concentric contraction) movement. These coordinate muscles to work together to achieve the sport motion.

positive addictions—Addictions that improve the quality of life, such as the urge to exercise.

postprandial lipemia—The presence of fat in the blood after a meal.

power—The rate of doing work. Power = (force × distance) / time. Since (force × distance) = work, power = work / time. In a similar fashion, since velocity = distance / time, power = force × velocity.

precontemplative stage—Stage of behavior change where a person is not considering an activity.

preparation stage—Stage of behavior change where a person is exhibiting some activity.

process-oriented goal—Goals that are described by the process of achieving them.

progression—How we gradually increase the overall training load.

progressive resistance training—This is a strength training method in which the overload is constantly increased to facilitate adaptation. Since the body adapts to exercise, it needs to be constantly challenged in order to continue to grow and change.

prospective research studies—Research studies that follow a population or a subset of the population for a period of time, often many years.

protein—Organic compound formed from amino acids; forms muscle tissue, hormones, and enzymes.

psychoneuroimmunology (PNI)—A field of study that explores links between the brain and nervous system and the immune system, or between thoughts and emotions and sickness and health.

psychosomatic illness—A physical ailment caused or exacerbated by a state of mind.

pulse—The wave that travels down the artery after each contraction of the heart (see heart rate).

purposeful or meaningful physical activity—An activity that is done in the normal course of activities of daily living that accomplishes a necessary or meaningful task.

race pace—This is the current speed that an athlete can maintain for a designated race length.

race pace–plus intervals—Intervals that are done at a speed slightly (1%–5%) faster than current race pace, but are generally done for a distance shorter than the race length.

rapid eye movement (REM)—A stage of sleep associated with dreams.

rating of perceived exertion (RPE)—A subjective rating scale of intensity of exercise.

reaction time—The time from a stimulus, such as a starting gun, until the beginning of a movement.

relapse—Temporarily returning to an old behavior when attempting to adopt a new behavior.

relative fitness—The percentage of maximal aerobic capacity that you can sustain (i.e., the percentage of $\dot{V}O_2$max that people can sustain for events of different duration). This can be defined using either LT1 or LT2 (lactate thresholds 1 and 2) in comparison with $\dot{V}O_2$max.

relative intensity (of physical activity)—The percent of aerobic power utilized during exercise, usually expressed as percent of maximal heart rate or percent of $\dot{V}O_2$max.

relaxation response—Proven method to achieve relaxation.

repetition—The number of times an exercise is repeated between rest periods.

repetition maximum (RM)—The maximum number of times one can lift a given weight (1 RM is the most a person can lift one time).

residual lung volume—The air remaining in the lung after a maximal exhalation. This can be measured in the lab using a simple rebreathing technique. It is an important measurement for accurate determination of percent body fat when using hydrostatic weighing.

respiration—Intake of oxygen (from the atmosphere into the lungs, and then to the blood and to the tissues) and exhalation of carbon dioxide (from tissues to the blood, to the lungs, and to the atmosphere).

respiratory compensation point—The exercise intensity at which ventilation (L of air/ min) rises disproportionably to increasing work and corresponds to the second lactate threshold. This point is also referred to as *breakaway ventilation*. This rapid rise in ventilation (respiratory rate and depth) provides a perceptible signal indicating that the person is flirting with excess anaerobic effort and exhaustion, and should ease off.

resting energy expenditure—The energy a person uses while quietly sitting. This is generally about 1.2 cal/min, but depends on genetics, body size, age, sex, body fat percent, and other factors.

retrospective research studies—Studies that look at past history.

rhabdomyolysis (exertional rhabdomyolysis)—This is a condition in which strenuous exercise (especially in heat and when dehydrated) may result in damaged skeletal muscle tissue releasing the breakdown products into the bloodstream. Rhabdomyolysis muscle damage may be caused by a number of other factors, including medications, drug abuse, and infections.

ribonucleic acid (RNA)—A cellular compound that carries messages from the nucleus (DNA) to the rest of the cell (messenger RNA) or transfers amino acids to the ribosome for protein synthesis (transfer RNA).

ribosome—A cellular organelle that synthesizes protein from amino acids.

risk ratio—The risk of disease (or other incident) compared to some norm. Thus, if a population has a risk ratio of 4, it suggests that it is more at risk for that issue (such as heart disease) compared to some normative group (such as active people with normal weight).

sarcopenia—Loss of muscle mass with age and inactivity.

seasonal periodization—Also called *year-round periodization*, this plans the training year into periods with specific goals. The four periods are generally off-season, preseason, early competitive season, and peak competitive season.

self-actualization—The full realization of one's potential (simple definition).

self-concept—Our knowledge, assumptions, and feelings about ourselves.

self-efficacy—The belief in one's capabilities to organize and execute the sources of action required to manage prospective situations and to succeed in specific situations.

set-point theory—A theory, with good scientific basis, that our metabolism attempts to maintain our current weight within a fairly tight range.

shin splints—Pain on the front portion of the shinbones that can be caused by inflammation of the tibialis anterior muscle, its membrane, or the bone it attaches to, or by a spasm of the inflamed muscle.

simple sugar—Basic 6-carbon ($C_6H_{12}O_6$) sugars such as glucose, fructose, along with sugars formed from joining two 6-carbon sugar molecules into a 12-carbon sugar such as sucrose (refined sugar, composed of molecules of glucose and fructose). Simple sugars are pure carbohydrates that contain energy but few nutrients (i.e., vitamins and minerals).

skinfold—A method to estimate percent body fat using measurements of subcutaneous fat obtained by measuring specific sites for thickness of skin plus fat. Equations are then used that correlate specific skinfold measurements with hydrostatic weight to determine percent body fat.

slow-twitch (slow, oxidative) muscle fibers—Muscle fibers with lower force output, more aerobic capacity and better endurance that contract more slowly than fast-twitch fibers.

somatopsychic—The effect of the body (soma) on the mind.

specificity—The concept that specific overloads (intensity, duration, and frequency), as well as the specific system or muscle that is overloaded will result in specific adaptations (i.e., you get what you train for).

speed of movement—Reaction time plus movement time.

standard deviation—A measure of the variation within a group or population. One standard deviation refers to the plus or minus range within which 67% of the population should fall.

state anxiety—A transitory emotional response to a specific situation, characterized by feelings of tension, apprehension, and nervousness.

static balance—The ability to maintain balance while stationary.

static strength—Same as isometric strength: The maximal force one can exert against an immovable object.

static stretching—Stretching using slow movements to reach a point of stretch, holding the position (for 10 seconds), and relaxing. You may repeat the stretch or perform very light bobbing.

stitch—Side pain, usually blamed on food or fluid in the digestive system, may be due to tugging of ligaments that attach the gut to the diaphragm.

strength—Ability of muscle to exert force.

stroke—When a blood clot forms in the brain, causing ischemia (reduced blood flow), which results in reduced oxygen to a portion of the brain. If the blood flow is restricted for a period of time, brain cells will die in the ischemic area.

stroke volume—The amount of blood pumped by each beat of the heart. Stroke volume depends on exercise state, aerobic fitness, body size, and other factors. On average, it is about 70 ml per beat.

subcutaneous fat—Fat stored in a layer just below the skin.

synapse—Junction between neurons. May also be used as a verb to indicate the act of transferring a nervous impulse between neurons.

systolic—Refers to the period of time during which the heart is contracting.

systolic blood pressure—Highest blood pressure in arteries during the contracting period of the heartbeat.

tendon—Tough tissue that connects muscle to bone.

tension—The condition of being strained or stretched.

testosterone—An anabolic (growth-stimulating) hormone that helps stimulate the growth of muscle. Testosterone decreases with overtraining.

threshold—The minimal level required to elicit a response or a transition point (lactate threshold).

thrombus—Blood clot.

tidal volume—Volume of air per breath.

training plateau—When increased training load does not result in improved performance; performance seems to plateau regardless of training increases.

training stimulus—The type of exercise that elicits the desired adaptation to training.

training zone—The heart-rate zone within which training is likely to produce the desired effect.

trait anxiety—A relatively stable level of anxiety proneness, a predisposition to respond to threats with elevated anxiety.

triglyceride—Human's form of stored fat in both adipose and muscle tissue. Triglycerides are composed of three chains of fatty acids (the smallest fat unit) attached to a glycerol molecule.

type 2 diabetes—Non-insulin-dependent diabetes mellitus (NIDDM), or adult-onset diabetes, is a disease characterized by high blood glucose as a result of insulin resistance (low sensitivity of insulin receptors to the hormone insulin) and, as the disease progresses, insulin deficiency.

variable (or accommodating) resistance—A machine or system that matches resistance to the capability of the muscle group.

vasoconstriction—Constriction of blood vessels.

velocity—Rate of movement or speed.

ventilation (V)—The amount of air inhaled per minute. Ventilation is the product of respiratory rate (or frequency, f) and the volume of air per breath (tidal volume, or TV), so $V = f \times TV$.

ventricle—Chamber of the heart that pumps blood to the lungs (right ventricle) or to the rest of the body (left ventricle).

vigorous-intensity activities—Those performed at a relative intensity of >60% of $\dot{V}O_2$max or absolute intensity of >6 METs.

visceral fat—Abdominal fat, stored in and around the viscera. High visceral fat stores put a person at higher risk for a number of chronic diseases, especially heart disease.

visualization—The process of beginning to see yourself as the new person that you are becoming.

vitamin—A vital nutrient required in tiny amounts that humans cannot make themselves and must obtain from the diet.

warm-up—A preperformance activity used to increase muscle temperature and to rehearse skills.

weekly periodization—Weekly systematic variation in physical training stress during a training season. Weeks are generally classified as average stress, high stress (20%–50% harder than an average week), and low stress (20%–50% easier than an average week).

weight training—Progressive exercise using weight for resistance.

wellness—A conscious and deliberate approach to an advanced state of physical, psychological, and spiritual health.

wet bulb globe temperature (WBGT)—A measurement used to provide a simple and accurate indication of the effect of environmental factors on active people. The index uses dry bulb and wet bulb thermometers to assess air temperature and relative humidity. The black copper globe thermometer indicates radiant heat as well as air movement. The several temperatures are weighted to indicate their relative contribution to the total heat stress.

windchill—The effect of wind speed on heat loss; the cooling effect of temperature and wind.

work capacity—The ability to accomplish productive goals without undue fatigue and without becoming a hazard to oneself or one's coworkers.

References

Aagaard, P., and J.L. Andersen. 2010. Effects of strength training on endurance capacity in top-level endurance athletes. *Scandinavian Journal of Medicine and Science in Sports* 20 (Suppl 2):39–47. Review.

Achten, J., M. Gleeson, and A. Jeukendrup. 2002. Determination of the exercise intensity that elicits maximal fat oxidation. *Medicine and Science in Sports and Exercise* 34:92–97.

Adams, W.C., E.M. Bernauer, D.B. Dill, and J.B. Bomar Jr. 1975. Effect of equivalent sea level and altitude training on $\dot{V}O_2$max and running performance. *Journal of Applied Physiology* 39:262–268.

Ainsworth, B., W. Haskell, A. Leon, D. Jacobs Jr., H. Montoye, J. Sallis, and R. Paffenbarger. 1993. Compendium of physical activities: Classification of energy costs of human physical activities. *Medicine and Science in Sports and Exercise* 25:71–80.

Alberti, K.G.M.M., R.H. Eckel, S.M. Grundy, P.Z. Zimmet, J.I. Cleeman, K.A. Donato, J. Fruchart, W. P.T. James, C.M. Loria, S.C. Smith, Jr. 2009. Harmonizing the metabolic syndrome: A joint interim statement of the International Diabetes Federation Task Force on Epidemiology and Prevention; National Heart, Lung, and Blood Institute; American Heart Association; World Heart Federation; International Atherosclerosis Society; and International Association for the Study of Obesity. *Circulation* 120:1640-1645.

Alderman, B., and D. Landers. 2004. The influence of cardiorespiratory fitness and hostility on cardiovascular reactivity in mental stress. *Medicine and Science in Sports and Exercise* 36:S91.

Amako, M., T. Oda, K. Masuoka, H. Yokoi, and P. Campisi. 2003. Effects of static stretching on prevention of injuries for military recruits. *Military Medicine* 168:442–446.

American College of Sports Medicine (ACSM). 2005. *ACSM guidelines for exercise testing and prescription.* 7th ed. Baltimore: Williams and Wilkins.

Amoroso, P., K. Reynolds, J. Barnes, and D. White. 1996. *Tobacco and injury.* Natick, MA: U.S. Army Research Institute for Environmental Medicine, Technical Report 91–96.

Anderson, T., and J. Kearney. 1982. Effects of three resistance training programs on muscular strength and absolute and relative endurance. *Research Quarterly for Exercise Science and Sport* 53:1–7.

Ardell, D. 1984. *The history and future of wellness.* Pleasant Hills, CA: Diablo Press.

Armstrong, L. 2000. *Performance in extreme environments.* Champaign, IL: Human Kinetics.

Armstrong, R. 1984. Mechanisms of exercise-induced delayed-onset muscular soreness: A brief review. *Medicine and Science in Sports and Exercise* 16:529–538.

Asahina, S., K. Asano, H. Horikawa, T. Hisamitsu, and M. Sato. 2003. Enhancement of beta-endorphin levels in rat hypothalamus by exercise. *Japanese Journal of Physical Fitness and Sports Medicine* 52:159–166.

Aspenes, T., T. Nilsen, E. Skaug, G. Birthheussen, O. Ellingsen, L. Vatten, and U. Wishloff. 2011. Peak oxygen uptake and cardiovascular risk factors in 4,631 healthy women and men. *Medicine and Science in Sports and Exercise* 43:1465–1473.

Åstrand, P.O., and K. Rodahl. 1970. *Textbook of work physiology: Physiological bases of exercise.* 2nd ed. New York: McGraw-Hill.

Avins, A., and J. Neuhaus. 2000. Do triglycerides provide meaningful information about heart disease risk? *Archives of Internal Medicine* 160:1937–1944.

Baechle, T., R. Earle, and D. Wathen. 2000. Resistance training. In *Essentials of strength training and conditioning,* ed. T. Baechle and R. Earle. Champaign, IL: Human Kinetics.

Balady, G. 2002. Survival of the fittest—more evidence. *New England Journal of Medicine* 346:852–854.

Balady, G., B. Chaitman, D. Driscoll, C. Foster, E. Froelicher, N. Gordon, R. Pate, J. Rippe, and T. Bazzarre. 1998. Recommendations for cardiovascular screening, staffing, and emergency policies at health/fitness facilities. *Medicine and Science in Sport and Exercise* 30:1009–1018.

Balke, B. 1963. *A simple field test for the assessment of physical fitness.* Report no. 63-66. Oklahoma City: Civil Aeronautic Research Institute, Federal Aviation Agency.

Bandura, A. 1986. Social foundations of thought and action: A social cognitive theory. Englewood Cliffs, NJ, Prentice Hall.

Barham, J. 1960. A comparison of the effectiveness of isometric and isotonic exercise when performed at different frequencies per week. Unpublished doctoral dissertation, Louisiana State University, Baton Rouge.

Barnard, R.J., G.W. Gardner, N. Diaco, and A.A. Kattus. 1972. Ischemic response to sudden strenuous exercise. Paper presented at the annual meeting of the American College of Sports Medicine, Philadelphia.

Barton-Davis, E., D. Shoturma, and H. Sweeney. 1999. Contribution of satellite cells to IGF-I induced hypertrophy of skeletal muscle. *Acta Physiologica Scandinavica* 167:301–305.

Barzalai, N., G. Atzmon, C. Schecter, E. Schaefer, A. Cupples, R. Lipton, S. Cheng, and A. Shuldiner. 2003. Unique lipoprotein phenotype and genotype associated with exceptional longevity. *Journal of the American Medical Association* 290:2030–2040.

Bauer, D., I. Varahram, G. Proest, and U. Halter. 2001. Benefits from aerobic exercise in patients with major depression: A pilot study. *British Journal of Sports Medicine* 35:114–117.

Beck, B., and C. Snow. 2003. Bone health across the lifespan: Exercising our options. *Exercise and Sports Science Reviews* 31:117–122.

Bekinschtein, P., C.A. Oomen, L.M. Saksida, and T.J. Bussey. 2011. Effects of environmental enrichment and voluntary exercise on neurogenesis, learning and memory, and pattern separation: BDNF as a critical variable? *Seminars in Cell and Development Biology.* 22(5):536-542.

Bell, G., D. Syrotuik, T. Martin, R. Burnham, and H. Quinney. 2000. Effects of concurrent strength and endurance training on skeletal muscle properties and hormone concentrations in humans. *European Journal of Applied Physiology* 81:418–427.

Benson, H. 1975. *The relaxation response.* New York: Harper and Row.

Bisson, L.F., C.E. Butzke, and S.E. Ebeler. 1995. The role of moderate ethanol consumption in health and human nutrition. *American Journal of Enology and Viticulture* 46(4):449–462.

Blair, S.N. 2009. Physical inactivity: The biggest public health problem of the 21st century. *British Journal of Sports Medicine* 43:1–2.

Blair, S.N., and H. Kohl. 1988. Physical activity or physical fitness: Which is more important for health? *Medicine and Science in Sports and Exercise* 20:S8.

Blair, S.N., H. Kohl, C. Barlow, R. Paffenbarger, L. Gibbons, and C. Macera. 1995. Changes in physical fitness and all-cause mortality: A prospective study of healthy and unhealthy men. *Journal of the American Medical Association* 273:1093–1098.

Blair, S.N., H. Kohl, R. Paffenbarger, D. Clark, K. Cooper, and L. Gibbons. 1989. Physical fitness and all-cause mortality: A prospective study of healthy men and women. *Journal of the American Medical Association* 262:2395–2401.

Blair, S.N., M. LaMonte, and M. Nichaman. 2004. The evolution of physical activity recommendations: How much is enough? *American Journal of Clinical Nutrition* 79:913–920.

Blaschke, F., D. Bruemmer, F. Yin, Y. Takata, W. Wang, M. Fishbein, T. Okura, J. Higaki, K. Graf, E. Fleck, W. Hsueh, and R. Law. 2004. C-reactive protein induces apoptosis in human coronary vascular smooth muscle cells. *Circulation* 110:579–587.

Blomqvist, C.G., and B. Saltin. 1983. Cardiovascular adaptations to physical training. *Annual Review of Physiology* 45:169–185.

Blumenthal, J., A. Sherwood, E. Gullette, M. Babyak, R. Waugh, A. Georgiades, L. Craighead, D. Tweedy, M. Feinglos, M. Appelbaum, J. Hayano, and A. Hinderliter. 2000. Exercise and weight loss reduce blood pressure in men and women with mild hypertension. *Archives of Internal Medicine* 160:1947–1958.

Boileau, R., B. McKeown, and W. Riner. 1984. Cardiovascular and metabolic contributions to the maximal aerobic power of the arms and legs. *International Journal of Sports Cardiology* 4:67–75.

Booth, F., and M. Chakravarthy. 2002. Cost and consequences of sedentary living: New battleground for an old enemy. *President's Council on Physical Fitness and Sports Research Digest*, 3rd ser., no. 16.

Booth, F., S. Gordon, C. Carlson, and M. Hamilton. 2000. Waging war on modern chronic diseases: Primary prevention through exercise. *Journal of Applied Physiology* 88:774–787.

Borensztajn, J. 1975. Effect of exercise on lipoprotein lipase activity in rat heart and skeletal muscle. *American Journal of Physiology* 229:394–400.

Borg, G. 1973. Perceived exertion: A note on history and methods. *Medicine and Science in Sports and Exercise* 5:90–93.

Bortz, W.M. 2010. Disuse and aging. *Journals of Gerontology: Series A Biological Sciences.* 65(4):382-385.

Bortz, W.M., D.H. Wallace, and D. Wiley. 1999. Sexual function in 1,202 aging males: differentiating aspects. *Journals of Gerontology: Series A Biological Sciences* 54(5):M237-241.

Bouchard, C., P. An, T. Rice, J. Skinner, J. Wilmore, J. Gagnon, L. Perusse, A. Leon, and D. Rao. 1999. Familial aggregation of $\dot{V}O_2$max response to exercise training: Results from the Heritage Family Study. *Journal of Applied Physiology* 87:1003–1008.

Bouchard, C., M. Boulay, J. Simoneau, G. Lorrie, and L. Pierrise. 1988. Heritability and trainability of aerobic and anaerobic performance: An update. *Sports Medicine* 5:69–73.

Bouchard, C., W. Holimann, H. Venrath, G. Herkenrath, and H. Schlussel. 1966. Minimal amount of physical training for the prevention of cardiovascular disease. Paper presented at the 16th World Conference for Sports Medicine, Hanover, Germany.

Bravata, D., L. Sanders, J. Huang, H. Krumholz, I. Olkin, C. Gardner, and D. Bravata. 2003. Efficacy and safety of low-carbohydrate diets: A systematic review. *Journal of the American Medical Association* 289:1837–1850.

Breslow, L., and J. Enstrom. 1980. Persistence of health habits and their relationship to mortality. *Preventive Medicine* 9:469–483.

Brill, P., C. Macera, D. Davis, S. Blair, and N. Gordon. 2000. Muscular strength and physical function. *Medicine and Science in Sports and Exercise* 32:412–416.

Brook, R.D., B. Franklin, W. Cascio, Y. Hong, G. Howard, M. Lipsett, R. Luepker, M. Mittleman, J. Samet, S.C. Smith Jr., and I. Tager. 2004. Air pollution and cardiovascular disease: A statement for healthcare professionals from the Expert Panel on Population and Prevention Science of the American Heart Association. *Circulation* 109:2655–2671.

Brown, R., and C. Cox. 1998. Effects of high fat versus high carbohydrate diets on plasma lipids and lipoproteins in endurance athletes. *Medicine and Science in Sports and Exercise* 30:1677–1683.

Brownell, K. 1995. Exercise and obesity treatment: Psychological aspects. *International Journal of Obesity* 19:S122–125.

Brownell, K., M. Greenwood, E. Stellar, and E. Shrager. 1986. The effects of repeated cycles of weight loss and regain in rats. *Physiology and Behavior* 38:459–464.

Brownell, K., and J. Rodin. 1994. Medical, metabolic, and psychological effects of weight cycling. *Archives of Internal Medicine* 154:1325–1330.

Brynteson, P., and W. Sinning. 1973. The effects of training frequencies on the retention of cardio-vascular fitness. *Medicine and Science in Sports and Exercise* 5:29–33.

Bussau, V., T. Fairchild, A. Rao, P. Stelle, and P. Fournier. 2002. Carbohydrate loading in human muscle: An improved 1 day protocol. *European Journal of Applied Physiology* 87:290–295.

Calle, E., C. Rodriquez, K. Walker-Thurmond, and M. Thun. 2003. Overweight, obesity, and mortality from cancer in a prospectively studied cohort of U.S. adults. *New England Journal of Medicine* 348:1625–1638.

Calle, E., M. Thun, J. Petrelli, C. Rodriguez, and C. Heath. 1999. Body mass index and mortality in a prospective cohort of U.S. adults. *New England Journal of Medicine* 341:1097–1105.

Campbell, W., M. Crim, V. Young, and W. Evans. 1994. Increased energy requirements and changes in body composition with resistance training in older adults. *American Journal of Clinical Nutrition* 60:167–175.

Carey, T., J. Garrett, A. Jackman, C. McLaughlin, J. Fryer, D. Smucker, P. Curtis, J. Darter, G. DeFriese, A. Evans, N. Hadler, G. Hunter, J. Joines, W. Kalsbeek, T. Konrad, R. McNutt, T. Rickets, and D. Taylor. 1995. The outcomes and cost of care for acute low-back pain among patients seen by primary-care practitioners, chiropractors, and orthopaedic surgeons. *New England Journal of Medicine* 333:913–917.

Carpenter, D., and B. Nelson. 1999. Low back strengthening for the prevention and treatment of low back pain. *Medicine and Science in Sports and Exercise* 31:18–24.

Cattell, R.B., H.W. Eber, and M.M. Tatsuoka. 1970. *Handbook for the sixteen personality factor questionnaire*. Champaign, IL: Institute for Personality and Ability Testing.

Centers for Disease Control and Prevention (CDC). 2009. Deaths and Mortality. www.cdc.gov/nchs/fastats.deaths.htm. Accessed August 16, 2012.

———. 2011a. Obesity Prevalence data. www.cdc.gov/nchs/data/series/sr_10/sr10_252.pdf. Accessed August 16, 2012.

———. 2011b. Physical Inactivity Estimates, by County. www.cdc.gov/Features/dsPhysicalInactivity. Accessed August 16, 2012.

———. 2011c. Overweight and Obesity-Adult Obesity Facts. www.cdc.gov/obesity/data/adult.html. Accessed August 18, 2012.

———. 2011d. *National Vital Statistics Reports*. www.cdc.gov/nchs/data/nvsr/nvsr59/nvsr59_04.pdf. Accessed September 13, 2012.

————. 2012. Barriers to Physical Activity. www.cdc.gov/nccdphp/dnpa/physical/life/barries_quiz.pdf. Accessed August 16, 2012.

Chang, P., D. Ford, L. Meoni, N. Wang and M. Klag. 2002. Anger in young men and subsequent premature cardiovascular disease. *Archives of Internal Medicine* 162:901–906.

Chapman, R., J. Stray-Gunderson, and B. Levine. 1998. Individual variation in response to altitude training. *Journal of Applied Physiology* 85:1448–1456.

Chenoweth, D. 2005. The economic costs of physical inactivity, obesity and overweight in California adults: Health care, worker's compensation and lost productivity. www.cdph.ca.gov/HealthInfo/healthyliving/nutrition/Documents/CostofObesityToplineReport.pdf.

Choi, H., K. Atkinson, W. Karlson, W. Willett, and C. Curhan. 2004. Purine-rich foods dairy and protein intake, and the risk of gout in men. *New England Journal of Medicine* 350:1093–1103.

Church, T. 2011. Exercise in obesity, metabolic syndrome, and diabetes. *Progress in Cardiovascular Diseases* 53(6):412–418.

Clarkson, P., and S. Sayers. 2008. Intersubject variability in developing exertional muscle damage. *Skeletal Muscle Damage and Repair*, ed. P. Tiidus, 185–191. Champaign, IL: Human Kinetics.

Clarkson, P., E. Hoffman, E. Zambraski, H. Gordish-Dressman, A. Kearns, M. Hubal, B. Harmon, and J. Devaney. 2005. ACTN3 and MLCK genotype associations with exertional muscle damage. *Journal of Applied Physiology* 99:564–569.

Coggan, A., and B. Williams. 1995. Metabolic adaptations to endurance training: Substrate metabolism during exercise. In *Exercise metabolism*, ed. M. Hargraves, 177–210. Champaign, IL: Human Kinetics.

Comfort, A. 1979. *The biology of senescence*. New York: Elsevier.

Consolazio, C.F., R.E. Johnson, and L.J. Pecora. 1963. *Physiological measurements of metabolic functions in man*. New York: McGraw-Hill.

Cooper, K. 1968. *Aerobics*. New York: Bantam Books.

Cordain, L., R.W. Gotshall, and S.B. Eaton. 1998. Physical activity, energy expenditure and fitness: An evolutionary perspective. *International Journal of Sports Medicine* 9:328–335.

Cordes, K., and B. Sharkey. 1995. Physiological comparison of protective clothing variations. *Medicine and Science in Sports and Exercise* 27:S153.

Cotman, C., and C. Engesser-Cesar. 2002. Exercise enhances and protects brain function. *Exercise and Sports Science Reviews* 30:75–79.

Coyle, E. 1995. Substrate utilization during exercise in active people. *American Journal of Clinical Nutrition* 61:S968–979.

Coyle, E., M. Hemmert, and A. Coggan. 1986. Effects of detraining on cardiovascular responses to exercise: Role of blood volume. *Journal of Applied Physiology* 60:95–99.

Cracchiolo, J.R., T. Mori, S.J. Nazian, J. Tan, H. Potter, and G.W. Arendash. 2007. Enhanced cognitive activity—over and above social or physical activity—is required to protect Alzheimer's mice against cognitive impairment, reduce Abeta deposition, and increase synaptic immunoreactivity. *Neurobiology of Learning and Memory* 88(3):277-94.

Crews, D., M. Lochbaum, and D. Landers. 2004. Aerobic physical activity effects on psychological well-being in low-income Hispanic children. *Perceptual and Motor Skills* 98:319–324.

Crothers, L.M., T.J. Kehle, M.A. Bray, and L.A. Theodore. 2009. Correlates and suspected causes of obesity in children. *Psychology in the Schools* 48:787–796.

Cureton, T.K. 1969. *The physiological effects of exercise programs upon adults*. Springfield, IL: Charles C Thomas.

Danesh, J., J. Wheeler, G. Hirschfield, S. Eda, G. Eirksdottir, A. Rumley, G. Lowe, M. Pepys, and V. Goudnason. 2004. C-reactive protein and other circulating markers of inflammation in the predictin of coronary heart disease. *New England Journal of Medicine* V350:1387-1397.

Dansinger, M., J. Gleason, J. Griffith, H. Selker, and E. Schaefer. 2005. Comparison of the Atkins, Ornish, Weight Watchers, and Zone diets for weight loss and heart disease risk reduction. *Journal of the American Medical Association* 293:43–53.

de Bruin M., P. Sheeran, G. Kok, A. Hiemstra, J.M. Prins, H.J. Hospers, and G.J. van Breukelen. 2012. Self-regulatory processes mediate the intention-behavior relation for adherence and exercise behaviors. *Health Psychology* Mar 5. [Epub ahead of print]

DeLorme, T., and A. Watkins. 1951. *Progressive resistance exercise*. New York: Appleton-Century-Crofts.

Demopoulos, H., J. Santomier, M. Seligman, D. Pietrogro, and P. Hogan. 1986. Free radical pathology: Rationale and toxicology of antioxidants and other supplements in sports medicine and exercise science. In *Sport, health, and nutrition: 1984 proceed-*

ings of the Olympic Scientific Congress, ed. F. Katch, 139–189. Champaign, IL: Human Kinetics.

Department of Health, Education, and Welfare: Vital Statistics of the United States. 1977. National Center for Health Statistics, DHEW Publication PHS 80-1104 (vol. 2, sec. 5).

Despres, J. 2004. Visceral fat and the metabolic syndrome: Effect of activity intervention. Paper presented at the annual meeting of the American College of Sports Medicine, Indianapolis.

Deschenes, M. 2005. Effects of aging on muscle fiber type and size. Sports Medicine 34:809–824.

deVries, H.A., and G.M. Adams. 1972. Electromyographic comparison of single doses of exercise and meprobromate as to effects on muscular relaxation. American Journal of Physical Medicine 51:130–141.

deVries, H., and T. Housh. 1994. Physiology of exercise. Madison, WI: Brown and Benchmark.

Dintiman, G., and R. Ward. 2003. Sportspeed, 3rd ed. Champaign, IL: Human Kinetics.

Docktor, R., and B.J. Sharkey. 1971. Note on some physiological and subjective reactions to exercise and training. Perceptual and Motor Skills 32:233–234.

Doe, J. 2009. WHO Statistical Information System (WHOSIS). Geneva: World Health Organization.

Dokken, B.B., and T.S. Tsao. 2007. The physiology of body weight regulation: Are we too efficient for our own good? Diabetes Spectrum 20(3):166–170.

Dorado, C., J.A. Calbet, A. Lopez-Gordillo, S. Alayon, and J. Sanchis-Moysi. 2012. Marked effects of pilates on the abdominal muscles: a longitudinal magnetic resonance imaging study. Medicine and Science in Sports and Exercise 44(8):1589-94.

Drygas, W., T. Kostka, A. Jegier, and H. Kunski. 2000. Long-term effects of different physical activity levels on coronary heart disease risk factors in middle-aged men. International Journal of Sports Medicine 21:235–241.

Egger, G.J., N. Vogels, and K.R. Westerterp. 2001. Estimating historical changes in physical activity levels. Medical Journal of Australia 175(11-12):635–636.

Ehrlich, N. 1971. Acquisition rates of competitors and performers: A note on the theory of athletic performance. Perceptual and Motor Skills 33:10–66.

Eichner, R. 1995. Contagious infections in competitive sports. Sports Science Exchange 8(3):1–4.

Eisenmann, J.C. 2007. Aerobic fitness, fatness and the metabolic syndrome in children and adolescents. Acta Paediatrica 96(12):1723–1729.

Enos, W.F., J.C. Beyer, and R.H. Holmes. 1955. Pathogenesis of coronary disease in American soldiers killed in Korea. Journal of the American Medical Association 158:912–917.

Epel, E., E. Blackburn, J. Lin, F. Dhabhar, N. Alder, J. Morrow, and R. Cawthon. 2004. Accelerated telomere shortening in response to life stress. Proceedings of the National Academy of Sciences 101:17312–17315.

Ernst, E. 1993. Regular exercise reduces fibrinogen levels: A review of longitudinal studies. British Journal of Sports Medicine 27:175–176.

Esparza, J., C. Fox, I. Harper, L. Schulz, M. Valencia, and E. Ravussin. 2000. Daily energy expenditure in Mexican and USA Pima Indians: Low physical activity as a possible cause of obesity. International Journal of Obesity 24:55–59.

Estabrooks, P. 2000. Sustaining exercise participation through group cohesion. Exercise and Sports Science Reviews 28:63–67.

Evans, W. 2000. Vitamin E, vitamin C, and exercise. American Journal of Clinical Nutrition 72:S647–652.

Farias, M.M., A.M. Cuevas, and F. Rodriguez. 2011. Set-point theory and obesity. Metabolic Syndrome and Related Disorders 9(2):85–89.

Ferreira, I., J. Twisk, W. VanMechelen, H. Kemper, and C. Stehouwer. 2002. Amsterdam growth and health longitudinal study. European Journal of Clinical Investigation 32:723–731.

Fiatarone, M., E. O'Neill, N. Doyle Ryan, K. Clements, G. Solares, M. Nelson, S. Roberts, J. Kehayias, L. Lipsitz, and W. Evans. 1994. Exercise training and nutritional supplementation for physical frailty in very elderly people. New England Journal of Medicine 330:1769–1775.

Fincham, J.E. 2011. The expanding public health threat of obesity and overweight. International Journal of Pharmacy Practice 19(3):214–216.

Finkelstein, E.A., J.G. Trogdon, D.S. Brown, B.T. Allaire, P.S. Dellea, and S.J. Kamal-Bahl. 2008. The lifetime medical cost burden of overweight and obesity: Implications for obesity prevention. Obesity (Silver Springs) 16(8):1843–1848.

Fleck, S., and W. Kraemer. 1997. Designing resistance training programs. Champaign, IL: Human Kinetics.

Flegal, K., M. Carroll, C. Ogden, and C. Johnson. 2002. Prevalence and trends in obesity among U.S. adults, 1999–2000. Journal of the American Medical Association 288:1723–1727.

Fletcher, G.F., G.J. Balady, E.A. Amsterdam, B. Chaitman, R. Eckel, J. Fleg, V.F. Froelicher, A.S. Leon,

I.L. Piña, R. Rodney, D.A. Simons-Morton, M.A. Williams, and T. Bazzarre. 2001. Exercise standards for testing and training: A statement for healthcare professionals from the American Heart Association. *Circulation* 104:1694–1740.

Flodmark, C.E., I. Lissau, L.A. Moreno, A. Pietrobelli, and K. Widhalm. 2004. New insights into the field of children and adolescents' obesity: The European perspective. *International Journal of Obesity* 28:1189–1196.

Focht, B., and H. Hausenblas. 2001. Influence of quiet rest and acute aerobic exercise performed in a naturalistic environment on selected psychological responses. *Journal of Sports and Exercise Psychology* 23(2):108–121.

Folk, G.E. 1974. *Environmental physiology.* Philadelphia: Lea & Febiger.

Foster, C., L. Hector, R. Welsh, M. Schrager, M. Green, and A. Snyder. 1995. Effects of specific versus cross-training on running performance. *European Journal of Applied Physiology and Occupational Physiology* 70:367–372.

Foster, G., H. Wyatt, J. Hill, B. McGukin, C. Brill, B. Mohammed, P. Szapary, D. Rader, J. Edman, and S. Klein. 2003. A randomized trial of a low carbohydrate diet for obesity. *New England Journal of Medicine* 348:2082–2090.

Foster-Powell, K., and J. Miller. 1995. International tables of glycemic index. *American Journal of Clinical Nutrition* 62:S871–890.

Frederick, E.C. 1973. *The running body.* Mountain View, CA: World Publications.

Friedenreich, C., K. Courneya, and H. Bryant. 2001. Influence of physical activity in different life periods on the risk of breast cancer. *Epidemiology* 12:604–612.

Friedenreich, C., S. McGregor, K. Courneya, S. Angyalfi, and F. Elliott. 2004. Case-control study of lifetime total physical activity and prostate cancer risk. *American Journal of Epidemiology* 159:740–749.

Friedman, M., and R. Rosenman. 1973. Instantaneous and sudden death. *Journal of the American Medical Association* 22:1319–1328.

Fries, J., and L. Crapo. 1981. *Vitality and aging.* San Francisco: W.H. Freeman.

Frisch, R., G. Wyshak, N. Albright, T. Albright, I. Schiff, K. Jones, J. Witschi, E. Shiang, E. Koff, and M. Marguglio. 1985. Lower prevalence of breast cancer and cancers of the reproductive system among former college athletes compared to non-athletes. *British Journal of Cancer* 52:885–891.

Froelicher, V.F. 1984. *Exercise testing and training.* Chicago: Year Book Medical.

Frontera, W., and X. Bigard. 2002. The benefits of strength training in the elderly. *Science and Sports* 17:109–116.

Gardner, J.W. 2002. Death by water intoxication. *Military Medicine* 167(5):432–434.

Gaskill, S., R. Serfass, D. Bacharach, and J. Kelly. 1999. Responses to training in cross-country skiers. *Medicine and Science in Sports and Exercise* 31:1211–1217.

Gaskill S., A. Walker, C. Bouchard, T. Rankinen, D. Rao, J. Skinner, J. Wilmore, and A. Leon. 2005. Rating of perceived exertion is a stable marker of exercise intensity during training in previously sedentary individuals: The HERITAGE Family Study. Northwest American College of Sports Medicine Proceedings, 3:4.

Gaskill, S., A. Walker, R. Serfass, C. Bouchard, J. Gagnon, D. Rao, J. Skinner, J. Wilmore, and A. Leon. 2001. Changes in ventilatory threshold with exercise training in a sedentary population: The Heritage Family Study. Abstract. *Medicine and Science in Sports and Exercise* 33:S3.

Gaskill, S.E., A. Miller, and L. Wambold. 2012. Moderate-to-vigorous physical activity is related to 3rd- to 12th-grade academic achievement. In-Press.

Gaziano, J., J. Buring, J. Breslow, S. Goldhaber, B. Rosner, M. Vandenburgh, W. Willett, and C. Hennekens. 1993. Moderate alcohol intake, increased levels of high-density lipoprotein and its subfractions, and decreased risk of myocardial infarction. *New England Journal of Medicine* 329:1829–1834.

Gaziano, J.M., and C.M. Gibson. 2006. Potential for drug-drug interactions in patients taking analgesics for mild-to-moderate pain and low-dose aspirin for cardioprotection. *American Journal of Cardiology* 97(9A):23–29.

Gill, J., and A. Hardman. 2000. Postprandial lipemia: Effects of exercise and restriction of energy intake compared. *American Journal of Clinical Nutrition* 71:465–471.

Glasser, W. 1976. *Positive addiction.* New York: Harper and Row.

Gledhill, N., D. Warburton, and V. Jamnik. 1999. Haemoglobin, blood volume, cardiac function, and aerobic power. *Canadian Journal of Applied Physiology* 24:54–65.

Glowacki, S., S. Martin, A. Maurer, W. Baek, J. Green, and S. Crouse. 2004. Effects of resistance, endurance, and concurrent exercise on training outcomes in men. *Medicine and Science in Sports and Exercise* 36:2119–2127.

Going, S. 1996. Densitometry. In *Human body composition*, ed. A. Roche, S. Heymsfield, and T. Lohman, 3–24. Champaign, IL: Human Kinetics.

Gordon, E.E. 1967. Anatomical and biochemical adaptations of muscle to different exercises. *Journal of the American Medical Association* 201:755–758.

Gordon, P., J. Senf, and D. Campos-Outcalt. 1999. Is the annual complete physical examination necessary? *Archives of Internal Medicine* 159:909–910.

Graham, T., and K. Adamo. 1999. Dietary carbohydrate and its effect on metabolism and substrate stores in sedentary and active individuals. *Canadian Journal of Applied Physiology* 24:393–415.

Greenberg, J. 2011. *Behavior in organizations* (10th ed). Upper Saddle River, New Jersey: Pearson.

Greenleaf, J.E., C.J. Greenleaf, D. VanDerveer, and K.J. Dorchak. 1976. *Adaptation to prolonged bedrest in man: A compendium of research.* Washington, DC: National Aeronautics and Space Administration.

Griffin, K. 2004. Health report: No more knife guys. *AARP The Magazine*, Nov–Dec:32–98.

Gruber, J. 1986. Physical activity and self-esteem development in children: A meta-analysis. *American Academy of Physical Education Papers* 19:30–48.

Grundy, S., J. Cleeman, C. Bairey Merz, H. Brewer, L. Clark, D. Hunninghake, R. Pasternak, S. Smith, and N. Stone. 2004. Implications of recent clinical trials for the National Cholesterol Education Program adult treatment panel III guidelines. *Circulation* 110:227–239.

Gwinup, G. 1970. *Energetics.* New York: Bantam.

Hale, B., and J. Raglin. 2002. State anxiety responses to acute resistance training and step aerobic exercise across 8 weeks of training. *Journal of Sports Medicine and Physical Fitness* 42:108–112.

Haltom, R., R. Kraemer, R. Sloan, E. Herbert, K. Frank, and J. Tryniecki. 1999. Circuit weight training and its effects on excess postexercise oxygen consumption. *Medicine and Science in Sports and Exercise* 31:1613–1618.

Hass, C., L. Garzarella, D. DeHoyos, and M. Pollock. 2000. Single verses multiple sets in long-term recreational weightlifters. *Medicine and Science in Sports and Exercise* 32:235–242.

Hays, N., R. Starling, X. Liu, D. Sullivan, T. Trappe, J. Fluckey, and W. Evans. 2004. Effects of an ad libitum low fat, high carbohydrate diet on body weight, body composition, and fat distribution in older men and women: A randomized controlled trial. *Archives of Internal Medicine* 164:210–217.

Hendrix, W., and R. Hughes. 1997. Relationship of trait, Type A behavior, and physical fitness variables to cardiovascular reactivity and coronary heart disease risk potential. *American Journal of Health Promotion* 11:264–271.

Hettinger, T., and E.A. Müller. 1953. Muscle strength and training. *Arbeitsphysiologie* 15:111–126.

Hickson, R. 1980. Interference of strength development by simultaneously training for strength and endurance. *Journal of Applied Physiology* 45:255–263.

Hill, J., and E. Melanson. 1999. Overview of the determinants of overweight and obesity: Current evidence and research issues. *Medicine and Science in Sports and Exercise* 31:S515–621.

Hill, S.R., F.C. Goetz, and H.M. Fox. 1956. Studies on adrenocortical and psychological responses to stress in man. *Archives of Internal Medicine* 97:269–298.

Holloszy, J.O. 1967. Biochemical adaptations in muscle: Effects of exercise on mitochondrial oxygen uptake and respiratory enzyme activity in skeletal muscle. *Journal of Biological Chemistry* 242:2278–2282.

Holloszy, J.O., G. Dalsky, P. Nemeth, B. Hurley, W. Martin, and J. Hagberg. 1986. Utilization of fat as a substrate during exercise: Effect of training. In *Biochemistry of exercise IV*, ed. B. Saltin, 183–190. Champaign, IL: Human Kinetics.

Hood, D., M. Takahashi, M. Connor, and D. Freyssenet. 2000. Assembly of the cellular powerhouse: Current issues in muscle mitochondrial biogenesis. *Exercise and Sports Science Reviews* 28:68–73.

Hulver, M., and J. Houmar. 2003. Plasma leptin and exercise: Recent findings. *Sports Medicine* 33:473–482.

Ikai, M. 1970. Training of muscle strength and power in athletes. Paper presented at Fédération Internationale de Médecine du Sport Congres, Oxford, England.

Ikai, M., and A.H. Steinhaus. 1961. Some factors modifying the expression of human strength. *Journal of Applied Physiology* 16:157–163.

Ismail, A.H., and R.J. Young. 1977. Effects of chronic exercise on the personality of adults. In *The marathon*, ed. P. Milvy. New York: New York Academy of Sciences.

Issekutz, B., and H. Miller. 1962. Plasma free fatty acids during exercise and the effect of lactic acid. *Proceedings of the Society of Experimental Biology and Medicine* 110:237–239.

Ivy, J., W. Goforth, W. Damon, T. McCauley, E. Parsons, and B. Price. 2002. Early post-exercise muscle glycogen recovery is enhanced with a carbohydrate-protein supplement. *Journal of Applied Physiology* 93:1337–1344.

Ivy, J., T. Zderic, and D. Fogt. 1999. Prevention and treatment of non-insulin-dependent diabetes mellitus. In *Exercise and sports science reviews*, Vol. 27, ed. J. Holloszy, 1–36. Indianapolis: American College of Sports Medicine.

Jackson, C., and A. Dickinson. 1988. Adaptations of skeletal muscle to strength or endurance training. In *Advances in sports medicine and fitness*, ed. W. Grana, J. Lombardo, B. Sharkey, and J. Stone, 45–59. Chicago: Year Book Medical.

Jackson, C., and B. Sharkey. 1988. Altitude training and human performance. *Sports Medicine* 6:279–284.

Jackson, J., B.J. Sharkey, and L.P. Johnston. 1968. Cardiorespiratory adaptations to training at specified frequencies. *Research Quarterly* 39:295–300.

Jacobson, E. 1938. *Progressive relaxation*. Chicago: University of Chicago Press.

James, W.P.T. 1995. A public health approach to the problem of obesity. *International Journal of Obesity Related Metabolism Disorders* 19:S37–S45.

Janssen, I., P. Katzmarzyk, and R. Ross. 2002. Body mass index, waist circumference, and health risk. *Archives of Internal Medicine* 162:2074–2079.

Jenkins, D., R. Taylor, and T. Wolever. 1982. The diabetic diet, dietary carbohydrate and differences in digestibility. *Diabetologia* 23:477–485.

Jensen, M., M. Brant-Zawadzki, N. Obuchowski, M. Modic, D. Malkasian, and J. Ross. 1994. Magnetic resonance imaging of the lumbar spine in people without back pain. *New England Journal of Medicine* 331:69–73.

Johnsgard, K. 1985. The motivation of the long distance runner. *Journal of Sports Medicine* 25:135–143.

Jones, A. 2002. Running economy is negatively related to sit-and-reach test performance in international-standard distance runners. *International Journal of Sports Medicine* 23:40–43.

Kanehisa, H., and M. Miyashita. 1983. Specificity of velocity in strength training. *European Journal of Applied Physiology* 52:104–110.

Kang, J., J. Hoffman, H. Walker, E. Chaloupka, and A. Utter. 2003. Regulating intensity using perceived exertion during extended exercise periods. *European Journal of Applied Physiology* 89:475–482.

Kanter, M. 1995. Free radicals and exercise: Effects of nutritional antioxidant supplements. In *Exercise and sports science reviews*, ed. J. Holloszy. Baltimore: Williams & Wilkins.

Kasari, D. 1976. The effects of exercise and fitness on serum lipids in college women. Unpublished master's thesis, The University of Montana.

Katzmarzyk, P.T., J. Gagnon, A.S. Leon, J.S. Skinner, J.H. Wilmore, D.C. Rao, and C. Bouchard. 2001. Fitness, fatness, and estimated coronary heart disease risk: The HERITAGE family study. *Medicine and Science in Sports and Exercise* 33(4):585–590.

Kay A.D., and Blazevich A.J. 2012. Effect of acute static stretch on maximal muscle performance: a systematic review. *Medicine and Science in Sports and Exercise* 44(1):154-64.

Kemi, O., P. Haram, U. Wisloff, and O. Ellingsen. 2004. Aerobic fitness is associated with cardiomyocyte contractile capacity and endothelial function in exercise training and detraining. *Circulation* 109:2897–2904.

Kemmler, W., D. Lauber, J. Weineck, J. Hensen, W. Kalender, and K. Engelke. 2004. Benefits of 2 years of intense exercise on bone density, physical fitness, and blood lipids in early postmenopausal women. *Archives of Internal Medicine* 164:1084–1091.

Kempen, K., W. Saris, and K. Westerterp. 1995. Energy balance during an 8-week restricted diet with and without exercise in obese women. *American Journal of Clinical Nutrition* 62:722–729.

Kenrick, M.M., M.F. Ball, and J.J. Canary. 1972. Exercise and fat loss in obese patients. Paper presented at the annual meeting of the American Academy of Physical Medicine and Rehabilitation, San Juan, Puerto Rico.

Kenyon, G. 1968. Six scales for assessing attitudes toward physical activity. *Research Quarterly* 37:566–574.

Keul, J. 1971. Myocardial metabolism in athletes. In *Muscle metabolism during exercise*, ed. B. Pernow and B. Saltin. New York: Plenum.

Keys, A., J. Brožek, A. Henschel, O. Mickelsen, and H.L. Taylor. 1950. *The biology of human starvation*. St. Paul, MN: University of Minnesota Press.

Kivimaki, M., P. Leino-Arjas, R. Luukkonen, H. Riihimaki, J. Vahtera, and J. Kirjonen. 2002. Work stress and risk of cardiovascular mortality. *British Medical Journal* 325:857–860.

Kline, G., J. Pocari, R. Hintermeister, P. Freedson, A. Ward, R. McCarron, J. Ross, and J. Rippe. 1987. Estimation of $\dot{V}O_2$max from a one-mile track walk, gender, age, and body weight. *Medicine and Science in Sports and Exercise* 19:253–259.

Klissouras, V. 1976. Heritability of adaptive variation. *Journal of Applied Physiology* 31:338–344.

Knab, A.M., R.A. Shanely, K.D. Corbin, F. Jin, W. Sha, and D.C. Nieman. 2011. A 45-minute vigorous exercise bout increases metabolic rate for 14 hours. *Medicine and Science in Sports and Exercise* 43(9): 1643–1648.

Knoops, K., L. deGroot, D. Kromhout, A. Perrin, O. Moreiras-Varela, A. Menotti, and W. vanStaveren. 2004. *Journal of the American Medical Association* 292:1433–1439.

Kobasa, S. 1979. Stressful life events, personality and health: An inquiry into hardiness. *Journal of Personality and Social Psychology* 37:1–11.

Komi, P. 1992. Stretch-shortening cycle. In *Strength and power in sport*, ed. P. Komi. Oxford: Blackwell Scientific.

Komi, P., and E.R. Buskirk. 1972. Effect of eccentric and concentric muscle conditioning on tension and electrical activity of human muscle. *Ergonomics* 15:417–422.

Kong, D. 2004. Aspirin in cardiovascular disorders: What is the optimal dose? *American Journal of Cardiovascular Drugs* 4:151–158.

Kramer, J., M. Stone, H. Obryant, M. Conley, R. Johnson, D. Nieman, D. Honeycutt, and T. Hoke. 1997. Effects of single vs. multiple sets of weight training: Impact of volume, intensity and variation. *Journal of Strength and Conditioning Research* 11:143–147.

Kuh, D., J. Bassey, R. Hardy, A. Sayer, M. Wadsworth, and C. Cooper. 2002. Birth weight, childhood size, and muscle strength in adult life: Evidence from a birth cohort study. *American Journal of Epidemiology* 156(7):627–633.

Kull, M. 2003. Physical activity and mental health: Relationship between depressiveness, psychological disorders and physical activity levels in women. *Biology of Sport* 20:129–138.

Lail, A., J. Marino, A. Russo, R. Serrano, A. Lamonte, J. Wygard, and R. Otto. 2004. The effect of six weeks of balance intervention on trained senior males. *Medicine and Science in Sports and Exercise* 36:S358.

Lakka, T., D. Laaksonen, H. Lakka, N. Mannikko, L. Niskanen, R. Rauramaa, and J. Salonen. 2003. Sedentary lifestyle, poor cardiovascular fitness, and the metabolic syndrome. *Medicine and Science in Sports and Exercise* 35:1279–1286.

Lakka, T., J. Venalainen, R. Rauramaa, R. Salonen, J. Tuomilehto, and J. Salonen. 1994. Relation of leisure-time physical activity and cardiorespiratory fitness to the risk of acute myocardial infarction in men. *New England Journal of Medicine* 330:1549–1554.

Landers, D., and S. Petruzzello. 1994. Physical activity, fitness and anxiety. In *Physical activity, fitness and health*, ed. C. Bouchard, R. Shephard, and T. Stevens. Champaign, IL: Human Kinetics.

Larson, E., L. Wang, J. Bowen, W. McCormick, L. Teri, P. Crane, and W. Kukull. 2006. Exercise is associated with reduced risk for incident dementia among persons 65 years of age and older. *Annals of Internal Medicine* 144:73–81.

Leaf, A. 1973. Getting old. *Scientific American* 229:45–55.

Lee, C., A. Jackson, and S. Blair. 1998. U.S. Weight Guidelines: Is it also important to consider cardiorespiratory fitness? *International Journal of Obesity* 22:S2–7.

Lee, I-Min, C. Hsieh, and R. Paffenbarger. 1995. Exercise intensity and longevity in men: The Harvard alumni health study. *Journal of the American Medical Association* 273:1179–1184.

Leibel, R., M. Rosenbaum, and J. Hirsch. 1995. Changes in energy expenditure resulting from altered body weight. *New England Journal of Medicine* 332:621–628.

Leitzmann, M., E. Rimm, W. Willett, D. Spiegelman, F. Grodstein, M. Stampfer, G. Colditz, and E. Giovannucci. 1999. Recreational physical activity and the risk of cholecystectomy in women. *New England Journal of Medicine* 341:777–784.

Lemon, P. 1995. Do athletes need more protein and amino acids? *International Journal of Sports and Nutrition* 5:S39–61.

Leon A., S. Gaskill, C. Bouchard, J. Gagnon, D. Rao, J. Skinner, J. Wilmore, T. Rice, S. Mandel, and J. Bergeron. 2002. Variability in the response of HDL cholesterol to exercise training in the HERITAGE Family Study. *International Journal of Sports Medicine* 23:1–9.

Leonard, J., J. Hofer, and N. Pritikin. 1974. *Live longer now*. Mountain View, CA: World Sports Library.

Lieber, C. 1976. The metabolism of alcohol. *Scientific American* 229:45–55.

Locke, E., and G. Latham. 1985. The application of goal setting to sports. *Journal of Sports Psychology* 7:205–222.

Lopez, S.A., R. Vial, L. Balart, and G. Arroyave. 1974. Effects of exercise and physical fitness on serum lipids and lipoproteins. *Atherosclerosis* 20:1–9.

Lubell, A. 1988. Blacks and exercise. *Physician and Sportsmedicine* 16:162–176.

Macera, C., D. Jones, M. Yore, S. Ham, H. Kohl, C. Kimsey, and D. Buchner. 2003. Prevalence of physical activity, including lifestyle activities among adults—United States, 2000–2001. Centers for Disease Control, *Morbidity and Mortality Weekly Report* 52:764–769.

Mackinnon, L. 1992. *Exercise and immunology*. Champaign, IL: Human Kinetics.

Malina, R., and C. Bouchard. 1991. *Growth, maturation, and physical activity*. Champaign, IL: Human Kinetics.

Malmivaara, A., U. Hakkinen, T. Aro, M. Heinrichs, L. Koskenniemi, E. Kuosma, S. Lappi, R. Paloheimo, C. Servo, V. Vaaranen, and S. Hernberg. 1995. The treatment of acute low back pain: Bed rest, exercises, or ordinary activity? *New England Journal of Medicine* 332:351–355.

Manninen, P., M. Heliovaara, H. Riihimaki, and O. Suomalainen. 2002. Physical workload and the risk or severe osteoarthritis. *Scandinavian Journal of Work Environment and Health* 28:25–32.

Manson, J., F. Hu, J. Rich-Edwards, G. Colditz, M. Stampfer, W. Willet, F. Speizer, and C. Hennekens. 1999. A prospective study of walking as compared with vigorous exercise in the prevention of coronary heart disease in women. *New England Journal of Medicine* 341:650–658.

Manson, J., W. Willett, M. Stampfer, G. Colditz, D. Hunter, S. Hankinson, C. Hennekens, and F. Speizer. 1995. Body weight and mortality among women. *New England Journal of Medicine* 333:677–685.

Marcus, B., and L. Forsyth. 2003. *Motivating people to be physically active*. Champaign, IL: Human Kinetics.

Markoff, R., P. Ryan, and T. Young. 1982. Endorphins and mood changes in long-distance running. *Medicine and Science in Sports and Exercise* 14(1):11–15.

Maslow, A.H. 1954. *Motivation and personality*. New York: Harper.

Massey, B.H., R.C. Nelson, B.J. Sharkey, and T. Comden. 1965. Effects of high-frequency electrical stimulation on the size and strength of skeletal muscle. *Journal of Sports Medicine* 5:136–144.

Matejek, N., E. Weimann, C. Witzel, G. Molenkamp, S. Schwidergall, and H. Bohles. 1999. Hypoleptinaemia in patients with anorexia nervosa and in elite gymnasts with anorexia athletica. *International Journal of Sports Medicine* 20:451–456.

Mayer, J., and B.A. Bullen. 1974. Nutrition, weight control and exercise. In *Science and medicine of exercise and sport*, ed. W.R. Johnson and E.R. Buskirk. New York: Harper and Row.

McArdle, W., F. Katch, and V. Katch. 1994. *Essentials of exercise physiology*. Philadelphia: Lea & Febiger.

McAuley, E., and B. Blissmer. 2000. Self-efficacy determinants and consequences of physical activity. In *Exercise and sports science reviews*, Vol. 28, ed. D. Seals, 85–88. Indianapolis: American College of Sports Medicine.

McCarthy, J., M. Pozniak, and J. Agre. 2002. Neuromuscular adaptations to concurrent strength and endurance training. *Medicine and Science in Sports and Exercise* 34:511–519.

Mehrotra, A., A. Zaslavsky, and J. Ayanian. 2007. Preventive health examinations and preventive gynecological examinations in the United States. *Archives of Internal Medicine* 167(17):1876–1883.

Meyers, J. 2003. Exercise and cardiovascular health. *Circulation* 107:e2–e5.

Miller, D., and P. Payne. 1968. Longevity and protein intake. *Experimental Gerontology* 3:231–235.

Miller, E., R. Pastor-Barriuso, D. Dalal, R. Riemersma, L. Appel, and E. Guallar. 2005. Meta-analysis: High dosage of vitamin E supplementation may increase all-cause mortality. *Annals of Internal Medicine* 142:37–46.

Miller, W.R., and S. Rollnick. 1991. *Motivational interviewing: Preparing people to change addictive behavior.* New York: Guilford.

Mitchell, J.H., W. Reardon, D.I. McCloskey, and K. Wildnethal. 1977. Possible roles of muscle receptors in the cardiovascular response to exercise. In *The marathon*, ed. P. Milvy, 232–252. New York: New York Academy of Sciences.

Mokdad, A., J. Marks, D. Stroup, and J. Gerberding. 2004. Actual causes of death in the United States, 2000. *Journal of the American Medical Association* 291:1238–1245.

Móle, P.A., L.B. Oscai, and J.O. Holloszy. 1971. Adaptation of muscle to exercise: Increase in levels of palmityl CoA synthetase, carnitine palmityltransferase, and palmityl CoA dehydrogenase, and in the capacity to oxidize fatty acids. *Journal of Clinical Investigation* 50:2323–2329.

Móle, P.A., J. Stern, C. Schultz, E. Bernauer, and B. Holcomb. 1989. Exercise reverses depressed metabolic rate produced by severe caloric restriction. *Medicine and Science in Sports and Exercise* 21:29–33.

Molz, A., B. Heyduck, H. Lill, E. Spanuth, and L. Rocker. 1993. The effect of different exercise intensities on the fibrinolytic system. *European Journal of Applied Physiology and Occupational Physiology* 67:298–304.

Montani, J.P., A.K. Viecelli, A. Prévot, and A.G. Dulloo. 2006. Weight cycling during growth and beyond as a risk factor for later cardiovascular diseases: The 'repeated overshoot' theory. *International Journal of Obesity* 30:S58–S66.

Morgan, W.P. 1979. Negative addiction in runners. *Physician and Sportsmedicine* 7:57–70.

———. 2001. Prescription of physical activity: A paradigm shift. *Quest* 53:366–382.

Morgan, W., P. O'Conner, A. Ellickson, and P. Bradley. 1988. Personality structure, mood states and performance in elite male distance runners. *International Journal of Sport Psychology* 19:247–263.

Morrey, M., and D. Hensrud. 1999. Risk of medical events in a supervised health and fitness facility. *Medicine and Science in Sports and Exercise* 31:1233–1236.

Morris, J., and M. Crawford. 1958. Coronary heart disease and physical activity of work. *Journal of the British Medical Association* 2:1485–1496.

Morris, J.N., and P. Raffle. 1954. Coronary heart disease in transport workers. *British Journal of Industrial Medicine* 11:260–272.

Motl, R., A. Birnbaum, M. Kubik, and R. Dishman. 2004. Naturally occurring changes in physical activity are inversely related to depressive symptoms during early adolescence. *Psychosomatic Medicine* 66:336–342.

Mozaffarian, D., T. Hao, E.B. Rimm, W.C. Willett, and F.B. Hu. 2011. Changes in diet and lifestyle and long-term weight gain in women and men. *New England Journal of Medicine* 364(25):2392–2404.

Nadel, F.R., ed. 1977. *Problems with temperature regulation during exercise.* New York: Academic Press.

National Heart, Lung, and Blood Institute. 2012. What are blood pressure and prehypertension? www.nhlbi.gov/hbp/hbp/whathbp.htm. Accessed September 13, 2012.

Neary, J., G. Wheeler, I. Maclean, D. Cumming, and H. Quinney. 1994. Urinary free cortisol as an indicator of exercise training stress. *Clinical Journal of Sports Medicine* 4:160–165.

Nelson, M., M. Fiatarone, C. Morganti, I. Trice, R. Greenberg, and W. Evans. 1994. Effects of high-intensity strength training on multiple risk factors for osteoporotic fractures: A randomized controlled trial. *Journal of the American Medical Association* 272:1909–1914.

Nesser T., S. Chen, R. Serfass, and S. Gaskill. 2004. Development of upper body power in junior cross-country skiers. *Journal of Strength and Conditioning Research* 18(1):63–71.

Nevill, A., M. Burrows, R. Holder, S. Bird, and D. Simpson. 2003. Does lower-body BMD develop at the expense of upper-body BMD in female runners? *Medicine and Science in Sports and Exercise* 35:1733–1739.

Newham, D. 1988. The consequences of eccentric contractions and their relationship to delayed onset muscle pain. *European Journal of Applied Physiology* 57:353–359.

Nieman, D. 2003. Current perspectives on exercise immunology. *Current Sports Medicine Reports* 2:239–242.

Nieman, D., D. Henson, and S. McAnulty. 2002. Influence of vitamin C supplementation on oxidative and immune changes following an ultramarathon. *Journal of Applied Physiology* 92:1970–1977.

Nieman, D., D. Henson, S. McAnulty, L. McAnulty, J. Morrow, A. Ahmed, and C. Heward. 2004. Vitamin E and immunity after the Kona Triathlon World Championship. *Medicine and Science in Sports and Exercise* 36:1328–1335.

Nieman, D., and B. Pedersen. 1999. Exercise and immune function: Recent developments. *Sports Medicine* 27:73–80.

Nissen, S., E. Tuzcu, P. Schoenhagen, T. Crowe, W. Sasiela, J. Tsai, J. Orazem, R. Magorien, C. O'Shaughnessy, and P. Ganz. 2005. Statin therapy, LDL cholesterol, C-reactive protein, and coronary artery disease. *New England Journal of Medicine* 352:29–38.

North, T., P. McCullagh, and Z.V. Tran. 1990. Effects of exercise on depression. *Exercise and Sport Science Reviews* 18:379–415.

Nosaka, K., K. Sakamoto, M. Newton, and P. Sacco. 2001. How long does the protective effect on eccentric exercise-induced muscle damage last? *Medicine and Science in Sports and Exercise* 33:1490–1495.

O'Dougherty, M., A. Arikawa, B.C. Kaufman, M.S. Kurzer, and K.H. Schmitz. 2010. Purposeful exercise and lifestyle physical activity in the lives of young adult women: Findings from a diary study. *Women & Health* 49(8):642–661.

O'Malley, P., D. Jones, I. Feuerstein, and A. Taylor. 2000. Lack of correlation between psychological factors and subclinical coronary artery disease. *New England Journal of Medicine* 343:1298–1304.

Ornish, D. 1993. *Eat more, weigh less.* New York: Harper Collins.

Ornstein, R., and D. Sobel. 1989. *Healthy pleasures.* New York: Addison-Wesley.

Oscai, L.B., and J.O. Holloszy. 1969. Effects of weight changes produced by exercise, food restriction or overeating on body composition. *Journal of Clinical Investigation* 48:2124–2128.

Owen, N., G. Healy, C. Matthews, and D. Dunstan. 2010. Too much sitting: The population health science of sedentary behavior. *Exercise and Sport Sciences Review* 38:105–113.

Paffenbarger, R. 1994. Forty years of progress: Physical activity, health and fitness. In *American College of Sports Medicine 40th anniversary lectures*, 93–109. Indianapolis.

Paffenbarger, R., R. Hyde, and A. Wing. 1986. Physical activity, all-cause mortality, and longevity of college alumni. *New England Journal of Medicine* 314:605–613.

———. 1990. Physical activity and physical fitness as determinants of health and longevity. In *Exercise, fitness, and health*, ed. C. Bouchard, R.J. Shephard, T. Stephens, J.R. Sutton, and B.D. McPherson. Champaign, IL: Human Kinetics.

Parekh, R., D.A. Care, and C.R. Tainter. 2012. Rhabdomyolysis: advances in diagnosis and treatment. *Emergency Medical Practices.* 14(3):1-15.

Parfitt, G., and C. Gledhill. 2004. The effect of choice of exercise mode on psychological responses. *Psychology of Sport and Exercise* 5:111–117.

Passmore, R., and J. Durnin. 1955. Human energy expenditure. *Physiology Review* 35:801–824.

Pate, R., M. Pratt, S. Blair, W. Haskell, C. Macera, C. Bouchard, D. Buchner, W. Ettinger, G. Heath, A. King, A. Kriska, A. Leon, B. Marcus, J. Morris, R. Paffenbarger, K. Patrick, M. Pollock, J. Rippe, J. Sallis, and J. Wilmore. 1995. Physical activity and public health: A recommendation from the Centers for Disease Control and Prevention and the American College of Sports Medicine. *Journal of the American Medical Association* 273:402–407.

Patel, T., and K. Goldberg. 2004. Use of aspirin and ibuprofen compared with aspirin alone and the risk of myocardial infarction. *Archives of Internal Medicine* 164:852–856.

Pedersen, B., J. Helge, E. Richter, T. Rohde, and B. Kiens. 2000. Training and natural immunity: Effects of diets rich in fat or carbohydrate. *European Journal of Applied Physiology* 82:98–103.

Petruzzello, S.J. 2012. Doing what feels good (and avoiding what feels bad)—A growing recognition of the influence of affect on exercise behavior: A comment on Williams et al. *Annals of Behavioral Medicine.* On-line DOI: 10.1007/s12160-012-9374-5.

Pette, D. 1984. Activity induced fast to slow transitions in mammalian muscle. *Medicine and Science in Sports and Exercise* 16:517–528.

Piers, L., M. Soares, L. McCormack, and K. O'Dea. 1998. Is there evidence for an age-related reduction in metabolic rate? *Journal of Applied Physiology* 85:2196–2204.

Pimentel, A., C. Gentile, H. Tanaka, D. Seals, and P. Gates. 2003. Greater rate of decline in maximal aerobic capacity with age in endurance-trained than in sedentary men. *Journal of Applied Physiology* 94:2406–2413.

Plunkett, B., and W. Hopkins. 1995. The cause and treatment of the side pain "stitch." *Medicine and Science in Sports and Exercise* 27:S23.

Pollock, M.L. 1973. The quantification of endurance training programs. In *Exercise and sports sciences reviews*, Vol. 1, ed. J.H. Wilmore. New York: Academic Press.

Pollock, M.L., J. Dimmick, H. Miller, Z. Kendrick, and A. Linnerud. 1975. Effects of mode of training on cardiovascular function and body composition of middle-aged men. *Medicine and Science in Sports and Exercise* 7:139–145.

Powel, K., and R. Paffenbarger. 1985. Workshop on epidemiologic and public health aspects of physical activity and exercise: A summary. *Public Health Reports* 100:118–126.

President's Council on Physical Fitness and Sport. 1975. *An introduction to physical fitness.* Washington, DC: President's Council on Physical Fitness and Sport.

Pritikin, N. 1979. *The Pritikin program for diet and exercise.* New York: Bantam.

Prochaska, J.O., C.C. DiClemente, and J.C. Norcross. 1992. In search of how people change. *American Psychologist* 47:1102–1104.

Puchkoff, J., L. Curry, J. Swan, B. Sharkey, and B. Ruby. 1998. The effects of hydration status and blood glucose on mental performance during extended exercise in the heat. *Medicine and Science in Sports and Exercise* 30:S284.

Purcher, J., and C. Leferve. 1996. *The urban transport crisis in Europe and North America*. London: Macmillan Press Ltd.

Putman, C., X. Xu, E. Gillies, I. MacLean, G. Bell. 2004. Effects of strength, endurance and combined training on myosin heavy chain content and fiber-type distribution in humans. *European Journal of Applied Physiology* 92:376–384.

Radcliffe, J., and R. Farentinos. 1985. *Plyometrics: Explosive power training*. Champaign, IL: Human Kinetics.

Ratey, J.J., and E. Hagerman. 2008. *SPARK: The revolutionary new science of exercise and the brain*. New York: Little, Brown and Company.

Rejeski, W., K. Neal, M. Wurst, P. Brubaker, and W. Ettinger Jr. 1995. Walking, but not weight lifting, acutely reduces systolic blood pressure in older sedentary men and women. *Journal of Aging and Physical Activity* 3:163–177.

Rhea, M., B. Alvar, L. Burkett, and S. Ball. 2003. A meta-analysis to determine the dose response for strength development. *Medicine and Science in Sports and Exercise* 35:456–464.

Ridker, P., C. Hennekens, J. Buring, and N. Rifai. 2000. C-reactive protein and other markers of inflammation in the prediction of cardiovascular disease in women. *New England Journal of Medicine* 342:836–843.

Rising, R., I. Harper, A. Fontvielle, R. Ferraro, M. Spraul, and E. Ravussin. 1994. Determinants of total daily energy expenditure: Variability in physical activity. *American Journal of Clinical Nutrition* 59:800–804.

Robertson, R. 2004. *Perceived exertion for practitioners*. Champaign, IL: Human Kinetics.

Rosenstock, I.M. 1966. Why people use health services. *Milbank Memorial Fund Quarterly* 44(3):94–127.

Ross, R., H. Pedwell, and J. Rissanen. 1995. Effects of energy restriction and exercise on skeletal muscle and adipose tissue in women as measured by magnetic resonance imaging. *American Journal of Clinical Nutrition* 61:1179–1185.

Roth, D., and D. Holmes. 1985. Influence of physical fitness in determining the impact of stressful life events on physical and psychological health. *Psychosomatic Medicine* 47:164–173.

Roth, E.M., ed. 1968. *Compendium of human responses to the aerospace environment III*. Washington, DC: National Aeronautics and Space Administration.

Ruby, B., and R. Robergs. 1994. Gender differences in substrate utilization during exercise. *Sports Medicine* 17:393–410.

Ruby, B., D. Schoeller, and B. Sharkey. 2001. Evaluation of total energy expenditure (doubly-labeled water) across different measurement periods during arduous work. *Medicine and Science in Sports and Exercise* 33:S274.

Ruby, B., S. Gaskill, D. Heil, B. Sharkey, B. Hansen, and D. Lankford. 2002. Changes in salivary IgA during arduous wildfire suppression relative to work-shift length. *Medicine and Science in Sports and Exercise* 34:S195.

Ruby, B.C., S.E. Gaskill, D. Lankford, D. Slivka, D. Heil, and B. Sharkey. 2003. Carbohydrate feedings increase self-selected work rates during arduous wildfire suppression. *Medicine and Science in Sports and Exercise* 35(5):S210.

Ruby, B.C., S.E. Gaskill, D.P Heil, S.G. Harger, and B.J. Sharkey. 2004. Liquid and solid carbohydrate feedings increase self-selected work rates during arduous wildfire suppression. *Medicine and Science in Sports and Exercise* 36(5): S219.

Ryan, A., R. Pratley, D. Elahi, and A. Goldberg. 1995. Resistive training increases fat-free mass and maintains RMR despite weight loss in postmenopausal women. *Journal of Applied Physiology* 79:818–823.

Ryder, H.W., H.J. Carr, and R. Herget. 1976. Future performance in footracing. *Scientific American* 234:109–116.

Sachs, G., D. Weeks, K. Melchers, and D. Scott. 2003. The gastric biology of *Heliobactor pylori*. *Annual Review of Physiology* 65:349–369.

Sallis J.F., and M.F. Hovell. 1990. Determinants of exercise behavior. *Exercise and Sport Sciences Review*. 18:307-30.

Sallis J.F., B.G. Simons-Morton, E.J. Stone, C.B. Corbin, L.H. Epstein, N. Faucette, R.J. Iannotti, J.D. Killen, R.C. Klesges, C.K. Petray, T.W. Roland, and W. Taylor. 1992. Determinants of physical activity and interventions in youth. *Medicine and Science in Sports Exercise* 24(6 Suppl):S248-57.

Saltin, B. 1977. The interplay between peripheral and central factors in the adaptive response to exercise and training. In *The marathon*, ed. P. Milvy, 224–231. New York: New York Academy of Sciences.

Saltin, B., G. Blomqvist, J.H. Mitchell, R.L. Johnson Jr., K. Wildenthal, and C.B. Chapman. 1968. Response to exercise after bed rest and after training. *Circulation* 38(Suppl. 7):1–78.

Sanghavi Goal, M., E. McCarthy, R. Phillips, and C. Wee. 2004. Obesity among U.S. immigrant subgroups by duration of residence. *Journal of the American Medical Association* 292:2860–2867.

Schauer, P.R., S.R. Kashyap, K. Wolski, S.A. Brethauer, J.P. Kirwan, C.E. Pothier, S. Thomas, B. Abood, S.E. Nissen, and D.L. Bhatt. 2012. Bariatric surgery versus intensive medical therapy in obese patients with diabetes. *New England Journal Medicine* 366:1567–1576.

Schulze, M., J. Manson, D. Ludwig, G. Colditz, M. Stampfer, W. Willett, and F. Hu. 2004. Sugar-sweetened beverages, weight gain, and incidence of type 2 diabetes in young and middle-aged women. *Journal of the American Medical Association* 292:927–934.

Seals, D. 2003. Habitual exercise and the age-associated decline in large artery compliance. *Exercise and Sport Sciences Reviews* 31:68–72.

Selye, H. 1956. *The stress of life.* New York: McGraw-Hill.

Sharkey, B.J. 1970. Intensity and duration of training and the development of cardiorespiratory endurance. *Medicine and Science in Sports and Exercise* 2:197–202.

———. 1974. *Physiological fitness and weight control.* Missoula, MT: Mountain Press.

———. 1984. *Training for cross-country ski racing.* Champaign, IL: Human Kinetics.

———. 1986. *Coaches guide to sport physiology.* Champaign, IL: Human Kinetics.

———. 1987. Functional vs. chronological age. *Medicine and Science in Sports and Exercise* 19:174–178.

———. 1990. *Physiology of fitness.* Champaign, IL: Human Kinetics.

———. 1991. *New dimensions in aerobic fitness.* Champaign, IL: Human Kinetics.

Sharkey, B.J., and P. Davis. 2008. *Hard work: Defining physical work performance requirements.* Champaign, IL: Human Kinetics.

Sharkey, B.J., and S. Gaskill. 2006. *Sport physiology for coaches.* Champaign, IL: Human Kinetics.

Sharkey, B.J., and S. Gaskill. 2007. *Fitness and Health, Sixth Edition.* Champaign, IL: Human Kinetics.

Sharkey, B.J., and D. Greatzer. 1993. Specificity of exercise, training and testing. In *ACSM's resource manual for guidelines for exercise testing and prescription*, ed. L. Durstine, A. King, P. Painter, and J. Roitman, 82–92. Philadelphia: Lea & Febiger.

Sharkey, B.J., and J.P. Holleman. 1967. Cardiorespiratory adaptations to training at specified intensities. *Research Quarterly* 38:398–404.

Sharkey, B.J., C. Simpson, R. Washburn, and R. Confessore. 1980. HDL cholesterol. *Running* 5:38–41.

Sharkey, B.J., D. Wilson, T. Whiddon, and K. Miller. 1978, September. Fit to work? *Journal of Health, Physical Education and Recreation* 18–21.

Simoes, E., T. Byers, R. Coates, M. Serdula, A. Mokdad, and G. Heath. 1995. The association between leisure-time physical activity and dietary fat in American adults. *American Journal of Public Health* 85:240–244.

Singh, A., L. Uijtdewilligen, J.W. Twisk, W. van Mechelen, and M.J.Chinapaw. 2012. Physical activity and performance at school: A systematic review of the literature including a methodological quality assessment. *Archives of Pediatric and Adolescent Medicine* 166(1):49–55.

Siscovick, D., R. LaPorte, and J. Newman. 1985. The disease-specific benefits and risks of physical activity and exercise. *Public Health Reports* 100:180–188.

Siscovick, D., N. Weiss, R. Fletcher, and T. Lasky. 1984. The incidence of primary cardiac arrest during vigorous exercise. *New England Journal of Medicine* 311:874–877.

Slattery, M. 2004. Physical activity and colorectal cancer. *Sports Medicine* 34:239–252.

Sleamaker, R. 1989. *Serious training for serious athletes.* Champaign, IL: Human Kinetics.

Smith, M., and B. Sharkey. 1984. Altitude training: Who benefits? *Physician and Sportsmedicine* 12:48–62.

Smith, R., and O. Rutherford. 1995. The role of metabolites in strength training. 1. A comparison of eccentric and concentric contractions. *European Journal of Applied Physiology and Occupational Physiology* 71:332–336.

Spalding, T., L. Lyon, and B. Hatfield. 2004. Relative efficacy of aerobic training and stress management in lowering cardiovascular activity during psychological stress. *Medicine and Science in Sports and Exercise* 36:S88.

Spiegel, K., E. Tasali, P. Penev, and E. Van Cauter. 2004. Brief communication: Sleep curtailment in healthy young men is associated with decreased leptin levels, elevated ghrelin levels, and increased hunger and appetite. *Annals of Internal Medicine* 141:846–850.

Spirduso, W. 1995. *Physical dimensions of aging.* Champaign, IL: Human Kinetics.

Stampfer, M., F. Hu, J. Manson, E. Rimm, and W. Willett. 2000. Primary prevention of coronary heart disease in women through diet and lifestyle. *New England Journal of Medicine* 343:16–22.

Stanhope, K. 2012. Role of fructose-containing sugars in the epidemics of obesity and metabolic syndrome. *Annual Review of Medicine* 63:329–343.

Steed, J., G. Gaesser, and A. Weltman. 1994. Rating of perceived exertion and blood lactate concentration during submaximal running. *Medicine and Science in Sports and Exercise* 26:797–803.

Steinberg, G. 2003. Acute and chronic effects of leptin on skeletal muscle fatty acid metabolism. *Canadian Journal of Applied Physiology* 28:210.

Stephens, T. 1988. Physical activity and mental health in the United States and Canada: Evidence from four population surveys. *Preventive Medicine* 17:35–47.

Stone, W., and D. Klein. 2004. Long-term exercisers: What can we learn from them? *ACSM's Health and Fitness Journal* 8:11–14.

Strawbridge, W., S. Deleger, R. Roberts, and G. Kaplan. 2002. Physical activity reduces the risk of subsequent depression for older adults. *American Journal of Epidemiology* 156:328–334.

Stray-Gunderson, J. 1986. The effect of pericardiectomy on maximal oxygen consumption and cardiac output in untrained dogs. *Circulation Research* 58:523–529.

Stubbs, R., D. Hughes, A. Johnstone, G. Horgan, N. King, and J. Blundell. 2004. A decrease in physical activity affects appetite, energy, and nutrient balance in lean men feeding ad libitum. *American Journal of Clinical Nutrition* 79:62–69.

Stunkard, A., T. Foch, and V. Hrubec. 1986. A twin study of human obesity. *Journal of the American Medical Association* 256:51–54.

Stunkard, A.J., T.A.I. Sørensen, C. Hanis, T.W. Teasdale, R. Chakraborty, W.J. Schull, and F. Schulsinger. 1986. An adoption study of human obesity. *New England Journal of Medicine* 314:193–198.

Sundet, J., P. Magnus, and K. Tambs. 1994. The heritability of maximal aerobic power: A study of Norwegian twins. *Scandinavian Journal of Medical Science in Sports* 4:181–185.

Suzuki, T. 1967. Effects of muscular exercise on adrenal 17-hydroxycorticosteroid secretion in the dog. *Endocrinology* 80:1148–1151.

Swinburn, B., and E. Ravussin. 1993. Energy balance or fat balance? *American Journal of Clinical Nutrition* 57:S766–771.

Taylor, C., and N. Miller. 1993. Principles of health behavior change. In *ACSM's resource manual for guidelines for exercise testing and prescription*, ed. L. Durstine, A. King, P. Painter, and J. Roitman. Philadelphia: Lea & Febiger.

Tenenbaum, G., and R. Singer. 1992. Physical activity and psychological benefits. Position statement of the International Society of Sport Psychology. *Physician and Sportsmedicine* 20:179–184.

Thacker, S., J. Gilchrist, D. Stroup, and C. Kimsey. 2004. The impact of stretching on sports injury risk: A systematic review of the literature. *Medicine and Science in Sports and Exercise* 36:371–378.

Thompson, D., J. Edelsberg, G. Colditz, A. Bird, and G. Oster. 1999. Lifetime health and economic consequences of obesity. *Archives of Internal Medicine* 159:2177–2183.

Thompson, P.D., D. Buchner, I.L. Piña, G.J. Balady, M.A. Williams, B.H. Marcus, K. Berra, S.N. Blair, F. Costa, B. Franklin, G.F. Fletcher, N.F. Gordon, R.R. Pate, B.L. Rodriguez, A.K. Yancey, and N.K. Wenger. 2003. AHA scientific statement: Exercise and physical activity in the prevention and treatment of atherosclerotic cardiovascular disease. *Circulation* 107:3109–3116.

Thune, I., T. Brenn, E. Lund, and M. Gaard. 1997. Physical activity and the risk of breast cancer. *New England Journal of Medicine* 336:1269–1275.

Tipton, K., and R. Wolfe. 2004. Protein and amino acids for athletes. *Journal of Sports Sciences* 22:65–79.

Treuth, M., G. Hunter, and T. Kekes-Szabo. 1995. Reduction in intraabdominal adipose tissue after strength training in older women. *Journal of Applied Physiology* 78:1425–1431.

Trichopoulou, A., C. Gnardellis, A. Laagiou, V. Benetou, A. Naska, and D. Trichopoulou. 2001. Physical activity and energy intake selectively predict the waist-to-hip ratio in men but not in women. *American Journal of Clinical Nutrition* 74:574–578.

Trikalinos, T.A., A.A. Alsheikh-Ali, A. Tatsioni, B.K. Nallamothu, and D.M. Kent. 2009. Percutaneous coronary interventions for non-acute coronary artery disease: A quantitative 20-year synopsis and a network meta-analysis. *Lancet* 373:911–918.

Trudeau, F. and R. Shephard. 2008. Associations of physical fitness and academic performance among schoolchildren. *International Journal of Behavioral Nutrition and Physical Activity* 5:10–15.

Tsang, W., and C. HuiChan. 2004. Effects of exercise on joint sense and balance in elderly men: Tai chi versus golf. *Medicine and Science in Sports and Exercise* 36:658–667.

Tudor-Locke, C., J. Williams, J. Reis, and D. Pluto. 2004. Utility of pedometers for assessing physical activity—construct validity. *Sports Medicine* 34:281–291.

Tutko, T., and U. Tosi. 1976. *Sports psyching*. New York: Hawthorn.

Tuzac, M. 1999. Heart disease prevention must begin in teen years. Paper presented at the annual meeting of the American Heart Association, Dallas, TX.

U.S. Department of Agriculture (USDA), and U.S. Department of Health and Human Services (USDHHS). 2011. *Dietary guidelines for Americans, 2010*. www.cnpp.usda.gov/DGAs2010-PolicyDocument.htm.

U.S. Department of Health and Human Services (USDHHS), and Public Health Service. 1991. *Healthy People 2000: National health promotion and disease prevention objectives (DHHS #91-50212)*. Washington, DC: U.S. Government Printing Office.

U.S. Department of Health and Human Services (USDHHS). 2008. Physical Activity Guidelines for Americans. www.health.gov/paguidelines. Accessed August 17, 2012.

U.S. Department of Health, Education, and Welfare, Public Health Service (USDHEW). 1979. *Smoking and health: A report of the surgeon general. Interaction between smoking and occupational exposure*. Washington, DC: U.S. Government Printing Office.

Urquhart, D., J. Tobing, F. Hanna, P. Berry, A. Wluka, C. Ding, and F. Cicuttini. 2011. What is the effect of physical activity on the knee joint? A systematic review. *Medicine and Science in Sports and Exercise* 43:432–442.

Vaillant, G. 2001. *Aging well*. New York: Little, Brown.

Vailodash, B. 2000. The effects of 22 weeks of cycle training on body weight, heart rate, fitness and diet. Unpublished thesis, The University of Minnesota.

Van Aaken, E. 1976. *Van Aaken method*. Mountain View, CA: World Publications.

Van Linge, B. 1962. The response of muscle to strenuous exercise. *Journal of Bone and Joint Surgery* 44:711–721.

VanderVliet, P., Y. Vanden-Auweele, J. Knapen, R. Rzewnicki, P. Onghena, and H. VanCoppenolle. 2004. The effect of fitness training on clinically depressed patients: An intra-individual approach. *Psychology of Sport and Exercise* 5:153–167.

VanLangendonck, L., J. Lefevre, A. Claessens, M. Thomis, R. Phillippaerts, K. Delvaux, R. Lysens, R. Renson, B. Vanreusel, B. VandenEynde, J. Dequeker, and G. Beunen. 2003. Influence of participation in high-impact sports during adolescence and adulthood on bone mineral density in middle-aged men. *American Journal of Epidemiology* 158:525–533.

VanSchuylenbergh R., B. VandenEynde, and P. Hespel. 2004. Effects of air ventilation during stationary exercise testing. *European Journal of Applied Physiology* 92:263–266.

Vasan, R., M. Larson, E. Leip, J. Evans, C. O'Donnell, W. Kannel, and D. Levy. 2001. Impact of high-normal blood pressure on the risk of cardiovascular disease. *New England Journal of Medicine* 345:1291–1297.

Vega deJesus, R., and S. Siconolfi. 1988. Fat mobilization and utilization during exercise at lactates of 2 and 4 mm. *Medicine and Science in Sports and Exercise* 20 (Suppl. 71).

Vogt, M. and H. Hoppeler. 2010. Is hypoxia training good for muscles and exercise performance? *Progress in Cardiovascular Diseases* 52(6):525–533.

Voight B.F., G.M. Peloso, M. Orho-Melander, R. Frikke-Schmidt, M. Barbalic, et al. 2012. Plasma HDL cholesterol and risk of myocardial infarction: A mendelian randomisation study. *Lancet* 380(9841):572-580.

Volek, J. 2003. Influence of nutrition on responses to resistance training. *Medicine and Science in Sports and Exercise* 36:689–696.

Votruba, S., R. Atkinson, M. Hirvonen, and D. Schoeller. 2002. Prior exercise increases subsequent utilization of dietary fat. *Medicine and Science in Sports and Exercise* 34:1757–1765.

Wajswelner, H., B. Metcalf, and K. Bennell. 2012. Clinical Pilates versus general exercise for chronic low back pain: randomized trial. *Medicine and Science in Sports and Exercise* 44(7):1197-205.

Walker, J., G. Heigenhauser, E. Hultman, and L. Spriet. 2000. Dietary carbohydrate, muscle glycogen content, and endurance performance in well-trained women. *Journal of Applied Physiology* 88:2151–2158.

Warburton, D., M. Haykowsky, H. Quinney, D. Blackmore, K. Teo, D. Taylor, J. McGavock, and D. Humen. 2004. Blood volume expansion and cardiorespiratory function: Effects of training modality. *Medicine and Science in Sports and Exercise* 36:991–1000.

Washburn, R., B. Sharkey, J. Narum, and M. Smith. 1982. Dryland training for cross-country skiers. *Ski Coach* 5:9–12.

Watson, P., A. Srivastava, and F. Booth. 1983. Cytochrome C synthesis rate is decreased in the 6th hour of hindlimb immobilization in the rat. In *Biochemistry of exercise*, Vol. 13, ed. J. Knutgen, J. Vogel, and J. Poortmans, 378–384. Champaign, IL: Human Kinetics.

Wei, M., J. Kampert, C. Barlow, M. Nichaman, L. Gibbons, R. Paffenbarger, and S. Blair. 1999. Relationship between low cardiorespiratory fitness and mortality in normal weight, overweight, and obese men. *Journal of the American Medical Association* 282:1547–1553.

Weinberg, R., and D. Gould. 2003. *Foundations of sport and exercise psychology*. Champaign, IL: Human Kinetics.

Welle, S. 2002. Cellular and molecular basis of age-related sarcopenia. *Canadian Journal of Applied Physiology* 27:19–41.

Wenger, C. 1988. Human heat acclimatization. In *Human performance physiology and environmental medicine at terrestrial extremes*, ed. K. Pandolf, M. Sawka, and R. Gonzalez. Indianapolis: Benchmark.

Wenger, H., and G. Bell. 1986. The interaction of intensity, duration and frequency of exercise training in altering cardiorespiratory fitness. *Sports Medicine* 3:346–356.

Wessell, R. and C. Edwards. 2012. Principles of longevity and aging: Interventions to enhance older adulthood. *Journal of Education and Developmental Psychology* 2:01. [Epub ahead of publication].

Whaley, M., J. Kampert, H. Kohl, and S. Blair. 1999. Physical fitness and clustering of risk factors associated with the metabolic syndrome. *Medicine and Science in Sports and Exercise* 31:287–293.

Whiddon, T.R., B.J. Sharkey, and R.J. Steadman. 1969. Exercise, stress and blood clotting in men. *Research Quarterly* 40:431–434.

Willardson, J.M. 2007. Core stability training: Applications to sports conditioning programs. *Journal of Strength and Conditioning Research* 21(3):979–985.

Willett, W. 2001. *Eat, drink and be healthy*. New York: Simon and Schuster.

Williams, P. 1974. *Low back and neck pain*. Springfield, IL: Charles C Thomas.

Willis, J., and L. Campbell. 1992. *Exercise psychology*. Champaign, IL: Human Kinetics.

Wilmore, J.H. 1983. *Athletic training and physical fitness*. Boston: Allyn & Bacon.

Wilson, P.K., W. Castelli, and W. Kannel. 1987. Coronary risk prediction in adults (the Framingham Study). *American Journal of Cardiology* 59:91–94.

Wing, R.R., W. Lang, T.A. Wadden, M. Safford, W.C. Knowler, A.G. Bertoni, J.O. Hill, F.L. Brancati, A. Peters, and L. Wagenknecht. 2011. Benefits of modest weight loss in improving cardiovascular risk factors in overweight and obese individuals with type 2 diabetes. *Diabetes Care* 34:1481–1486.

Witvrouw, E., N. Mahieu, L. Danneels, and P. McNair. 2004. Stretching and injury prevention: An obscure relationship. *Sports Medicine* 34:443–449.

Womack, C., P. Nagelkirk, and A. Coughlin. 2003. Exercise-induced changes in coagulation and fibrinolysis in healthy populations and patients with cardiovascular disease. *Sports Medicine* 33:795–807.

Wood, P. 1975. Middle-aged joggers show healthy lipoprotein pattern. *Medical Tribune* 38:27.

Wood, R., R. Reyes, M. Welsch, J. Favaloro-Sabatier, M. Sabatier, C. Lee, L. Johnson, and P. Hooper. 2001. Concurrent cardiovascular and resistance training in healthy older adults. *Medicine and Science in Sports and Exercise* 33:1751–1758.

Wootan, M. and N. Hailpern. 2005. Obesity and other diet- and inactivity-related diseases: national impact, costs, and solutions. *National Alliance for Nutrition and Activity*. www.cspinet.org/nutrition-policy/NANA advocates_national_policies.pdf. Accessed August 18, 2012.

Wright, J., J. Kennedy-Stephenson, C. Wang, M. McDowell, and C. Johnson. 2004. Trends in intake of energy and macronutrients—United States, 1971–2000. Centers for Disease Control and Prevention, *Morbidity and Mortality Weekly Report* 53:80–82. www.cdc.gov/mmwr.

Young, A. 1988. Human adaptation to cold. In *Human performance physiology and environmental medicine at terrestrial extremes*, ed. K. Pandolf, M. Sawka, and R. Gonzalez. Indianapolis: Benchmark.

Zauner, C.W., J.J. Burt, and D.F. Mapes. 1968. The effect of strenuous and mild premeal exercise on postprandial lipemia. *Research Quarterly* 39:395–401.

Zhang, K., M. Sun, A. Kovera, J. Albu, F. PiSunyer, and C. Boozer. 2002. Sleeping metabolic rate in relation to body mass index and body composition. *International Journal of Obesity* 26:376–383.

Zuti, W.B., and L. Golding. 1976. Comparing diet and exercise as weight reduction tools. *Physician and Sportsmedicine* 4:59–62.

Index

Note: The italicized *f* and *t* following page numbers refer to figures and tables, respectively.

About the Authors

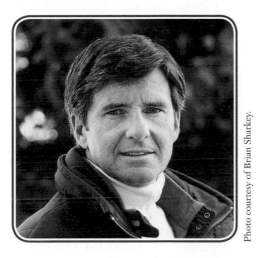

Photo courtesy of Brian Sharkey.

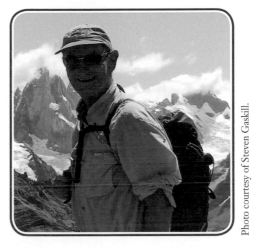

Photo courtesy of Steven Gaskill.

Brian J. Sharkey, PhD, has nearly 40 years of experience as a leading fitness researcher, educator, and author. Sharkey served as director of the University of Montana's Human Performance Laboratory for many years and remains associated with the university and lab as professor emeritus. He also served as a consultant with the U.S. Forest Service in the areas of fitness, health, and work capacity.

Sharkey is a fellow and past president of the American College of Sports Medicine and has served on the board of trustees. He served on the NCAA committee on competitive safeguards and medical aspects of sports, where he chaired the Sports Science and Safety subcommittee, which uses research and data on injury to improve the safety of intercollegiate athletes. Sharkey also coordinated the U.S. Ski Team Nordic Sportsmedicine Council. In 2009, Sharkey received the Fire Safety Award from the International Association of Wildland Firefighters.

Sharkey and his wife, Ann, reside in Missoula, Montana. He enjoys hiking, paddling, cycling, and both cross-country and downhill skiing.

Steven E. Gaskill, PhD, is a professor in the department of health and human performance at the University of Montana. His research interests include the relationship of physical activity to cognitive functioning in children; submaximal aerobic fitness and its relationship to work capacity and chronic disease; and long-duration work and exercise fitness as related to fitness, fatigue, immune function, and cognitive performance. Gaskill has published more than 40 articles in refereed journals, presented his research at numerous conferences, and authored three books.

Gaskill worked for the U.S. ski team for 10 years as head coach of the Nordic combined (ski jumping and cross-country skiing) and cross-country teams and as director of the coaches' educational programs. He has coached at three Olympic Games, and 20 skiers who have trained under him have competed in the Olympics. In 1992, the U.S. Ski Association named him the U.S. Cross-Country Coach of the Year.

Gaskill enjoys backpacking, tennis, mountain biking, cross-country skiing, fishing, and mountaineering. Serious about the active life, he continues to be active year round with his wife, Kathy.

Sharkey and Gaskill also coauthored *Sport Physiology for Coaches* (Human Kinetics, 2006) and *Fitness and Work Capacity* (National Wildfire Coordinating Group, 2009).